Electroceuticals

Arshad Majid
Editor

Electroceuticals

Advances in Electrostimulation Therapies

Springer

Editor
Arshad Majid
Sheffield Institute for Translational
Neuroscience, Department of Neuroscience,
Faculty of Medicine, Dentistry & Health
University of Sheffield
Sheffield, South Yorkshire,
United Kingdom

ISBN 978-3-319-28610-5 ISBN 978-3-319-28612-9 (eBook)
DOI 10.1007/978-3-319-28612-9

Library of Congress Control Number: 2017930687

Printed on acid-free paper

This Springer imprint is published by Springer Nature
The registered company is Springer International Publishing AG
The registered company address is Gewerbestrasse 11, 6330 Cham, Switzerland

Preface

Electroceuticals is a term that has recently come into use and encompasses the rapidly growing fields of bioelectrical and bioelectronics medicine. In broad and general terms, electroceuticals covers the therapeutic use of electrical stimulation to influence and modify biological functions or pathological processes in the body. Strictly speaking, this field is not new. Electrical stimulation has been used over the last 50 years for therapeutic benefits. For example, electroconvulsive therapy has been successfully employed for decades to treat pharmacologically resistant depression. However, over the last 20 years, there has been an exponential rise in research activity focused on electroceuticals, and exciting new areas of discovery and development have emerged which may offer alternatives to the traditional pharmaceutical options. The increasing sophistication and miniaturization of technology coupled with rapid advances in understanding of the function of electrical pathways in the body has made it increasingly feasible to modify electrical pathways for therapeutic gain.

This has also been reflected in the increased interest that research funding bodies such as the National Institute of Health (NIH) in the USA and pharmaceutical companies like GlaxoSmithKline (GSK) have taken in this area. The NIH has established a US$248 million fund to map the electrical wiring of the body and advance the development of new therapeutics. Similar efforts have been initiated by GSK.[1] Other initiatives like the NIH-funded human connectome project also promise to unravel the structural and functional connectivity of the human brain in health and disease.[2]

In this book, we present areas where electroceuticals research has made exciting progress toward therapy development. These include clinical neural implants such as cochlear implants to restore hearing, deep brain stimulators to treat movement disorders, and stimulation of the pharynx and of peripheral nerves to assist in dysphagia and gait disorders.

More recent varieties of electroceuticals include the electrical stimulation of the vagus nerve to modulate the immune system in order to provide relief from rheumatoid arthritis, prevent epileptic seizures, treat heart failure, aid recovery from brain trauma, and treat inflammatory bowel disease and gut motility disorders. Equally exciting is the potential that electroceuticals may enhance memory and consciousness.

Electroceuticals is a broad and rapidly growing field, and it is not possible to cover all the progress that is being made. However, we believe that this publication will give the reader new insights into the progress that has been made in this field. Each chapter in this book has been written by experts with an international reputation in their specialty who discuss the development of electroceuticals in their disease areas. They have included discussion on the historical background, research developments, current uses, and future prospects.

The regulatory approval process is of course an important consideration for all therapy development. However, I have chosen not to include chapters on the regulatory process as it varies according to jurisdiction and it would not be possible to cover all the jurisdictions of potential readers of this book.

Despite the rapid progress that has already been made, we stand at the dawn of a new era that will surely see huge developments over the coming decades, not only in treatments of diseases but also in enhancing human function.

References

1. Reardon, S. Electroceuticals spark interest. Nature. 2014;511:18.
2. $40 Million awarded to trace human's brain connections. https://www.nih.gov/news-events/news-releases/40-million-awarded-trace-human-brains-connections. 2010. Accessed 31Jul 2016.

About the Editor

Arshad Majid is a Professor of Cerebrovascular Neurology and Consultant Neurologist at the University of Sheffield and the Royal Hallamshire Hospital. Professor Majid graduated in Medicine from the University of Glasgow, Scotland. He trained in Neurology at the University of Pennsylvania and did fellowship training in Stroke Research at Washington University in St. Louis. He did additional fellowship training in Endovascular Surgical Neuroradiology at the Medical College of Wisconsin. He then served as the founding Director of the Division of Cerebrovascular Diseases at Michigan State University and was also the founding Medical Director of the William and Claire Dart Stroke Center at Sparrow Health System in Lansing, Michigan. He has published extensively in international peer-reviewed journals and presented at national and international meetings. His research has been funded by the NIH, the American Heart Association, the NIHR (UK), and the industry.

Contents

Contributors

Arshad Majid, BSc (Hons) MBChB FRCP (Glasg) DAPN Sheffield Institute for Translational Neuroscience, Department of Neuroscience, Faculty of Medicine, Dentistry & Health, University of Sheffield, Sheffield, UK

Bruno Bonaz, MD, PhD Clinique Universitaire d'Hépato-Gastroentérologie, Centre Hospitalier Universitaire Grenoble Alpes, Grenoble, France

University Grenoble Alpes, Grenoble Institut des Neurosciences, Grenoble, France

Lu Bu, BS, MBA Cyberonics, Inc, Department of Clinical and Medical Affairs, Houston, TX, USA

Natasha Calder Green, MA, ELS Cyberonics, Department of Global Medical Affairs, Houston, TX, USA

Simon Carr, MD, FRCS (ORL-HNS) Royal Hallamshire Hospital, Department of ENT, Sheffield, UK

Kelvin L. Chou, MD University of Michigan, Department of Neurology, Ann Arbor, MI, USA

Ana Ciurea, PhD Carol Davila University of Medicine and Pharmacy, Neurology Department, Bucharest, Romania

University of Bucharest, Physics Department, Bucharest, Romania

Jean Ciurea, PhD Neurosurgery Department, Bagdasar-Arseni Hospital, Bucharest, Romania

Didier Clarençon, PhD University Grenoble Alpes, Grenoble Institut des Neurosciences, Grenoble, France

Institut de Recherche Biomedicale des Armees, Paris, France

Pam Enderby, PhD, DSc (Hon), MSc, FRCSLT University of Sheffield, School of Health and Related Research, Sheffield, UK

Michael Faltys SetPoint Medical Corporation, Valencia, CA, USA

Christopher Heath, MD Sheffield Institute for Translational Neuroscience, University of Sheffield, Sheffield, UK

April Jones, BS Cyberonics, New Products and Clinical Engineering, Houston, TX, USA

Frieda Koopman, MD Academic Medical Center, University of Amsterdam, Clinical Immunology and Rheumatology, Amsterdam, The Netherlands

Yaakov A. Levine, PhD SetPoint Medical Corporation, Valencia, CA, USA

Harvey Leung, PhD Sheffield Institute for Translational Neuroscience, University of Sheffield, Sheffield, UK

Daniel Levanthal, MD, PhD University of Michigan Health Systems/VA Ann Arbor Healthcare System, Department of Neurology, Ann Arbor, MI, USA

Emily L. Levin, MD University of Michigan Hospital and Health Systems, Department of Neurosurgery, Ann Arbor, MI, USA

Manjit S. Matharu, FRCP, PhD Headache Group, Institute of Neurology and The National Hospital for Neurology and Neurosurgery, London, UK

Thomas H. Mercer, PhD, FBASES Queen Margaret University, Centre for Health Activity and Rehabilitation Research, Department of Rehabilitation Sciences, Musselburgh, UK

Sarah Miller, MRCP Headache Group, Institute of Neurology and The National Hospital for Neurology and Neurosurgery, London, UK

Ioan Opris, PhD Miami Project to Cure Paralysis, Department of Neurological Surgery, University of Miami, Miami, FL, USA

Wake Forest School of Medicine, Department of Physiology and Pharmacology, Winston Salem, NC, USA

Parag G. Patil, MD, PhD University of Michigan, Department of Neurosurgery, Ann Arbor, MI, USA

Sonia Pellissier, PhD Universite Savoie Mont-Blanc, Laboratoire Interuniversitaire de Pschologie, Personnalite, Cognition, et Changement Social, Grenoble Institute of Neurosciences, Chambéry, France

Sue Pownall, PhD, BSc (Hons), FRCSLT Sheffield Teaching Hospital NHS Foundation Trust, Department of Speech and Language Therapy, Royal Hallamshire Hospital, Sheffield, UK

Emma J. Radcliffe, Bsc (Hons) University of Manchester, Institute of Cardiovascular Sciences, 3.06 Core Technology Faculty, Manchester, UK

Jaydip Ray, MS, PhD FRCS (ORL-HNS) Department of ENT, Royal Hallamshire Hospital, Sheffield, UK

Jessica Redgrave, MD Sheffield Institute for Translational Neuroscience, University of Sheffield, University of Sheffield, Sheffield, UK

Valérie Sinniger, PhD University Hospital, Grenoble Alpes, Department of Hepatogastroenterology, Institute of Neurosciences, Grenoble, France

Monty Silverdale, MD, PhD Salford Royal NHS Foundation Trust, Department of Neurology, Greater Manchester, UK

Jesse M. Simon, MS SetPoint Medical, Valencia, CA, USA

Valerie Sinniger, PhD Grenoble Alpes, Hepatogastroenterology Department, Institute of Neurosciences, Universite Joseph Fourier-Site Sante, Grenoble, France

Lise Sproson, MSc, BMedSci (Hon), MRCSLT Sheffield Teaching Hospital NHS Foundation Trust, Department of Speech and Language Therapy, Royal Hallamshire Hospital, Sheffield, UK

Paul-Peter Tak, MD, PhD Department of Medicine, University of Cambridge, Cambridge, UK

Department of Rheumatology, Ghent University, Ghent, Belgium

Research & Development, GlaxoSmithKline, Stevenage, UK

Andrew W. Trafford, BVSc, Cert VA, PhD, MRCVS Manchester Academic Health Science Centre, Institute of Cardiovascular Science, Manchester, UK

Marietta L. van der Linden, PhD, MSc Queen Margaret University, Centre for Health Activity and Rehabilitation Research, Department of Rehabilitation Sciences, Musselburgh, UK

Clinton W. Wright, PharmD, BCPP Cyberonics, Department of Global Medical Affairs, Houston, TX, USA

Ralph Zitnik, MD SetPoint Medical Corporation, Valencia, CA, USA

Chapter 1
The Use of Electroceuticals and Neuromodulation in the Treatment of Migraine and Other Headaches

Sarah Miller and Manjit S. Matharu

Abstract Over recent years there has been increasing interest in the role of neurostimulation in the treatment of headache disorders. Currently both peripheral and central neuromodulation devices are available although evidence to support their use is still limited. Both non-invasive and invasive devices can be used for neurostimulation. Non-invasive peripheral stimulation options include supra-orbital stimulation (Cefaly® device) and vagal nerve stimulation (gammaCore® device), while invasive peripheral stimulation options include occipital nerve stimulation and sphenopalatine ganglion stimulation. Non-invasive central neurostimulation option involves single pulse transcranial magnetic stimulation (SpringTMS® device), while invasive central neurostimulation can be carried out using ventral tegmental area deep brain stimulation. Neurostimulation therapies offer a promising approach to otherwise medically intractable or difficult to treat headache disorders with each device having specific roles within the treatment pathway.

Keywords Electroceuticals • Nuromodulationl • Migraine • Headaches

Introduction

Primary headache conditions are benign, reoccurring headaches not caused by any underlying structural issue or disease. The primary headaches are subdivided into phenotypes based on the International Classification of Headache Disorders (ICHD-III beta) [1]. The main divisions are migraine and the trigeminal autonomic cephalalgias (TACs). Migraine is a recurrent headache disorder manifesting in attacks of pain lasting between 4 and 72 h, which is accompanied by nausea, vomiting, light and noise sensitivity and aggravation of the pain with movement. The TACs are a group of disorders characterised by unilateral head pain occurring in association

S. Miller, MRCP • M.S. Matharu, FRCP, PhD (✉)
Institute of Neurology and The National Hospital for Neurology and Neurosurgery, Queen Square, London WC1N 3BG, UK
e-mail: m.matharu@uclmail.net

A. Majid (ed.), *Electroceuticals*, DOI 10.1007/978-3-319-28612-9_1

with prominent ipsilateral cranial autonomic features. The TACs include cluster headache, paroxysmal hemicrania, hemicrania continua and short-lasting unilateral neuralgiform headache attacks, which is further subdivided into SUNCT (short-lasting unilateral neuralgiform headache attacks with conjunctival injection and tearing) and SUNA (short-lasting unilateral neuralgiform headache attacks with autonomic symptoms). The most common primary headache is migraine with an estimated 15% of the population affected [2]. The TACs are less common with estimated prevalence of cluster headache of 1 in 500 [3], of paroxysmal hemicrania around 0.5 per 1000 [4] and that of hemicrania continua and SUNCT/SUNA not well defined but thought to be similar to that of paroxysmal hemicrania [4]. The clinical features, epidemiology and first-line treatment options are summarised in Table 1.1.

The above primary headache conditions can be classified by their frequency into either episodic or chronic forms. Chronic migraine is defined as a headache occurring on 15 or more days of the month (of which eight or more are migrainous) for a period of over 3 months. Chronic TACs are diagnosed when patients go a year without remission periods or with remission periods lasting less than 1 month [1]. Chronic headache is a global health issue affecting up to 4% of the population [5], with chronic migraine or cluster headache forming the majority of chronic headaches seen in neurology units. The estimated prevalence of chronic migraine is 2% and chronic cluster headache 0.02% [6]. Patients may have headaches that are chronic from onset or evolve from an episodic form.

Although advances in the management of headache disorders means that the majority can be managed with medical treatments, a significant minority will not tolerate or prove intractable to available preventative pharmacological treatments. Neurostimulation techniques with peripheral and central targets appear to offer a promising approach to treating such patients. Devices allowing acute treatment of attacks may be useful to those unable to use or who overuse acute medications such as triptans. The peripheral targets used include the occipital nerve, the supra-orbital nerves, the sphenopalatine ganglion and the vagus nerve. Current central targets are the ventral tegmental area and the cortex. In this chapter, the main focus is on the treatment of chronic migraine and chronic cluster headache as this is where the bulk of literature and experience lies. Some reference will be made to the treatment of episodic migraine and cluster headache where relevant.

Pathophysiology of Primary Headache Conditions

Migraine

Migraine is a complex neurological disorder that affects multiple cortical, subcortical and brainstem regions that regulate the autonomic, affective, cognitive and sensory functions. The pathophysiology of the condition involves different neural networks and pathways interacting together to generate the clinical features of migraine. The main pathways and mechanisms involved in migraine generation include (Fig. 1.1):

Table 1.1 Clinical features of the primary headache disorders

	Migraine	Cluster headache	Paroxysmal hemicrania	SUNCT/SUNA	Hemicrania continua
Frequency in general population	15% (2% chronic)	0.2%	Rare	Rare	Rare
Sex ratio	Female > male	Male > Female	Female = Male	Male > Female	Female > Male
Pain:					
Description	Throbbing, aching, squeezing	Stabbing, boring	Stabbing, boring, throbbing	Sharp, stabbing, neuralgiform	Background pain: dull, heavy Exacerbations: throbbing, aching, squeezing
Severity	Moderate to severe	Severe, excruciating	Severe, excruciating	Severe, excruciating	Mild to moderate background pain with severe exacerbations
Laterality	Unilateral or bilateral	Unilateral	Unilateral	Unilateral	Unilateral
Attack frequency	Variable	1 to 8 attacks a day	5–40 attacks a day	3–200 attacks a day	Continuous pain
Attack duration	Hours	15–180 min	2–30 min	5–240 s	Continuous pain
Periodicity	–	Circadian and circannual ++	Circadian and circannual +/–	–	–
Autonomic features[a]	Sometimes, mild	Yes	Yes	Yes	Yes, with exacerbations
Migrainous features[b]	Yes	Yes, may be mild	Yes, may be mild	Rare	Yes
Triggers					
Alcohol	Yes	Yes	No	No	No
Cutaneous touch	No	No	No	Yes	No
Indometacin response	None	None	Complete resolution	None	Complete resolution
Abortive treatment	Oral triptan, NSAID	Subcutaneous Sumatriptan, Oxygen	Nil	Nil	Nil
First-line prophylactic	Beta-Blockers, tricyclic antidepressant, topiramate	Verapamil, lithium, topiramate	Indometacin	Lamotrigine, oxcarbazepine	Indometacin

NSAID non-steroidal anti-inflammatory drugs, *SUNA* short-lasting unilateral neuralgiform headache attacks with autonomic features, *SUNCT* short-lasting unilateral neuralgiform headache attacks with conjunctival injection and tearing

[a]Autonomic features: One or more of ptosis, lacrimation, conjunctival injection, facial redness/sweating, eyelid/facial swelling, nasal stuffiness, rhinorrhea

[b]Migrainous features: One or more of nausea and/or vomiting, photophobia, phonophobia

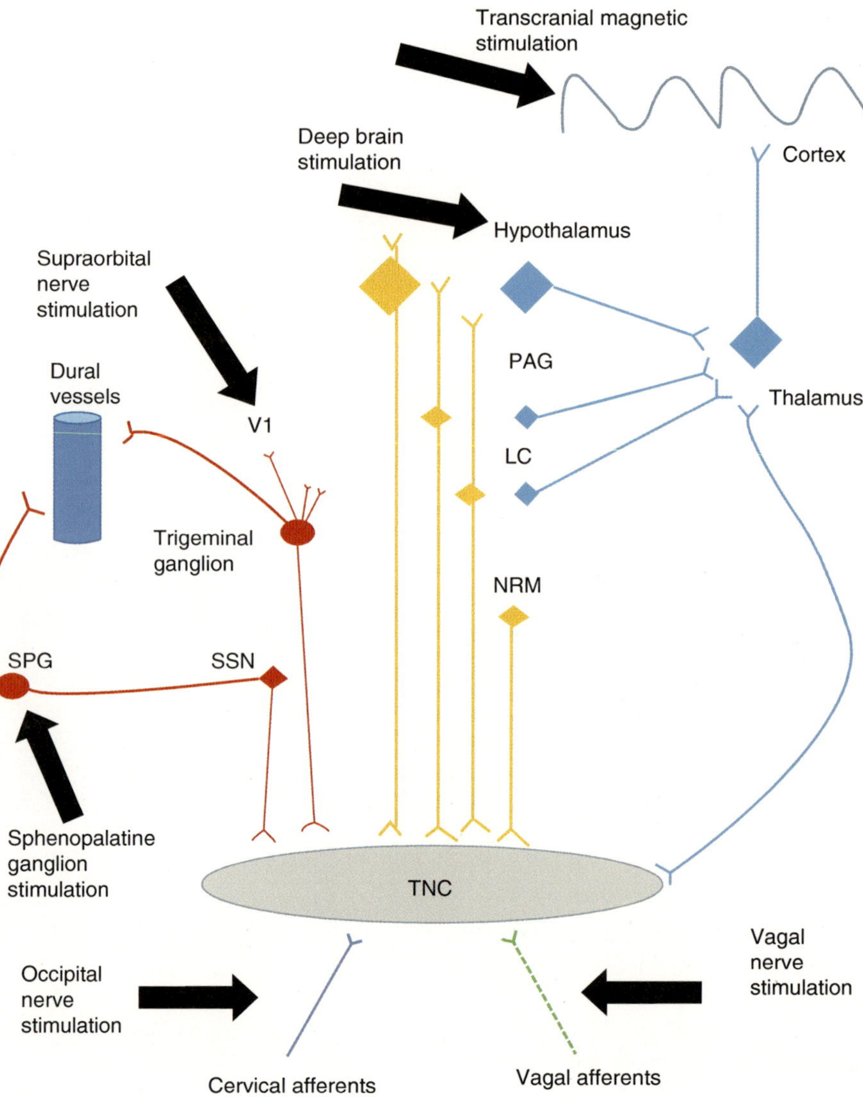

Fig. 1.1 Schematic of headache pain pathways and the targets for neurostimulation

- the trigeminovascular system including the large intracranial vessels,
- brain hyperexcitability and cortical spreading depression (CSD),
- the trigeminocervical complex consisting of the caudal trigeminal nucleus and the spinal roots of C1–C2.

The innervation of large intracranial vessels and the dura comes from the first division of the trigeminal nerve, a pathway known as the trigeminovascular system [7]. Activation of trigeminal nerve endings results in the release of neuro-inflammatory peptides such as calcitonin gene regulating peptide (CGRP), substance P and nitric oxide. These inflammatory mediators result in the activation of trigeminal nerve endings on adjacent blood vessels and a positive feedback loop is established via trigeminal brainstem connections to higher centres resulting in pain generation.

Trigeminal afferents pass caudally through the trigeminal ganglion to synapse in the trigeminal-cervical complex. This complex provides an anatomical and functional overlap of trigeminal afferents and cervical afferents from the level of the trigeminal nucleus caudalis to the level of C2 [8]. Stimulation of the cervical neurones at this level results in activation of trigeminal neurones, thus, nociceptive activation of either end of the pathway can result in both occipital and frontal pain. The trigeminal nucleus also makes connections with the thalamus via brainstem nuclei such as the periaqueductal gray, dorsal raphe nucleus and locus coeruleus.

There is evidence to support the concept that migraine sufferers have a sustained state of brain hyper-excitability [9]. Neurophysiological work shows increased visual evoked potentials and absence of habituation in migraineurs. Genetic causes of migraine have been linked to mutations leading to increased levels of synaptic glutamate, an excitatory neurotransmitter and transcranial magnetic stimulation studies has suggested reduced phosphene thresholds in migraineurs compatible with hyper-excitability. This excitability leads to a lowered threshold for the initiation of CSD. Cortical spreading depression, the physiological substrate of aura, consists of a wave of neuronal excitation spreading across the cortex followed by a reciprocal wave of neuronal inhibition [10]. Cortical spreading depression has been found to lead to the activation of the trigeminovascular system and potentially of brainstem regulatory centres, both of which can lead to pain generation.

Trigeminal Autonomic Cephalalgias

The pathophysiological constructs for TACs must account for the distinctive clinical characteristics of the disorders: the trigeminal distribution of pain, the ipsilateral autonomic features and the periodicity seen in cluster headache. Pain innervation of the head comes from branches of the first division of the trigeminal nerve. The links between the trigeminal system, the higher cervical nerve roots and brainstem structures are discussed above. The ipsilateral autonomic features are thought to arise from cranial parasympathetic activation and sympathetic hypofunctioning. The pathway controlling these symptoms is known as the trigeminoautonomic reflex. Experimental data suggests that stimulation of trigeminal afferents results in cranial autonomic outflow via this reflex [11]. In humans, the parasympathetic fibres involved in this reflex synapse in the sphenopalatine ganglion. Although the trigeminoautonomic reflex is active in other headache syndromes, it is the degree of activation in TACs that give the distinctive clinical features. Hypothalamic activation has been suggested on functional neuroimaging of TAC patients [12–15]. There is evidence of the role of hypothalamus in mediating anti-nociceptive and autonomic responses when intracranial pain structures are activated. In support of the role of the hypothalamus in pain processing in TACs, direct pathways between the hypothalamus and trigeminal nucleus have been mapped. Other supporting data for the importance of the hypothalamus in attack generation or pain control in TACs are the periodicity of cluster headache attacks that would suggest involvement of suprachiasmatic nucleus of the hypothalamus, where the "body clock" is sited, and the fact that hypothalamic peptides Orexin A and B elicit both pro- and anti-nociceptive effects on the trigeminal system [16].

The current hypothesis is that TACs are due to a central abnormality in hypothalamic processing with subsequent activation of the trigeminovascular and trigeminoautonomic pathways via the superior salivatory nucleus, sphenopalatine ganglion and trigeminal pathways.

Peripheral Neurostimulation Devices

Supraorbital Nerve Stimulation

The trigeminal system has a crucial role in generation of head pain. The supraorbital nerve is a branch of the frontal nerve (which in turn is a branch of the first division of the trigeminal nerve) and innervates the frontal sinus, upper eyelid and anterolateral part of the forehead and scalp. A transcutaneous supraorbital nerve stimulator has been developed as a potential treatment for headache and case reports also exist on the potential use of subcutaneous supraorbital nerve stimulation in isolation or alongside occipital nerve stimulator devices.

Evidence for the Use of Transcutaneous Supraorbital Nerve Stimulation

Transcutaneous supraorbital nerve stimulation involves the use of an external device to deliver an electrical current through the supraorbital nerves. The Cefaly® device is the only currently available external transcutaneous nerve stimulator. It is battery powered and worn on the forehead using a headband-like device. There is currently no evidence to support the use of transcutaneous nerve stimulation in chronic migraine or chronic cluster headache, either as an acute or preventative treatment. Some limited evidence of its possible use in episodic migraine is available.

Acute Treatment of Episodic Migraine

No controlled evidence for the use of transcutaneous supraorbital nerve stimulation in the acute treatment of episodic migraine has been published. However, a single pilot study of the Cefaly® device, reported that use of the device was associated with pain freedom in only 13% of treated cases and actually had no effect in 57% of attacks [17].

Preventative Treatment of Episodic Migraine

The evidence for transcutaneous supraorbital nerve stimulation in preventative treatment of episodic migraine comes from a small sham-controlled study of the Cefaly® device and manufacturer's post-marketing survey data [18, 19]. The sham-controlled study of 67 patients with episodic migraine using either a sham or active supraorbital nerve stimulator device for 3 months reported a significant drop of 30% in migraine days in the active group compared to 4.9% in the sham group [18]. Responder rates for the device were comparable to traditional migraine preventative agents such as propranolol [20]. The post-marketing survey incorporated data from 2313 subjects who used the transcutaneous supraorbital nerve stimulator for migraine prevention. Fifty three percent of subjects rated themselves "satisfied" and continued treatment after a 40-day trial period [19]. Although the therapeutic gain in migraine day reduction was lower at 12% than that seen in other migraine preventatives such as topiramate (25%), the lower levels of adverse events and higher rates of patient satisfaction with Cefaly® device may counterbalance this issue.

Evidence for the Use of Subcutaneous Supraorbital Nerve Stimulation

Subcutaneous supraorbital nerve stimulation is achieved by placing subdermal-subcutaenous electrodes on the forehead in the territory innervated by the supraorbital nerve [21]. The electrodes can be placed in isolation or in combination with occipital nerve electrodes. The only evidence for the use of subcutaneous supraorbital nerve stimulation comes from small open-label case series on the preventative treatment of chronic migraine and chronic cluster headache, most often in combination with occipital electrodes.

Preventative Treatment of Chronic Migraine

Two small series are available in the literature on the use of combined supraorbital and occipital nerve stimulation for the prevention of intractable chronic migraine. The first was by Reed et al. [22] and included seven patients receiving bilateral supraorbital and occipital electrodes. With a median follow-up of 15 months, all patients reported a more than 50% reduction in headache severity. Adverse events included lead migration, infection and allergy. Hann and Sharan performed a similar procedure on 14 patients [23]. With a mean follow-up of 31 months, ten patients had a more than 50% reduction in headache severity. Adverse events included lead migration, allodynia and infection and the group reported a reoperation rate of 36%.

Preventative Treatment of Chronic Cluster Headache

Current literature on subcutaneous supraorbital nerve stimulation for chronic cluster headache is limited to a total of six patients, one case report and one case series. Narouze and Kapural were the first to publish a case report of isolated supraorbital nerve stimulation for chronic cluster headache in 2007 [24]. Following the implant of a unilateral lead with programmes for both preventative and acute treatments, the patient had a complete remission of pain for over 14 months. When the stimulation was terminated, the attacks returned within 24 h. Interestingly, the device was also successfully used as an abortive treatment to terminate acute attacks. The second series of four chronic cluster headache patients with a mixture of unilateral and bilateral leads reported a more than 50% reduction in pain severity in all patients after a follow-up of 25 months [25]. Adverse events were high with two patients suffering electrode erosion through the skin and one a lead infection.

Safety of Supraorbital Nerve Stimulation

Transcutaneous supraorbital nerve stimulation appears to be a safe and well-tolerated treatment option. In the study from Magis et al. of 2313 participants using the Cefaly® device for the treatment of migraine only 4% of subjects reported any adverse events [19]. The most frequent adverse event was intolerable paraesthesia (30% of adverse events) but sleepiness during treatment (12%), skin irritation at the application site (5%) and worsening of headache with treatment (12%) were also reported.

Subcutaneous supraorbital nerve stimulation seems to have a similar risk profile to ONS. As the majority of patients reported in literature had both ONS and supraorbital electrodes, the adverse event data is discussed in ONS section.

The Possible Role of Supraorbital Nerve Stimulation (Table 1.2)

Transcutaneous supraorbital stimulation may be useful in the prevention of episodic migraine in those unable to tolerate or not responding to traditional pharmacotherapy. As yet, there is not enough evidence to support its use for chronic migraine, chronic cluster headache or acute treatment of either migrainous or cluster attacks. From the limited evidence available for invasive supraorbital nerve stimulation, routine use of this procedure to treatment primary headaches cannot be advocated as yet.

Vagal Nerve Stimulation

The vagus nerve contains both motor and sensory components and has a role in controlling autonomic responses as well as pain processing via its projections to higher pain control centres. The initial concept of vagal nerve stimulation as a

Table 1.2 Summary table of the possible roles of neurostimulation in primary headache disorders

	Supraorbital stimulation	Vagal nerve stimulation	Transcranial magnetic stimulation	Occipital nerve stimulation	Sphenopalatine ganglion stimulation	Deep brain stimulation
Device name	Cefaly	GammaCore	Spring TMS		Pulsante	
Treatment use						
Acute migraine attacks	X	√	√ (with and without aura)	X	X	X
Prevention of episodic migraine	√	X	X	X	X	X
Prevention of chronic migraine	X	X	X	√	X	X
Acute cluster attacks	X	X	X	X	√	X
Prevention of episodic cluster headache	X	√[a]	X	X	X	X
Prevention of chronic cluster headache	X	√	X	√	√ (studies on-going)	√
Other TACs	X	X	X	√ (prevention of chronic intractable TACs)	X	√ (prevention of chronic intractable TACs)

TACs trigeminal autonomic cephalalgias
[a]Usefulness may be dictated by length of episodic cluster bout, if bout lasts less than 3 months may be difficult to assess as treatment may take this long to have clear effect

headache treatment came following observations of migraine improvement in patients undergoing invasive vagal nerve stimulator implants for intractable epilepsy [26]. The use of invasive vagal nerve stimulation for headache has been limited to small case reports. The development of non-invasive transcutaneous vagal nerve stimulator devices such as the gammaCore®, a handheld device used on the neck, has led to a resurgence of interest in the role of vagal nerve modulation in primary headache.

Evidence for the Use of Transcutaneous Vagal Nerve Stimulation

Preventative Treatment of Chronic Cluster Headache

Available evidence for the possible use of transcutaneous vagal nerve stimulation comes from a study of the gammaCore® device, the Prevention and Acute Treatment of Chronic Cluster Headache (PREVA) trial [27]. This trial, consisting of 45 active and 47 control subjects, compared standard of care plus vagal nerve stimulation to standard care alone. Regular use of the gammaCore® device for 4 weeks was associated with a significant reduction in cluster attack frequency compared to control (6 vs. 2 less attacks a week). The 50% response rate was also higher in the active group (40% vs. 8%). Following a four-week extension phase, both the reduction in attack frequency and response rate were seen to increase (to 8 attacks a week less and a 46% responder rate) suggesting a prolonged period of use is required to gain maximal benefit. Following treatment, 50% reported satisfaction with the device and 65% would recommend treatment to others.

Acute Treatment of Chronic Cluster Headache

A small open-label series of 19 patients using the gammaCore® device reported that it was useful as an acute treatment with 47% of attacks terminated within 11 min [28]. Subsequently, the PREVA study also reported on the use of the gammaCore® device to abort cluster attacks [27]. The use of transcutaneous vagal nerve stimulation as an acute treatment in 75 of 92 participants had no effect on cluster headache attack duration or severity. The PREVA study results suggest that there is no role for the use of gammaCore® as an acute treatment in cluster headache.

Preventative Treatment of Chronic Migraine

The controlled trial evidence for the use of transcutaneous vagal nerve stimulation with the gammaCore® as a preventative treatment in chronic migraine is limited to a single trial of 59 patients [29]. The trial, comparing 2 months treatment with active treatment to treatment with a sham device, failed to show a difference in headache day reduction between the groups (reduction of 2 days per group). An open-label extension phase suggested a significant difference emerges with a longer duration of treatment but further studies are needed to validate this [30].

Acute Treatment of Migraine

There is no controlled data to support the use of transcutaneous vagal nerve stimulation with the gammaCore® device in the acute treatment of migraine. Open-label data is, however, available on a total of 27 patients with episodic migraine [31] and 48 with high frequency or chronic migraine [32]. In the episodic migraine cohort, a total of 80 attacks were treated and 22% of attacks achieved pain freedom within 2 h, a figure similar to that seen with Naproxen 500 mg but below the 67% reported with Sumatriptan100 mg [31, 33, 34]. The series of high frequency and chronic migraine reported by Barbanti et al. [32] included 131 attacks treated over a 2-week period. In this cohort, 23% were pain free at 2 h.

Evidence for the Use of Invasive Vagal Nerve Stimulation

Invasive vagal nerve stimulation is carried out primarily for intractable epilepsy and involves the implantation of an electrode over the left vagus nerve [35]. Following reports of pain relief in concurrent migraine attacks, some groups have used the implants for the treatment of intractable chronic migraine.

Preventative Treatment of Chronic Migraine

The outcomes of invasive vagal nerve stimulation in chronic migraine are limited to three series [36–38]. Mauskop reported on four patients treated with invasive vagal nerve stimulation, two of whom achieved substantial improvements [36]. Hord et al. found four patients with migraine within their cohort of 27 epilepsy patients undergoing invasive vagal nerve stimulation. All reported a decrease in migraine intensity and frequency, with one being rendered pain free [38]. The final series by Cecchini and colleagues (2009) reported on four patients implanted for chronic migraine with two reporting a more than 50% reduction in headache frequency.

Safety of Vagal Nerve Stimulation

Transcutaneous vagal nerve stimulation appears to be a safe treatment with no serious adverse events linked to the device recorded. Using data from the above studies [27, 31], the most common adverse events reported were facial muscle twitching, neck pain, rash or redness at the application site and worsening of the headache. In sham-controlled studies [27, 29], it was noted that similar proportions of active and control subjects reported adverse events and in fact, control subjects in the Silberstein et al. study [29] on chronic migraine prevention reported more adverse events of severe intensity than those in the active group.

The Possible Role of Vagal Nerve Stimulation (Table 1.2)

Available literature on transcutaneous vagal nerve stimulation using the gammaCore® device suggests that at present, it could be considered for the use of prevention of chronic cluster headache. There is, as yet, insufficient evidence for the use of transcutaneous vagal nerve stimulation for acute or preventative treatment of migraine and the acute treatment of cluster headache. From current evidence, there is not a role for invasive vagal nerve stimulation in the treatment of primary headaches.

Occipital Nerve Stimulation

The occipital region is innervated by the greater, lesser and least occipital nerves. The greater occipital nerve is a branch of the C2 spinal root and provides innervation to the occipito-parietal area around 6–8 cm wide ascending paramedially from the suboccipital region to the vertex [39]. There is an anatomical overlap between the cervical and trigeminal afferents from the level of the trigeminal nucleus caudalis to the level of C2 [8]. This overlap allows the stimulation of the occipital region to modulate pain in both trigeminal and cervical distributions. Occipital nerve stimulation (ONS) involves a non-destructive surgical process whereby electrodes are placed subcutaneously in the occipital region at the level of C1 and then wired to an implantable pulse generator (IPG) in the chest, abdomen or occasionally buttocks. Current batteries are rechargeable with a lifespan close to 10 years. Patients are able to adjust their own stimulation intensity levels using a hand-held remote control. Stimulation parameters of frequency, pulse width and voltage are adjusted to achieve continuous comfortable paraesthesia in the distribution of the greater occipital nerves. The optimum settings for ONS are not yet defined and there is a wide variation in the stimulation settings used across centres.

Evidence for the Use of Occipital Nerve Stimulation

ONS is most commonly used for chronic cluster and chronic migraine and so more extensive literature exists to support its use in these conditions. As with other neurostimulation techniques, the majority of published data on the use of ONS for primary headaches consists of open-label case series. However, randomised placebo-controlled trials have been conducted on the use of ONS in the prevention of chronic migraine. Smaller open-label series exist for the use of ONS in SUNCT/SUNA and hemicrania continua. Table 1.3 summarises the available

Table 1.3 Evidence from published case series for occipital nerve stimulation in primary headache conditions

Trial (first author, year)	Patients (n)	Average follow-up (months)	Response rate (proportion reporting at least 50% reduction in attack frequency)
Supraorbital nerve stimulation (+/− ONS) for chronic migraine			
Reed et al. [22]	7	17	100%
Hann and Sharan [23]	14	31	71%[a]
TOTAL	**21**	**16**	**86%**
ONS for chronic migraine			
Saper et al. [40]	75	3 months	39%[b]
Silberstein et al. [41] [Extended follow up, Dodick et al. [42]]	157 [157]	3 months [12 months]	17% [60%]
Brewer et al. [43]	12	34 months	42%
Lipton et al. [44]	125	3 months	N/A (−6 days week active group vs. −4 days week sham group, p = 0.29)
Mueller et al. [45]	3	7 months	100%[c]
Paemeleire et al. [46]	8	24 months	71%[d]
TOTAL	**380**	**12 months**	**42%** **[53%]**
ONS for chronic cluster headache			
Magis et al. [47, 48]	14	37	86%
Schwedt et al. [49]	3	19	33%
Brewer et al. [43]	5	41	80%
Burns et al. [50, 51]	14	18	36%
Fontaine et al. [52]	13	15	77%
Mueller et al. [45]	24	22 months	88%[c]
Mueller et al. [53]	10	12 months	90%[c]
TOTAL	**83**	**23 months**	**62%**
ONS for SUNCT/SUNA			
Lambru et al. [54]	9	38 months	89%
ONS for hemicrania continua			
Burns et al. [55]	6	14	67%

ONS occipital nerve stimulation, *SUNCT* short-lasting unilateral neuralgiform headache attacks with conjunctival injection and tearing, *SUNA* short-lasting unilateral neuralgiform headache attacks with autonomic features

[a]Clinical response defined as least 50% reduction in headache severity

[b]Clinical response defined as least 50% reduction in monthly headache days or greater than 3 point reduction verbal rating scale

[c]Definition of response not given/unclear, not included in response rate total

[d]Response defined by least 3 point reduction verbal rating scale; [ ] data from extended follow-up of the original Silberstein et al. [41] series

published case studies on ONS in primary headache. It is worth stressing the fact that there is no data to support the use of ONS in the acute treatment of any primary headache syndromes.

Preventative Treatment of Chronic Migraine

The outcomes of the three randomised placebo-controlled trials on ONS in chronic migraine have been somewhat mixed. The first trial conducted in 2009, the Precision Implantable Stimulator for Migraine (PRISM) study, reported on the outcomes of 125 subjects randomised to active or sham stimulation for 3 months [44]. Although full results are not yet available, preliminary data failed to show a significant reduction in migraine days between treatment groups. The second trial, the occipital nerve stimulation for the treatment of intractable chronic migraine headache (ONSTIM) study, published in 2011, was a randomised controlled study of 61 subjects comparing active adjustable stimulation (28 patients), pre-set "sham" stimulation (16 patients) and standard medical treatment (17 patients) [40]. A positive clinical response (defined as a 50% reduction in headache days or greater than 3-point reduction in pain scores) was seen in 39% of the active adjustable stimulation group, 6% in the sham-stimulation group and 0% in the medical group. The most recent study from Silberstein et al. published in 2012 reported on 157 patients comparing active stimulation (105 patients) to sham stimulation (52 subjects) [41]. The primary outcome measure of clinical responders (the proportion of patients achieving a 50% or more reduction in pain scores) showed no significant difference between groups (17% vs. 14%). However, significant differences between the groups were seen in the reduction of headache days (27% vs. 15%) and in the proportion of patients achieving a 30% or more reduction in pain scores (38% vs. 19%). As the International Headache Society have issued clinical trial guidelines stating that, due to the intractable and highly disabling nature of chronic migraine, a 30% reduction in outcome measures should be considered as clinically relevant [56], these findings can be interpreted as a positive outcome of ONS for chronic migraine. A meta-analysis of the pooled data has found that ONS was associated with a reduction of 3 migraine days per month after 3 months of active treatment when compared to sham stimulation [57]. Interestingly, comments are made in the same systemic review that the poor and incomplete reporting of data has hindered greater interpretation of results. Open-label data on ONS in chronic migraine is summarised in Table 1.3 [45] and adverse event data that has been a cause for concern in some ONS series in Table 1.4.

Preventative Treatment of Chronic Cluster Headache

Although as of yet controlled data on the use of ONS in chronic cluster headache is not available, the available open-label data supports the potential efficacy of the treatment (Table 1.3) [53]. Over 90 patients have been reported in the literature and a pooled analysis suggests a mean reduction of daily attack frequency of 67% [65]. Numerous case series have been published (Table 1.3) and we will discuss some of the larger ones in more detail below. Individual case reports will not be explored.

The first published cohort of ONS in chronic cluster headache was in 2007 and involved the prospective study of eight patients treated with unilateral ONS lead

Table 1.4 Adverse reactions reported in published occipital nerve stimulation series

Author	Number patients	Duration follow-up (mean)	Hardware related complications		Surgical action required	Biological related complications		Surgical action required	Stimulation related complications		Surgical action required
Weiner and Reed [58]	13	2.4 years	Migration	1 (8%)	1 (8%)	Infection	1 (8%)	1 (8%)			
Popeney and Alo [59]	25	18.3 months	Migration Re-implantation post infection	9 (36%) 1 (4%)	0 (36%) 1 (4%)	Infection	1 (4%)	1 (4%)			
Fontaine et al. [52]	20	6 months–4 years (no mean given)	Migration Explantation (headache free) Battery failure	7 (35%) 1 (5%) 1 (5%)	7 (35%) 1 (5%) 1 (5%)	Infection	2 (10%)	1 (5%)			
Johnstone and Sundaraj [60]	7	25 months	Re-implantation post infection	2 (29%)	2 (29%)	Infection	2 (29%)	2 (29%)			
Slavin et al. [61]	10	22 months	Migration Explantation (headache free)	1 (10%) 1 (10%)	1 (10%) 1 (10%)	Infection Neck pain	1 (10%) 1 (10%)	1 (10%) 1 (10%)			
Magis et al. [62]	8	15.1 months	Migration Lead fracture/displacement Battery failure	1 (13%) 1 (13%) 4 (50%)	0 0 4 (50%)	IPG/Lead/Wound pain	2 (25%)	0	Undesirable changes in stimulation	1 (13%)	1 (13%)
Schwedt et al. [49]	15	3 year	Migration Battery failure	8 (53%) 5 (33%)	N/A N/A	IPG, Lead or Wound pain Neck stiffness Wound site complications	12 (80%) 5 (33%) 4 (27%)	N/A N/A N/A			

(continued)

Table 1.4 (continued)

Author	Number patients	Duration follow-up (mean)	Hardware related complications		Surgical action required	Biological related complications		Surgical action required	Stimulation related complications		Surgical action required
Burns et al. [51]	14	17.5 months	Migration Lead fracture/displacement Explantation (lack efficacy) Battery failure Additional electrode	3 (21%) 2 (14%) 1 (7%) 8 (57%) 1 (7%)	3 (21%) 2 (14%) 1 (7%) 6 (57%) 1 (7%)	Infection IPG, Lead or Wound pain Neck stiffness Wound site complications	3 (21%) 4 (29%) 1 (7%) 1 (7%)	0 0 0 0	Undesirable changes in stimulation	4(29%)	0
Lipton et al. [44] (Data from Sharan et al. [63])	125	12 week	Migration	7%	N/A	Infection IPG, Lead or Wound pain	15% 8%	N/A N/A			
Paemeleire et al. [46]	44	36 months	Migration Lead fracture/displacement	2 (5%) 9 (21%)	2 (5%) 9 (21%)	Infection IPG, Lead or Wound pain	2 (5%) 3 (7%)	0 3 (7%)			
Saper et al. [40]	51	3 month	Migration Lead fracture	12 (24%) 1 (2%)	N/A N/A	Infection IPG, Lead or Wound pain Neck stiffness Wound site complication	12 (24%) 5 (10%) 2 (4%) 4 (8%)	N/A N/A N/A N/A	Undesirable changes in stimulation 3 (6%)		N/A
Fontaine et al. [52]	13	14.6 months				Infection Wound site complication	1 (8%) 1 (8%)	1 (8%) 1 (8%)	Undesirable changes in stimulation	1 (8%)	0
Magis et al. [48]	15	36.8 months	Migration Battery failure	1 (7%) 9 (60%)	1(7%) 9 (60%)	Infection IPG, Lead or Wound pain	3 (20%) 5 (33%)	3 (20%) 0	Undesirable changes in stimulation	3 (20%)	1 (7%)

Brewer et al. [43]	26	8.5 years	Migration Explantation (headache free ×2, lack efficacy ×3) Battery failure Lead revisions	1 (4%) 5 (19%) 1 (4%) 15 (58%)	0 5 (19%) 0 15 (58%)	Infection	1 (4%)	1 (4%)			
Silberstein et al. [41]	157	12 weeks	Migration Lead fracture/displacement Erosion	20 (13%) 2 (1%) 7 (5%)	N/A N/A N/A	Infection IPG, Lead or Wound pain Wound site complication Allergy to surgical material	7 (5%) 23 (15%) 4 (3%) 4 (3%)	N/A N/A N/A N/A	Undesirable changes in stimulation	9 (6%)	N/A
Palmisani et al. [64]	23	36 months	Migration Fracture Erosion (all with associated infection) Explantation (lack efficacy)		3 (13%) 2 (9%) 3 (13%) 4 (17%)	Infection		2 (9%)	Undesirable changes in stimulation		2 (9%)
Dodick et al. [42]	157	52 weeks	Migration Lead fracture/displacement Skin erosion Battery failure	29 (19%) 7 (4%) 8 (5%) 8 (5%)	27 (17%) 7 (4%) 7 (4%) 7 (4%)	Infection IPG, Lead or Wound pain Wound site complication Allergy to surgical material	11 (7%) 38 (24%) 6 (3%) 5 (3%)	6 (4%) 12 (8%) 1 (1%) 2 (1%)	Undesirable changes in stimulation	17 (11%)	8 (5%)

IPG implantable pulse generator, *N/A* data not available from paper implantation ipsilateral to the side of pain [47]. After a mean follow-up period of 15 months, five patients were considered to be clinical responders with a reduction of more than 50% in daily attack frequency. In fact, all of these patients reported a more than 90% reduction in attack frequency and two remained pain-free for prolonged periods. There was a delay of at least 2 months following implant before clinical response emerged and attacks recurred or worsened within days to weeks of stimulation stopping – a feature that has been consistently reported in studies of ONS for primary headaches ever since. The group also reported that two patients with initial relief of their cluster attacks went on to develop new attacks on the opposite side to the ONS electrode. This phenomenon has been confirmed by other series and has led to recommendations that bilateral leads are placed in all patients. Although no serious adverse events were reported, lead migration and electrode displacement were observed (Table 1.4).

Burns et al. reported on a cohort of 14 medically intractable chronic cluster headache patients undergoing bilateral ONS implants [50, 51]. Following a median follow-up period of 18 months, 10 of the 14 patients reported an improvement. Of those with benefit, three had a more than 90% reduction in attack frequency and a further three had a reduction of between 40 and 60%. As in the previous series by Magis et al. [47], a delay of weeks was seen until clinical response and attacks were seen to return within days when the devices were turned off. Adverse events reported included lead migration in nearly a third of patients, superficial infection, painful paraesthesia and neck stiffness (Table 1.4).

In 2011, Fontaine and colleagues reported on their cohort of 13 chronic cluster headache patients undergoing ONS [52]. After a mean follow-up period of 15 months, a reduction of 68% was seen in mean attack frequency and a 50% improvement in attack frequency was seen in ten of the patients.

Magis et al. have examined long-term efficacy in their cohort with a mean follow-up time of 37 months [48]. Of the 15 patients implanted, 14 went on to long-term follow-up (one implant was removed due to infection). Eleven of the 14 patients reported a more than 90% reduction in attack frequency. Again, the authors commented on side shifting of attacks when unilateral stimulation was employed and adverse events were similar to their previous report. Other groups looking at long-term outcome have also reported sustained efficacy over periods of 20–33 months but patient numbers were very small; three in the series by Schwedt et al. and five in the series from Brewer et al. [43, 49].

Preventative Treatment of Other TACs

Published data on the use of ONS in SUNCT/SUNA is currently limited to a series of nine patients with median follow-up of 38 months [54]. Authors report that four patients became pain free following treatment and all others had a more than 80% improvement in attack frequency. As with ONS in chronic cluster headache, a time lag to clinical response was observed as was worsening of attacks within days to weeks of stimulation stopping. A total of ten patients with hemicrania continua treated with ONS in an open-label fashion are currently reported in the literature [43, 49, 55, 66]. All were treated with unilateral miniaturised stimulation devices no longer available for use. Although outcome measures differ across the four cohorts, it appears that at least five were counted as clinical responders (Table 1.3). There are no reports on the use of ONS in paroxysmal hemicrania as yet available in the literature.

Safety of Occipital Nerve Stimulation (Table 1.4)

Major concerns have been voiced over the adverse event data collected from the controlled and open-label studies of ONS in primary headache, particularly hardware related events. Adverse event data available in the literature is summarised in Table 1.4 [46, 58–61, 64]. Lead migration was reported in 24% of ONSTIM subjects, [40] 7% in the PRISM series [44] and in up to 19% of subjects in the extended phase of the Silberstein et al. cohort [42]. Open-label series has reported lead migration rates between 4 and 53% with the series from Brewer et al. reporting the need for lead revision in 58% of patients. A high rate of infection has also been reported in a number of series ranging from 4 to 29%. Many of the complications reported in the ONS literature are potentially serious and often require surgical intervention. However, data is emerging that adverse event rates can be dramatically reduced if ONS implants are conducted by well-trained, highly experienced surgical teams specialising in ONS surgery. A review of the adverse event data collected from the randomised study of Silberstein et al. showed that the incidence of surgery-related adverse events and the need for additional surgical procedures decreased with increased levels of surgical experience [63].

The Possible Role of Occipital Nerve Stimulation (Table 1.2)

As with all invasive neuromodulation treatments, ONS should be reserved for those with highly intractable medical refractory guidelines that have failed to respond to all other treatments. To stress this point, the European Headache Society has published clear guidelines on the use of invasive neurostimulation and this is summarised in Table 1.5. From current data, ONS could be considered for the preventative treatment of refractory chronic migraine and cluster headaches (and possibly other TACs) once they have failed all available pharmacological input. In order to minimise adverse events, patients should be assessed and treated in highly specialised units.

Sphenopalatine Ganglion Stimulation

The sphenopalatine ganglion (SPG) is an extracranial structure lying in the pterygopalatine fossa (PPF) containing both sympathetic and parasympathetic fibres. The SPG has connections, both direct and indirect, to many centres considered important

Table 1.5 Criteria for the use of invasive neurostimulation in primary headache

Patient must meet the International Headache Society criteria for chronic migraine or trigeminal autonomic cephalalgia
For chronic cluster headache, patients should have had daily or near daily attacks for at least 2 years prior to stimulation
Patients should have been under the care of a headache specialist team for at least 1 year
All reasonable drugs must have been tried at the correct doses and for sufficient durations unless contraindicated
All patients should have a psychological assessment prior to surgery
All co-existent conditions should be identified and treated where possible prior to surgery (e.g. depression, medication overuse)
Patients (and doctors) must have a realistic expectation of the surgical outcome
Patients should be followed up by the headache specialist team for at least 1 year
Prospective headache diaries recording headache attack frequency, severity and duration as well as analgesia intake must be kept
Appropriate quality of life measures, disability scores and self-assessments must be kept by the patient prior and post-operatively
Where possible the neurostimulator should only be switched off for efficacy assessment, ideally in a double-blind fashion
A clear record of adverse events is kept

Adapted from Martelletti et al. [67] and Leone et al. [68]

in nociception and the pathophysiology of cluster headache such as the trigeminovascular system, the superior salivatory nucleus and the hypothalamus. Given the anatomy of the SPG, it has been investigated as a potential target in the treatment of cluster headache. Sphenopalatine ganglion stimulation can be achieved using a Pulsante® device, which has controlled evidence for efficacy in chronic cluster headache. The Pulsante® device is a miniaturised implantable neurostimulator with integral lead and battery. The lead is placed within the PPF using minimally invasive surgery with a trans-oral approach and the patient then controls the device using a handheld remote control.

Evidence for the Use of Sphenopalatine Ganglion Stimulation

Sphenopalatine ganglion stimulation has been developed for use in chronic cluster headache. Evidence is limited to one randomised control study although further studies are currently ongoing.

Acute Treatment of Chronic Cluster Headache

A randomised sham-controlled trial of 28 patients used the Pulsante® device to treat acute cluster attacks with either full, sub-perception or sham stimulation levels [69]. Pain relief after 15 min of SPG stimulation was seen in a significantly higher number of full-stimulation treated attacks (67%) than either sub-perception level (7%)

or sham stimulation (7%). After 2 months of treating acute attacks, only 31% of the full-stimulation group were still using medication to abort attacks compared to 77% in the sham stimulation group.

Preventative Treatment of Chronic Cluster Headache

During the above controlled trial, it was observed that subjects using the Pulsante® device began to report a reduction in attack frequency over time. After the 2 months study period, 43% of subjects using the full-stimulation device to treat attacks regularly reported a more than 50% reduction in daily attack frequency suggesting that the device has a preventative effect [69]. Further study into the efficacy and optimal stimulation settings of SPG stimulation as a preventative treatment for chronic cluster headache is ongoing.

Safety of Sphenopalatine Ganglion Stimulation

In the available study, 81% of subjects reported a transient sensory disturbance within the maxillary nerve distribution post-operatively but this resolved within 3 months in the majority of cases [69]. Two patients reported lead migration and misplacement requiring surgical revision and one a post-operative infection requiring antibiotics.

The Possible Role of Sphenopalatine Ganglion Stimulation (Table 1.2)

Guidelines for the use of SPG stimulation in chronic cluster headache were published by a group of headache experts in 2014 [70]. At present, the treatment should be considered as an acute treatment, with potential additional preventative effects, in those with medically intractable chronic cluster headache who have failed all available pharmacological therapies. The Pulsante® device may be particularly useful for those with contraindications to Sumatriptan or in those with a high frequency of daily attacks.

Central Neurostimulation Devices

Deep Brain Stimulation of the Ventral Tegmental Area

Functional neuroimaging studies on primary headache conditions have suggested that during acute cluster attacks there are changes in the posterior hypothalamic region in TACs that are not present in migraine [12–15, 71]. Further work has shown that stimulation of the same area in cluster headache patients increases blood flow throughout areas of the central pain matrix [72]. In 2001, Leone et al. used this functional imaging data evidence to implant deep brain electrodes in what was described as the posterior hypothalamic region in a patient with highly refractory chronic cluster headache [73]. Detailed analysis of the anatomy of the region described in the literature and on imaging has suggested that the actual site of interest for deep brain stimulation (DBS) is the ventral tegmental area and not the posterior hypothalamus [74]. Stereotactic surgical techniques are used to place an electrode within the target area ipsilateral to the side of headache. The device is kept active at all times and patients have limited control over the settings.

Evidence for the Use of Ventral Tegmental Area Deep Brain Stimulation

On the basis of the above functional neuroimaging studies, DBS is considered a possible treatment for TACs and not migraine. Although there are now a number of open-label studies on the use of DBS for chronic cluster headache (Table 1.6) there is only one placebo-controlled trial available in the literature that, unfortunately, had deeply-flawed study design [79]. Given the rarity of the TACs and the invasive nature of DBS surgery, it is highly unlikely that high quality controlled studies will ever be conducted in this area. Deep brain stimulation has been proven ineffective in the acute treatment of cluster attacks [86].

Preventative Treatment of Chronic Cluster Headache

There are now over 50 patients with DBS for chronic cluster headache published in the literature with an overall response rate (50% reduction in attack frequency or pain score) of 71% (Table 1.6). A summary of the available open-label series is given in Table 1.6 [75–81] and the largest of these series are examined further below.

Schoenen et al. implanted DBS leads into six patients with chronic cluster headache [75]. After a mean follow-up of 14.5 months in four of the patients, two patients were pain free, one was having less than three attacks a month and one reported no effect. One patient selected for treatment did not undergo implant due to a severe anxiety attack suffered during the operation. The only fatal adverse event recorded with DBS for headache occurred in this series with a patient dying post-operatively due to an intracerebral bleed along the lead. This tragic outcome led to a review of the use of DBS and guidelines that stress that DBS should be considered only as a last resort in patients with no other treatment options [67]. Bartsch et al. [78] published a series of six patients in 2008 with a follow-up of up to 17 months. At follow-up, three patients were almost pain free but one further patient who originally reported a more than 90% improvement in attack frequency lost efficacy over time so that after 3 months they no-longer reported any benefit. In 2011, both Franzini et al. [76] and Seijo et al. [77] each published a series of six patients undergoing DBS for chronic cluster headache. In the cohort from Franzini, five patients were reported as being pain free after up to 22 months follow-up. In the Seijo series, all

Table 1.6 Available evidence from published case series for ventral tegmental area deep brain stimulation in primary TACs

Trial (first author, year)	Patients (n)	Average follow-up (months)	Response rate (proportion reporting least 50% reduction attack frequency)	Adverse events (n)
DBS for chronic cluster headache				
Schoenen et al. [75]	4 (6 implanted)	15 months	75%	Fatal intracerebral haemorrhage [1], severe anxiety attack at time of implant [1]
Franzini et al. [76]	5	12 months	100% pain free	
Seijo et al. [77]	5	33 months	100%	Meiosis [3], Cable rupture [2]
Bartsch et al. [78]	6	17 months	50%	Cable revision [1]
Fontaine et al. [79]	11	12 months	55%	Infection [1]
Leone et al. [80]	17	108 months	70%	Electrode migration [2], infection [4], intraventricular haemorrhage [1], seizure [1]
Starr et al. [81]	4	12 months	50%	Transient ischaemic attack [1]
TOTAL	***52***	***30 months***	***71%***	
DBS for SUNCT/SUNA				
Lyons et al. [82]	1	12 months	100%	Nil
Miller et al. [83]	6	10 months	83%	Nil
Bartsch et al. [84]	1	15 months	100%	Nil
Leone et al. [85]	1	10 months	100%	Nil
TOTAL	***9***	***12 months***	***96%***	

DBS deep brain stimulation, *SUNA* short-lasting unilateral neuralgiform headache attacks with autonomic features, *SUNCT* short-lasting unilateral neuralgiform headache attacks with conjunctival injection and tearing

patients reported a more than 50% reduction in attack frequency after mean follow-up of 33 months with two being pain free. This series commented on a number of clinically relevant observations such as the occurrence of a transient benefit or "stun period" for up to 2 weeks following implantation, a feature of the treatment that our group sees commonly but which is not widely discussed in the literature. Again, a delay of weeks to months was observed before clinical benefit was observed and attacks were noted to return within days to weeks when stimulation was stopped. In terms of adverse events, the group reports the most common complaints were of transient diplopia and dizziness related to changes in stimulation parameters.

The largest open-label series of 16 patients in 2013 is also that with the longest follow-up period. Leone et al. [80] reported that following a median follow-up of 9 years, six remained pain free and a further six had converted to episodic cluster headache. In five of the pain free patients, the stimulator had been switched off with long-term remission maintained. Adverse events in the cohort included a post-operative seizure, infection (in four patients), electrode displacement (in two patients) and a non-symptomatic intraventricular haemorrhage was seen in one patient.

Fontaine et al. performed a randomised sham-controlled crossover study on DBS for chronic cluster headache in 2010 [79]. In this study, 11 patients were enrolled to a protocol consisting of two crossover periods of either sham or active stimulation each lasting 1 month in duration followed by a one-year open-label extension period. There was no difference in attack frequency between active and sham groups at the end of the 2 months crossover period. However, by the end of the longer open-label phase, more than 50% of subjects reported a more than 50% reduction in attack frequency. The negative outcome of the randomised part of the study is now considered to be due to poor study design with the cross-over periods far too short to account for the consistent delay to response seen in the open-label studies. Adverse events in this cohort included infection of the system requiring removal of the hardware in one patient.

Preventative Treatment of SUNCT/SUNA

The only other literature currently available on the use of ventral tegmental area DBS involve cases of SUNCT/SUNA. In total there are three case reports [82, 84, 85] and a series of six patients with refractory SUNCT/SUNA treated with DBS [83]. All three case reports were of successful treatment with all reporting a more than 90% improvement in attack frequency. In the case series, attack frequency reduced by a median of 79% and five out of six patients were considered clinical responders (Table 1.6). These data need to be interpreted with caution as the numbers reported are small and there is likely to be reporting bias.

Safety of Ventral Tegmental Area Deep Brain Stimulation

The death of a patient in the Schoenen et al. cohort from an intracerebral haemorrhage has led to concerns regards the safety of DBS in headache [75]. Other reported adverse events include non-symptomatic intraventricular haemorrhage, infection sometimes necessitating removal of the DBS system and electrode displacement. Adverse events from available cohorts are summarised in Table 1.6. Due to the potential serious adverse events, guidelines for DBS patient selection have been produced emphasising that surgery should be offered as a last resort only in patients with TACs who have failed all other available treatments (Table 1.5) [67].

The Possible Role of Ventral Tegmental Area Deep Brain Stimulation (Table 1.2)

On the basis of currently available evidence, DBS should be considered for medically intractable chronic cluster headache (and potentially other TACs) that have proven resistant to all other treatments, including other forms of neurostimulation. Due to the risks of surgery, implants should only be undertaken in highly specialised units and guidelines state that patients should be managed by a multidisciplinary team including psychologists [80].

Transcranial Magnetic Stimulation

It has been proposed that patients with migraine have a state of abnormal brain hyperexcitability and this theory is supported by transcranial magnetic stimulation studies [7, 9]. This hyperexcitable cortex is proposed to have a lower threshold for activation of cortical spreading depression (CSD), a process linked to the generation of migraine aura and activation of meningeal and trigeminal nociceptors [10]. Transcranial magnetic stimulation has been shown in animal studies to inhibit CSD and reduce cortical hyperexcitability by modulating levels of dopamine and glutamate [9]. On the basis of animal studies, transcranial magnetic stimulation was investigated as a potential treatment for migraine with aura. The SpringTMS® device, a single-pulse transcranial magnetic stimulator was designed specifically for migraine treatment. The device applies a brief single magnetic pulse to the scalp and underlying cortex resulting in induced electrical field generation in the cortex, changes in neurotransmitter release and disturbance of CSD.

Acute Treatment of Episodic Migraine with and Without Aura

The evidence for the use of the SpringTMS® device in acute migraine comes from a small sham-controlled study and post-marketing surveys. The sham-controlled study involved 164 migraine with aura patients using the device as an acute treatment for migraine attacks [87]. Active treatment was associated with a significantly higher rate of pain-freedom than sham treatment at both 2 h (39% vs. 22%) and 24 h (29% vs. 16%). The therapeutic gain of transcranial magnetic stimulation for acute migraine treatment was calculated at 17%. An open-label post-marketing survey included data on the acute treatment of migraine with and without aura in 190 patients who used the device for 3 months [88]. At the end of follow-up, 105 patients had discontinued the treatment mainly due to lack of efficacy, cost or convenience. Of those completing the follow-up period, 62% were noted as reporting "some" reduction in migraine intensity and 59% "some" reduction in migraine duration.

Preventative Treatment of Episodic or Chronic Migraine

On the basis of currently available data, there is insufficient evidence to support the use of the SpringTMS® device in the preventative treatment of migraine.

Safety of Transcranial Magnetic Stimulation

A safety review of published literature on the use of transcranial magnetic stimulation for migraine shows that the treatment is low-risk and well tolerated [89]. The most commonly reported adverse events in the transcranial magnetic stimulator literature include dizziness and drowsiness during treatment. In the sham-controlled trial from Lipton et al. [87], prevalence of adverse events was low (14%) with no significant difference to the sham group (9%). The events reported included worsening of headache and complaints of paraesthesia with treatment. Importantly, no subjects discontinued treatment due to adverse events.

The Possible Role of Transcranial Magnetic Stimulation (Table 1.2)

Transcranial magnetic stimulation may have a role in the acute treatment of migraine with and without aura. Given its efficacy as an acute treatment, the SpringTMS® stimulation device may be of potential benefit in patients who are at risk of overusing acute medications or in whom acute medications are ineffective. At present, transcranial magnetic stimulation does not appear effective in the prevention of migraine.

Mechanisms of Action of Neurostimulation

Peripheral Neurostimulation

The mechanisms by which peripheral neurostimulation modulates an antinociceptive response is still poorly understood. All of the peripheral nerves utilised for neurostimulation project either to the trigeminovascular system (occipital nerve, vagal nerve) or trigeminoautonomic system (sphenopalatine ganglion) which then project to brainstem centres such as the locus coeruleus and periaqueductal gray and further project to higher centres such as the thalamus (Fig. 1.1). This complex network is referred to as "the pain matrix" and functional neuroimaging suggests its major components include the primary and secondary somatosensory cortices, thalamus, anterior and posterior insula, anterior cingulate gyrus and prefrontal cortex [72]. This theory has been examined using functional neuroimaging of patients undergoing occipital nerve stimulation for headache [90–92] and vagal nerve stimulation for depression [93].

Matharu et al. [90] used positron emission tomography (PET) imaging to study eight patients with chronic migraine who had reported benefit to ONS. Patients were studied in three states: pain-free and stimulation on, in pain with stimulation off and during partial stimulation with varying levels of pain. Significant changes were observed in the regional cerebral blood flow in the dorsal rostral pons, anterior cingulate cortex and cuneus that were related to patient pain scores and changes in the anterior cingulate gyrus and left pulvinar regions correlated to paraesthesia scores. Magis and colleagues studied ten ONS-treated chronic cluster headache patients and compared them to 39 healthy volunteers using PET imaging [92]. ONS patients were scanned at intervals varying between 0 and 30 months post-implant and with stimulation on and off. At time of imaging, three cluster patients were pain free and four more had a greater than 90% reduction in attack frequency. Compared to controls, several areas of the pain matrix showed hyperactivity including the ipsilateral hypothalamus, midbrain and ipsilateral lower pons. Activity in all of these areas normalised with ONS except for the hypothalamus. The anterior cingulate cortex was a possible marker of efficacy as it was seen to be hyperactive in ONS responders compared to non-responders.

Kovacs et al. [91] investigated the potential mechanisms of action in ONS in healthy volunteer studying changes on functional MRI (fMRI) when stimulation was on or off. Significant differences were seen in the activity of the hypothalamus, thalamus, orbitofrontal cortex, prefrontal cortex, periaqueductal gray, inferior parietal regions and cerebellum. Suppression of activity was noted in the somatosensory areas, the amygdala, the hippocampus and primary motor cortex.

The effects on fMRI of a sham-controlled transcutaneous vagal nerve stimulator designed for treatment of depression has been reported [93]. The stimulation device was placed in the left external auditory meatus on the inner side of the tragus, an area known to receive innervation from the vagal nerve. Following stimulation, a reduction in signal was seen in the parahippocampal gyrus, posterior cingulate cortex and right thalamus was observed. Increased signal was observed in the anterior cingulate gyrus. In the brainstem, a significant reduction was seen in signal from the locus coeruleus and solitary tract nucleus.

In summary, simulation of the peripheral nerves is thought to modulate the afferent impulses travelling to the brainstem and higher centres resulting in long-term neuroplastic changes in various regions of the brain, including those outside of the regions stimulated. The finding of persistent hyper-metabolism of the ipsilateral hypothalamus outside of an attack, even after successful ONS, may explain why attacks recur after stimulation is stopped.

Central Neuromodulation

Positron emission tomography studies have implicated the posterior hypothalamic region as being abnormally activated during attacks of cluster headache [14], SUNCT/SUNA [15] and PH [12]. Further anatomical clarification at a later date revealed this area to be the ventral tegmental area and not posterior hypothalamus [74]. This finding has not been replicated in migraine imaging. The imaging findings seem to reinforce the concept of the hypothalamus as an important area in pain regulation and attack generation in TACs. This theory led Leone and colleagues to implant a DBS lead in the area observed on PET imaging in 2000 [73]. Ten patients successfully treated with DBS for intractable chronic cluster headache underwent PET imaging to investigate the possible mechanisms behind DBS effect. After ventral tegmental area stimulation activation was observed in the thalamus, somatosensory cortex, cuneus, anterior cingulate cortex and trigeminal nucleus and ganglion and deactivation in the middle temporal gyrus, posterior cingulate cortex and anterior insula. All of these regions are structures involved in the neural circuits of the pain matrix discussed above and thus, similar to ONS, stimulation of the ventral tegmental area appears to result in long-term neuroplastic changes of descending pain processing pathways distant to the site of stimulation itself.

During transcranial magnetic stimulation treatment for migraine a magnetic field is applied to the scalp. This field penetrates the scalp and induces a current in the underlying cortex. The induced electric field alters the membrane potentials, resulting in either depolarisation or repolarisation of a neuronal population. In the treatment of migraine with aura, this current is hypothesised to disrupt CSD as has been observed in animal studies [94].

Conclusions

Primary headache disorders are among the most commonly encountered neurological disorders, yet effective evidence based treatments, particularly the chronic forms, are lacking. With low satisfaction rates for traditional preventative medications due to tolerability and efficacy there is a growing demand for new treatment options for headache patients. Neurostimulation is emerging as a promising treatment option modality particularly for medically intractable chronic migraine and chronic TACs or those with contraindications to other medication. Open-label data is providing evidence that they can improve quality of life in highly disabled chronic headache patients and they can offer hope to many more. However, the quality of current evidence is poor and the ultimate confirmation of any new therapeutic modalities should come from randomised controlled trials. This poses a problem with neurostimulation as the paraesthesia created during treatment with many of these devices creates limits on what would constitute adequate placebo. Another issue with sham stimulation is that the level of current below which clinical effect is lost has not been investigated. It is therefore possible that previous sham studies have been using active placebo rather than control, a situation that complicates interpretation of the data. From available efficacy data, neurostimulation treatments appear to have efficacy similar or below that of available preventative treatments. However, their adverse event and tolerability data (especially in non-invasive devices) is far superior to current medications. At present, the place for neurostimulation seems to lie in two clear patient groups. The first is those with medically intractable chronic headaches where the cost and risk of treatment may be offset by the potential benefit in those with otherwise limited options. The second group is those with contraindications or intolerance to medications. This is a situation where the non-invasive devices may show major potential benefit especially if they can provide effective acute relief. In the future, if robust evidence can be generated, neurostimulation will likely take a prominent place in the treatment regimes of headache. However, until such a time, patients must be selected carefully in line with current guidelines.

References

1. Headache Classification Committee of the International Headache Society. The International Classification of Headache Disorders, 3rd edition (beta version). Cephalalgia: Int J Headache. 2013;33(9):629–808.
2. Stewart WF, Shechter A, Rasmussen BK. Migraine prevalence. A review of population-based studies. Neurology. 1994;44(6 Suppl 4):S17–23.
3. Bjørn RM. Epidemiology and genetics of cluster headache. Lancet Neurol. 2004;3(5): 279–83.
4. Sjaastad O, Bakketeig LS. Cluster headache prevalence. Vaga study of headache epidemiology. Cephalalgia: Int J Headache. 2003;23(7):528–33.
5. World Health Organisation. Atlas of headache disorders and resources in the world 2011. A collaberation project of the World Health Organisation and Lifting the Burden. WHO Press, World Health Organization, 20 Avenue Appia, 1211 Geneva 27, Switzerland; 2011.
6. Scher AI, Stewart WF, Liberman J, Lipton RB. Prevalence of frequent headache in a population sample. Headache. 1998;38(7):497–506.
7. Burstein R, Noseda R, Borsook D. Migraine: multiple processes, complex pathophysiology. J Neurosci Off J Soc Neurosci. 2015;35(17):6619–29.
8. Kerr FW, Olafson RA. Trigeminal and cervical volleys. Convergence on single units in the spinal gray at C-1 and C-2. Arch Neurol. 1961;5:171–8.
9. Lipton RB, Pearlman SH. Transcranial magnetic simulation in the treatment of migraine. Neurotherapeutics. 2010;7(2):204–12.
10. Charles AC, Baca SM. Cortical spreading depression and migraine. Nat Rev Neurol. 2013;9(11):637–44.
11. Goadsby PJ, Edvinsson L. Human in vivo evidence for trigeminovascular activation in cluster headache. Neuropeptide changes and effects of acute attacks therapies. Brain J Neurol. 1994;117(Pt 3):427–34.
12. Matharu MS, Cohen AS, Frackowiak RS, Goadsby PJ. Posterior hypothalamic activation in paroxysmal hemicrania. Ann Neurol. 2006;59(3):535–45.
13. Matharu MS, Cohen AS, McGonigle DJ, Ward N, Frackowiak RS, Goadsby PJ. Posterior hypothalamic and brainstem activation in hemicrania continua. Headache. 2004;44(8): 747–61.
14. May A, Bahra A, Büchel C, et al. Hypothalamic activation in cluster headache attacks. Lancet. 1998;352:275–8.
15. May A, Bahra A, Buchel C, Turner R, Goadsby PJ. Functional magnetic resonance imaging in spontaneous attacks of SUNCT: short-lasting neuralgiform headache with conjunctival injection and tearing. Ann Neurol. 1999;46(5):791–4.
16. Bartsch T, Levy MJ, Knight YE, Goadsby PJ. Differential modulation of nociceptive dural input to [hypocretin] orexin A and B receptor activation in the posterior hypothalamic area. Pain. 2004;109(3):367–78.

17. Gerardy PY, Fabry D, Fumal A, Schoenen J. A pilot study on supra-orbital surface electrotherapy in migraine. Cephalalgia. 2009;29:101–78.
18. Schoenen J, Vandersmissen B, Jeangette S, Herroelen L, Vandenheede M, Gerard P, et al. Migraine prevention with a supraorbital transcutaneous stimulator: a randomized controlled trial. Neurology. 2013;80(8):697–704.
19. Magis D, Sava S, d'Elia TS, Baschi R, Schoenen J. Safety and patients' satisfaction of transcutaneous supraorbital neurostimulation (tSNS) with the Cefaly(R) device in headache treatment: a survey of 2,313 headache sufferers in the general population. J Headache Pain. 2013;14:95.
20. Linde K, Rossnagel K. Propranolol for migraine prophylaxis. Cochrane Database Syst Rev. 2004;(2):CD003225.
21. Asensio-Samper JM, Villanueva VL, Perez AV, Lopez MD, Monsalve V, Moliner S, et al. Peripheral neurostimulation in supraorbital neuralgia refractory to conventional therapy. Pain Pract: Off J World Institute Pain. 2008;8(2):120–4.
22. Reed K, Black S, Banta C, Will K. Combined occipital and supraorbital neurostimulation for the treatment of chronic migraine headaches: initial experience. Cephalalgia: Int J Headache. 2010;30(3):260–71.
23. Hann S, Sharan A. Dual occipital and supraorbital nerve stimulation for chronic migraine: a single-center experience, review of literature, and surgical considerations. Neurosurg Focus. 2013;35(3):E9.
24. Narouze SN, Kapural L. Supraorbital nerve electric stimulation for the treatment of intractable chronic cluster headache: a case report. Headache. 2007;47(7):1100–2.
25. Vaisman J, Markley H, Ordia J, Deer T. The treatment of medically intractable trigeminal autonomic cephalalgia with supraorbital/supratrochlear stimulation: a retrospective case series. Neuromodulation: J Int Neuromodulation Soc. 2012;15(4):374–80.
26. Sadler RM, Purdy RA, Rahey S. Vagal nerve stimulation aborts migraine in patient with intractable epilepsy. Cephalalgia: Int J Headache. 2002;22(6):482–4.
27. Gaul C, Diener HC, Silver N, Magis D, Reuter U, Andersson A, et al. Non-invasive vagus nerve stimulation for PREVention and Acute treatment of chronic cluster headache (PREVA): a randomised controlled study. Cephalalgia: Int J Headache. 2016;36:534–46.
28. Nesbitt AD, Marin JC, Tompkins E, Ruttledge MH, Goadsby PJ. Initial use of a novel noninvasive vagus nerve stimulator for cluster headache treatment. Neurology. 2015;84:1249–53.
29. Silberstein S, Neves Da Silva A, Calhoun A, Grosberg B, Lipton R, Cady R, et al. Non-Invasive Vagus Nerve Stimulation for Chronic Migraine Prevention in a Propective, Randomized, Sham-Controlled Pilot Study (the EVENT Study): Report from the Double-blind Phase. Headache: J Head Face Pain. 2014;54:1–74.
30. Silberstein S, Neves Da Silva A, Calhoun A, Grosberg B, Lipton RB, Cady R, et al. Chronic Migraine Prevention with non-invasive Vagus Nerve Stimulation in a Prospective Pilot Study (the EVENT Study): Report from the Open-label Phase. Headache: J Head Face Pain. 2014;54:1–74.
31. Goadsby P, Grosberg B, Mauskop A, Cady R, Simmons K. Effect of noninvasive vagus nerve stimulation on acute migraine: An open-label pilot study. Cephalalgia: Int J Headache. 2014;34(12):986–93.
32. Barbanti P, Grazzi L, Egeo G, Padovan AM, Liebler E, Bussone G. Non-invasive vagus nerve stimulation for acute treatment of high-frequency and chronic migraine: an open-label study. J Headache Pain. 2015;16:61.
33. Bellavance AJ, Meloche JP. A comparative study of naproxen sodium, pizotyline and placebo in migraine prophylaxis. Headache. 1990;30(11):710–5.
34. Cady RK, Sheftell F, Lipton RB, O'Quinn S, Jones M, Gayla Putnam D, et al. Effect of early intervention with sumatriptan on migraine pain: retrospective analyses of data from three clinical trials. Clin Ther. 2000;22(9):1035–48.
35. Krishna V, Sammartino F, King NK, So RQ, Wennberg R. Neuromodulation for epilepsy. Neurosurg Clin N Am. 2016;27(1):123–31.
36. Mauskop A. *Vagus* nerve stimulation relieves chronic refractory migraine and cluster headaches. Cephalalgia: Int J Headache. 2005;25(2):82–6.

37. Cecchini AP, Mea E, Tullo V, Curone M, Franzini A, Broggi G, et al. Vagus nerve stimulation in drug-resistant daily chronic migraine with depression: preliminary data. Neurol Sci: Off J Italian Neurol Soc Italian Soc Clin Neurophysiol. 2009;30(Suppl 1):S101–4.
38. Hord ED, Evans MS, Mueed S, Adamolekun B, Naritoku DK. The effect of vagus nerve stimulation on migraines. J Pain. 2003;4(9):530–4.
39. Poletti CE. C2 and C3 pain dermatomes in man. Cephalalgia: Int J Headache. 1991; 11(3):155–9.
40. Saper JR, Dodick DW, Silberstein SD, McCarville S, Sun M, Goadsby PJ. Occipital nerve stimulation for the treatment of intractable chronic migraine headache: ONSTIM feasibility study. Cephalalgia: Int J Headache. 2011;31(3):271–85.
41. Silberstein SD, Dodick DW, Saper J, Huh B, Slavin KV, Sharan A, et al. Safety and efficacy of peripheral nerve stimulation of the occipital nerves for the management of chronic migraine: results from a randomized, multicenter, double-blinded, controlled study. Cephalalgia: Int J Headache. 2012;32(16):1165–79.
42. Dodick DW, Silberstein SD, Reed KL, Deer TR, Slavin KV, Huh B, et al. Safety and efficacy of peripheral nerve stimulation of the occipital nerves for the management of chronic migraine: long-term results from a randomized, multicenter, double-blinded, controlled study. Cephalalgia: Int J Headache. 2015;35(4):344–58.
43. Brewer AC, Trentman TL, Ivancic MG, Vargas BB, Rebecca AM, Zimmerman RS, et al. Long-term outcome in occipital nerve stimulation patients with medically intractable primary headache disorders. Neuromodulation: J Int Neuromodulation Soc. 2013;16(6):557–62.
44. Lipton R, Goadsby PJ, Cady R, Aurora SK, Grosberg BM, Freitag F, et al. PRISM study: occipital nerve stimulation for treatment-refractory migraine. Cephalalgia. 2009;29(Suppl 1):30.
45. Mueller O, Diener HC, Dammann P, Rabe K, Hagel V, Sure U, et al. Occipital nerve stimulation for intractable chronic cluster headache or migraine: a critical analysis of direct treatment costs and complications. Cephalalgia: Int J Headache. 2013;33(16):1283–91.
46. Paemeleire K, Van Buyten JP, Van Buynder M, Alicino D, Van Maele G, Smet I, et al. Phenotype of patients responsive to occipital nerve stimulation for refractory head pain. Cephalalgia: Int J Headache. 2010;30(6):662–73.
47. Magis D, Allena M, Bolla M, De Pasqua V, Remacle JM, Schoenen J. Occipital nerve stimulation for drug-resistant chronic cluster headache: a prospective pilot study. Lancet Neurol. 2007;6(4):314–21.
48. Magis D, Gerardy PY, Remacle JM, Schoenen J. Sustained effectiveness of occipital nerve stimulation in drug-resistant chronic cluster headache. Headache. 2011;51(8):1191–201.
49. Schwedt TJ, Dodick DW, Hentz J, Trentman TL, Zimmerman RS. Occipital nerve stimulation for chronic headache–long-term safety and efficacy. Cephalalgia: Int J Headache. 2007;27(2): 153–7.
50. Burns B, Watkins L, Goadsby PJ. Treatment of medically intractable cluster headache by occipital nerve stimulation: long-term follow-up of eight patients. Lancet. 2007;369(9567): 1099–106.
51. Burns B, Watkins L, Goadsby PJ. Treatment of intractable chronic cluster headache by occipital nerve stimulation in 14 patients. Neurology. 2009;72(4):341–5.
52. Fontaine D, Christophe Sol J, Raoul S, Fabre N, Geraud G, Magne C, et al. Treatment of refractory chronic cluster headache by chronic occipital nerve stimulation. Cephalalgia: Int J Headache. 2011;31(10):1101–5.
53. Mueller OM, Gaul C, Katsarava Z, Diener HC, Sure U, Gasser T. Occipital nerve stimulation for the treatment of chronic cluster headache – lessons learned from 18 months experience. Cen Eur Neurosurg. 2011;72(2):84–9.
54. Lambru G, Shanahan P, Watkins L, Matharu MS. Occipital nerve stimulation in the treatment of medically intractable SUNCT and SUNA. Pain Physician. 2014;17(1):29–41.
55. Burns B, Watkins L, Goadsby PJ. Treatment of hemicrania continua by occipital nerve stimulation with a bion device: long-term follow-up of a crossover study. Lancet Neurol. 2008;7(11):1001–12.

56. Silberstein S, Tfelt-Hansen P, Dodick DW, Limmroth V, Lipton RB, Pascual J, et al. Guidelines for controlled trials of prophylactic treatment of chronic migraine in adults. Cephalalgia: Int J Headache. 2008;28(5):484–95.
57. Chen YF, Bramley G, Unwin G, Hanu-Cernat D, Dretzke J, Moore D, et al. Occipital nerve stimulation for chronic migraine–a systematic review and meta-analysis. PLoS One. 2015;10(3):e0116786.
58. Weiner RL, Reed KL. Peripheral neurostimulation for control of intractable occipital neuralgia. Neuromodulation: J Int Neuromodulation Soc. 1999;2(3):217–21.
59. Popeney CA, Alo KM. Peripheral neurostimulation for the treatment of chronic, disabling transformed migraine. Headache. 2003;43(4):369–75.
60. Johnstone CS, Sundaraj R. Occipital nerve stimulation for the treatment of occipital neuralgia-eight case studies. Neuromodulation: J Int Neuromodulation Soc. 2006;9(1):41–7.
61. Slavin KV, Nersesyan H, Wess C. Peripheral neurostimulation for treatment of intractable occipital neuralgia. Neurosurgery. 2006;58(1):112–9; discussion –9.
62. Magis D. Neuromodulation in migraine: state of the art and perspectives. Expert Rev Med Devices. 2015;12(3):329–39.
63. Sharan A, Huh B, Narouze S, Trentman T, Mogilner A, Vaisman J, et al. Analysis of adverse events in the management of chronic migraine by peripheral nerve stimulation. Neuromodulation: J Int Neuromodulation Soc. 2015;18(4):305–12.
64. Palmisani S, Al-Kaisy A, Arcioni R, Smith T, Negro A, Lambru G, et al. A six year retrospective review of occipital nerve stimulation practice–controversies and challenges of an emerging technique for treating refractory headache syndromes. J Headache Pain. 2013;14:67.
65. Magis D, Schoenen J. Advances and challenges in neurostimulation for headaches. Lancet Neurol. 2012;11(8):708–19.
66. Schwedt TJ, Dodick DW, Trentman TL, Zimmerman RS. Occipital nerve stimulation for chronic cluster headache and hemicrania continua: pain relief and persistence of autonomic features. Cephalalgia: Int J Headache. 2006;26(8):1025–7.
67. Martelletti P, Jensen RH, Antal A, Arcioni R, Brighina F, de Tommaso M, et al. Neuromodulation of chronic headaches: position statement from the European Headache Federation. J Headache Pain. 2013;14(1):86.
68. Leone M, Proietti Cecchini A, Mea E, D'Amico D, Tullo V, Grazzi L, et al. Therapeutic neurostimulation in chronic headaches: problems of patient selection. Neurol Sci: Off J Italian Neurol Soc Italian Soc Clin Neurophysiol. 2008;29(Suppl 1):S59–61.
69. Schoenen J, Jensen RH, Lanteri-Minet M, Lainez MJ, Gaul C, Goodman AM, et al. Stimulation of the sphenopalatine ganglion (SPG) for cluster headache treatment. Pathway CH-1: a randomized, sham-controlled study. Cephalalgia: Int J Headache. 2013;33(10):816–30.
70. Jurgens TP, Schoenen J, Rostgaard J, Hillerup S, Lainez MJ, Assaf AT, et al. Stimulation of the sphenopalatine ganglion in intractable cluster headache: expert consensus on patient selection and standards of care. Cephalalgia: Int J Headache. 2014;34:1100–10.
71. Bahra A, Matharu MS, Buchel C, Frackowiak RS, Goadsby PJ. Brainstem activation specific to migraine headache. Lancet. 2001;357(9261):1016–7.
72. May A. A review of diagnostic and functional imaging in headache. J Headache Pain. 2006;7(4):174–84.
73. Leone M, Franzini A, Bussone G. Stereotactic stimulation of posterior hypothalamic gray matter in a patient with intractable cluster headache. N Engl J Med. 2001;345:1428–9.
74. Matharu MS, Zrinzo L. Deep brain stimulation in cluster headache: hypothalamus or midbrain tegmentum? Curr Pain Headache Rep. 2010;14(2):151–9.
75. Schoenen J, Di Clemente L, Vandenheede M, Fumal A, De Pasqua V, Mouchamps M, et al. Hypothalamic stimulation in chronic cluster headache: a pilot study of efficacy and mode of action. Brain J Neurol. 2005;128(Pt 4):940–7.
76. Franzini A, Messina G, Cordella R, Marras C, Broggi G. Deep brain stimulation of the posteromedial hypothalamus: indications, long-term results and neurophysiological considerations. Neurosurg Focus. 2010;29(2):1–13.

77. Seijo F, Saiz A, Lozano B, Santamarta E, Alvarez-Vega M, Seijo E, et al. Neuromodulation of the posterolateral hypothalamus for the treatment of chronic refractory cluster headache: experience in five patients with a modified anatomical target. Cephalalgia: Int J Headache. 2011;31(16):1634–41.
78. Bartsch T, Pinsker MO, Rasche D, et al. Hypothalamic deep brain stimulation for cluster headache: experience from a new multicase series. Cephalalgia: Int J Headache. 2008;28:285–95.
79. Fontaine D, Lazorthes Y, Mertens P, Blond S, Geraud G, Fabre N, et al. Safety and efficacy of deep brain stimulation in refractory cluster headache: a randomized placebo-controlled double-blind trial followed by a 1-year open extension. J Headache Pain. 2010;11(1):23–31.
80. Leone M, Franzini A, Proietti Cecchini A, Bussone G. Success, failure, and putative mechanisms in hypothalamic stimulation for drug-resistant chronic cluster headache. Pain. 2013;154(1):89–94.
81. Starr PA, Barbaro NM, Raskin NH, Ostrem JL. Chronic stimulation of the posterior hypothalamus region for cluster headache: technique and 1-year results in four patients. J Neurosurg. 2007;106:999–1005.
82. Lyons MK, Dodick DW, Evidente VG. Responsiveness of short-lasting unilateral neuralgiform headache with conjunctival injection and tearing to hypothalamic deep brain stimulation. J Neurosurg. 2009;110(2):279–81.
83. Miller S, Rasul F, Lambru G, Lagrata S, Hariz GM, Zrinzo L, et al. Posterior hypothalamic region deep brain stimulation in shoer lasting unilateral neuralgiform headache with conjunctival injection and tearing (SUNCT). Cephalalgia: Int J Headache. 2013;33(8 Suppl):1–309.
84. Bartsch T, Falk D, Knudsen K, Reese R, Raethjen J, Mehdorn HM, et al. Deep brain stimulation of the posterior hypothalamic area in intractable short-lasting unilateral neuralgiform headache with conjunctival injection and tearing (SUNCT). Cephalalgia: Int J Headache. 2011;31(13):1405–8.
85. Leone M, Franzini A, D'Andrea G, Broggi G, Casucci G, Bussone G. Deep brain stimulation to relieve drug-resistant SUNCT. Ann Neurol. 2005;57(6):924–7.
86. Leone M, Franzini A, Broggi G, Mea E, Cecchini AP, Bussone G. Acute hypothalamic stimulation and ongoing cluster headache. Neurology. 2006;67:1844–5.
87. Lipton RB, Dodick DW, Silberstein SD, Saper JR, Aurora SK, Pearlman SH, et al. Single-pulse transcranial magnetic stimulation for acute treatment of migraine with aura: a randomised, double-blind, parallel-group, sham-controlled trial. Lancet Neurol. 2010;9(4):373–80.
88. Bhola R, Kinsella E, Giffin N, Lipscombe S, Ahmed F, Weatherall M, et al. Single-pulse transcranial magnetic stimulation (sTMS) for the acute treatment of migraine: evaluation of outcome data for the UK post market pilot program. J Headache Pain. 2015;16:535.
89. Dodick DW, Schembri CT, Helmuth M, Aurora SK. Transcranial magnetic stimulation for migraine: a safety review. Headache. 2010;50(7):1153–63.
90. Matharu MS, Bartsch T, Ward N, Frackowiak RS, Weiner R, Goadsby PJ. Central neuromodulation in chronic migraine patients with suboccipital stimulators: a PET study. Brain J Neurol. 2004;127(Pt 1):220–30.
91. Kovacs S, Peeters R, De Ridder D, Plazier M, Menovsky T, Sunaert S. Central effects of occipital nerve electrical stimulation studied by functional magnetic resonance imaging. Neuromodulation: Technol Neural Interface. 2011;14(1):46–57.
92. Magis D, Bruno MA, Fumal A, Gerardy PY, Hustinx R, Laureys S, et al. Central modulation in cluster headache patients treated with occipital nerve stimulation: an FDG-PET study. BMC Neurol. 2011;11:25.
93. Kraus T, Kiess O, Hosl K, Terekhin P, Kornhuber J, Forster C. CNS BOLD fMRI effects of sham-controlled transcutaneous electrical nerve stimulation in the left outer auditory canal – a pilot study. Brain Stimul. 2013;6(5):798–804.
94. Holland PR, Schembri CT, Fredrick J, Goadsby P. Transcranial magnetic stimulation for the treamtent of migraine aura? Cephalalgia: Int J Headache. 2009;29(1 suppl):22.

Chapter 2
VNS for Treatment of Inflammatory Joint Diseases

Yaakov A. Levine, Jesse M. Simon, Frieda Koopman, Michael Faltys, Ralph Zitnik, and Paul-Peter Tak

Abstract The cholinergic anti-inflammatory pathway regulates innate and adaptive immunity during normal physiological function, and activation of the pathway by electrical stimulation of the vagus nerve (VNS) can reduce pathological levels of inflammation in animal models of autoimmune disorders. A proof-of-concept human study of VNS in rheumatoid arthritis (RA) has shown that VNS can ameliorate inflammation in humans. Future clinical studies will employ a novel, application-specific investigational stimulation system. In concept, this system is capable of being evolved to function in a closed-loop manner, adjusting therapy delivery to the patient's level of disease activity.

Keywords Bioelectronic medicine • Electroceuticals • Vagus nerve stimulation • Rheumatoid arthritis • Cholinergic anti-inflammatory pathway • Tumor necrosis factor

Introduction

Rheumatoid arthritis (RA) is a chronic autoimmune disease affecting approximately 1% of the population, and is characterized by joint inflammation leading to structural damage and disability [1]. RA patients have elevated cardiovascular mortality

---

Conflicts Statement: P.P.T. has received consulting fees from SetPoint Medical Corporation and is currently an employee of GlaxoSmithKline, which holds an equity interest in SetPoint Medical Corporation. He is a on the Board of Directors for Galvani Biosciences, another electroceuticals firm.

Y.A. Levine, PhD • J.M. Simon, MS • M. Faltys • R. Zitnik, MD
SetPoint Medical Corporation, Valencia, CA, USA

F. Koopman, MD
Academic Medical Center, University of Amsterdam, Clinical Immunology and Rheumatology, Amsterdam, The Netherlands

P.-P. Tak, MD, PhD (✉)
Department of Medicine, University of Cambridge, Cambridge, UK

Department of Rheumatology, Ghent University, Ghent, Belgium

Research & Development, GlaxoSmithKline, Stevenage, UK
e-mail: P.P.Tak@amc.uva.nl

A. Majid (ed.), *Electroceuticals*, DOI 10.1007/978-3-319-28612-9_2

rates due to the exacerbating effect of systemic inflammation on atherosclerosis, and anti-inflammatory treatment may be associated with risk reduction [2–4]. Targeted small molecule and biologic therapies have greatly improved the care of RA patients, yet these drugs carry safety risk, are costly, and are ineffective or lose effect in a substantial proportion of patients, so there remains an unmet need for additional and alternative therapeutic approaches [5].

The central nervous system regulates innate and adaptive immunity through an “inflammatory reflex” which senses inflammation afferently, responding via its efferent arm termed the cholinergic anti-inflammatory pathway (CAP) [6]. The inflammatory reflex modulates responses to infection or tissue injury, and accelerates inflammation resolution. Similar reflexive neural modulation of inflammation is highly conserved across species evolutionarily, highlighting its importance as a physiological mechanism aiding host defense [7, 8].

The CAP can also be activated electrically or pharmacologically to reduce pathological inflammation in animal models [9–11]. This led us to postulate that active implantable medical devices of the kind in use for several years to deliver vagus nerve stimulation (VNS) for the treatment of refractory epilepsy might also be beneficial in RA patients and patients suffering from other similar chronic inflammatory disorders [12].

Herein we will review the biology of the CAP and results in animal models that led us to study the use of VNS in patients with RA, describe a novel, application-specific VNS system that will soon enter studies in RA, and speculate on ways that this implanted device might be modified in the future to create a “closed loop” system that could respond to changes in systemic inflammation in RA patients, automatically optimizing its stimulation parameters to accommodate the patient’s level of disease activity.

The Cholinergic Anti-inflammatory Pathway

Tracey and colleagues described the first use of electrical VNS to reduce systemic inflammation, demonstrating that Tumor Necrosis Factor (TNF) production and the physiological manifestations of endotoxemic shock in rodents were increased by vagotomy and reduced by electrical stimulation of the cervical vagus nerve. Using antisense oligonucleotide and targeted genetic disruption approaches, they also demonstrated that the CAP effect was mediated through specific alpha 7 nicotinic acetylcholine receptors (α7nAChR) on macrophages [13]. When these a7nAChR are liganded, macrophages produce reduced amounts of TNF and other cytokines in response to pro-inflammatory signals mediated by Toll-Like Receptor Ligands (TLR) such as bacterial lipopolysaccharide (LPS). It was later demonstrated that reducing the response to endotoxemia using neurostimulation of the CAP (NCAP) by VNS required an intact spleen, and selective anatomical lesion experiments showed that an intact neural pathway to the spleen from the cervical vagus through the celiac ganglion was also necessary for CAP

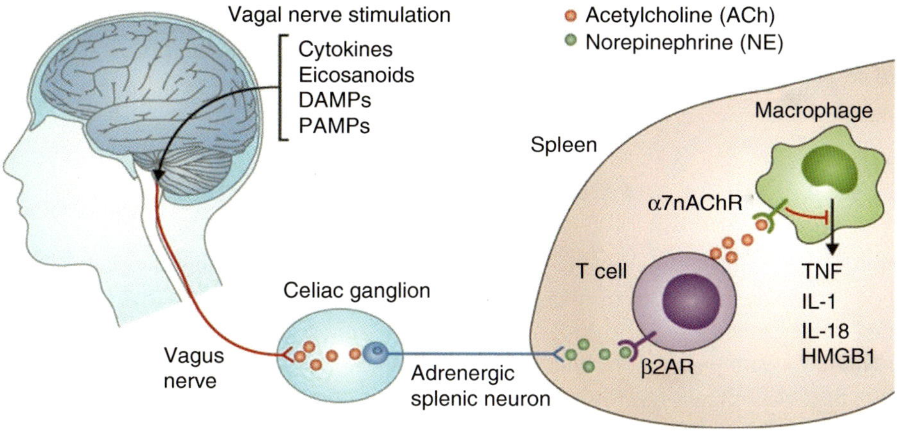

Fig. 2.1 The inflammatory reflex and the cholinergic anti-inflammatory pathway (CAP) act to physiologically modulate inflammation. Inflammatory meditators including cytokines, eiconsanoids, and damage- or pathogen-associated molecular pattern molecules (DAMPs, PAMPs) are sensed peripherally and in the central nervous system (CNS), and brainstem nuclei of the vagus nerve are reflexively activated to induce signaling through the efferent vagus. Alternatively, the vagus nerve can be stimulated electrically to activate the CAP. Neural signals travel through the celiac ganglion to the adrenergic splenic nerve, which terminates in close apposition to CAP-specific T cells bearing beta-2 adrenergic receptors (β2AR). In response to activation of the b2AR these T cells then secrete acetylcholine which ligands alpha 7 nicotinic acetylcholine receptors on nearby splenic macrophages, causing them to produce reduced levels of inflammatory mediators, thereby closing the reflex loop (With permission © Rockefeller University Press [9])

activation [14]. Within the spleen itself, nerve fiber synaptic vesicles are found in close apposition to TNF-secreting macrophages [15], and a recently described population of memory T cells [16]. These T cells bear surface beta adrenoceptors, and have the capacity to synthesize and secrete acetylcholine. This unique T cell population functions analogously to an intermediate neuron, sensing the adrenergic neurotransmitters released by the splenic nerve, and in turn transmitting the efferent signal to adjoining splenic macrophages by local secretion of acetylcholine. In the macrophage, and other immune cells, the a7nAChR does not appear to transduce signals through ion channels, as is the case in neuronal tissue. Instead, the NCAP effect is mediated at the subcellular level by alterations in the intracellular transcription factors Nuclear Factor- (NF) κb, Janus-Activated Kinase (JAK), Signal Transducer and Activator of Transcription (STAT), and Suppressor of Cytokine Signaling (SOCS) which transduce cellular signals that reduce cytokine production [17, 18], as well as inhibiting inflammasome activation by limiting stress-induced mitochondrial damage, and subsequent release of mitochondrial DNA [19].

These neuronal and immune cells function together to mediate the inflammatory reflex. As shown in Fig. 2.1, the presence of inflammation is sensed, and reflexively causes increased efferent vagal activity. The efferent vagus nerve synapses on the celiac ganglion and signals are further transmitted via the splenic nerve to splenic T cells, which then down regulate macrophage inflammatory mediator release. In this way the inflammatory reflex serves to maintain a physiologically appropriate level of response to infection, inflammation or tissue damage.

CAP Activation and the Immunopathology of Arthritis

Beyond its role in physiologic regulation of host responses, there is a substantial body of evidence that both pharmacologic and neural activation of the CAP have favorable effects on the dysregulated immunological processes that initiate and maintain systemic and synovial inflammation in RA. CAP activation affects the function of both spleen-resident and circulating immunocytes. In addition, cholinergic stimulation has inhibitory effects on the fibroblast-like synoviocyte (FLS), a resident cell of the synovium that is increasingly appreciated to play a critical local controlling role in the initiation and maintenance of joint inflammation [20].

Circulating monocytes produce TNF and other proinflammatory cytokines in response to in vitro exposure to bacterial LPS. After VNS or in vitro exposure to cholinergic agonists, the ability of these peripheral blood cells to release inflammatory mediators in response to LPS is reduced [21, 22]. Further, CAP activation is associated with reduced trafficking of effector immune cells into inflamed tissue. VNS reduced granulocytic infiltration to the muscularis mucosa in a model of inflammatory postoperative ileus [17], to the pancreas in pancreatitis [23], and to the lung following burn-induced acute lung injury [24]. Experiments using carrageenan-induced skin or joint inflammation demonstrated that VNS or pharmacologic CAP reduced neutrophil influx into tissue, driven by a reduction in surface expression of the adhesion molecule integrin component CD11b [25, 26]. Finally CAP affects the trafficking and function of B cells, which play a key role in RA pathogenesis. In response to VNS or cholinergic agonists, splenic marginal zone B cells exhibit reduced trafficking to the splenic red pulp and peri-follicular areas. This migratory arrest is driven by changes in CD11b, and is associated with reduced secretion of antibodies [27].

Among circulating immunocytes, regulatory T cells (Treg) are a specialized T cell population that functionally suppress other immunocytes in order to regulate the natural course of immune responses. Reductions in Treg number and function have been reported in a variety of autoimmune diseases, including RA, and loss of Treg function plays an important role in the progression of RA [28]. CAP activation modulates Treg number and function, as murine Treg suppressive activity is enhanced by nicotine, which ligands the a7nAChR, and this effect that is blocked by the nicotinic receptor antagonist α-bungarotoxin [29]. Further, in vitro culture of naïve Cluster of Differentiation (CD)4+CD62+ T cells with nicotine enhances the effect of cell activation-induced expression of Forkhead Box (Fox)P3, an important intracellular transcription factor associated with differentiation of naive T cells into Tregs, and nicotine also markedly increases the influx of CD4+CD25+FoxP3+ Tregs into the gut in oxalazone-induced colitis [30]. In rodent hapten-induced colitis, disease severity is worsened by vagotomy, which is correlated with reductions in Foxp3+ Tregs. Over time the proinflammatory effect of vagotomy wanes, accompanied by recovery of Treg numbers [31, 32]. In a model of post-hemorrhagic shock, CAP activation by vagus nerve stimulation prevented the decrease in lymph Treg numbers and the accompanying gut injury [33]. Finally, adoptive transfer of CD4+ choline acetytransferase (ChAT)+ splenocytes having demonstrable in vitro regulatory effects ameliorated disease in a T cell transfer colitis model [34]. In addition to effects on Tregs, CAP activity also affects T helper (Th) 1 cells: vagotomy increases and pharmacologic CAP agonists decrease in vitro T cell proliferation and production of the Th1 cytokines Interferon (IFN)-gamma, TNF and Interleukin (IL)-6 [35].

While the vagus nerve does not directly innervate the joint, the a7nAChR gene product is expressed in the synovium, and immunohistochemistry identifies a7nAChR that bind a-bungarotoxin both in the synovium and on isolated FLS. Expression of inhibitory RNA targeting the a7nAChR in FLS increased spontaneous FLS production of IL-8, demonstrating the functional significance of the receptor on the FLS [36]. Further, in FLS cultures, in vitro acetylcholine exposure dose- and time-dependently reduces IL-1 induced production of Il-6 ([37]). These studies demonstrate that cholinergic signaling; either through native acetylcholine or using pharmacologic agonists of the a7nAChR receptor may be an important mechanism by which local synovial inflammation can be reduced.

Taken together the observations on the effect of CAP activation on splenic and circulating immunocytes and FLS in the joint together lead to a model in which neural CAP activation exerts an anti-inflammatory effect by reducing production of systemically active cytokines, chemokines and antibodies by resident spleen cells, by increasing T regulatory cell number, and also by causing circulating cells which traverse the spleen to develop an altered phenotype with reduced expression of inflammatory mediators and adhesion molecules. As a result of this altered phenotype, trafficking of immune cells to inflamed tissue is reduced, and upon entering the diseased tissue these cells are less able to release mediators that both directly damage tissue, and induce other cells to migrate and cause damage secondarily. In the joint, the FLS can respond to acetylcholine or pharmacologic a7nAChR agonists by reducing production of cytokines and inflammatory mediators (Fig. 2.2).

Activation of the CAP Ameliorates Disease in the Collagen-Induced Arthritis Model

Tak and colleagues were the first to study the role of CAP in animal models of RA [12, 38–40]. The collagen-induced arthritis (CIA) model has been helpful historically in facilitating assessment of preclinical efficacy and guiding decisions on advancement of candidate RA drugs [41], and was similarly used to advance NCAP to human RA studies [42]. In this model autoimmunity against the joint is induced by repeated injections of collagen, often in the presence of an immune-activating compound such

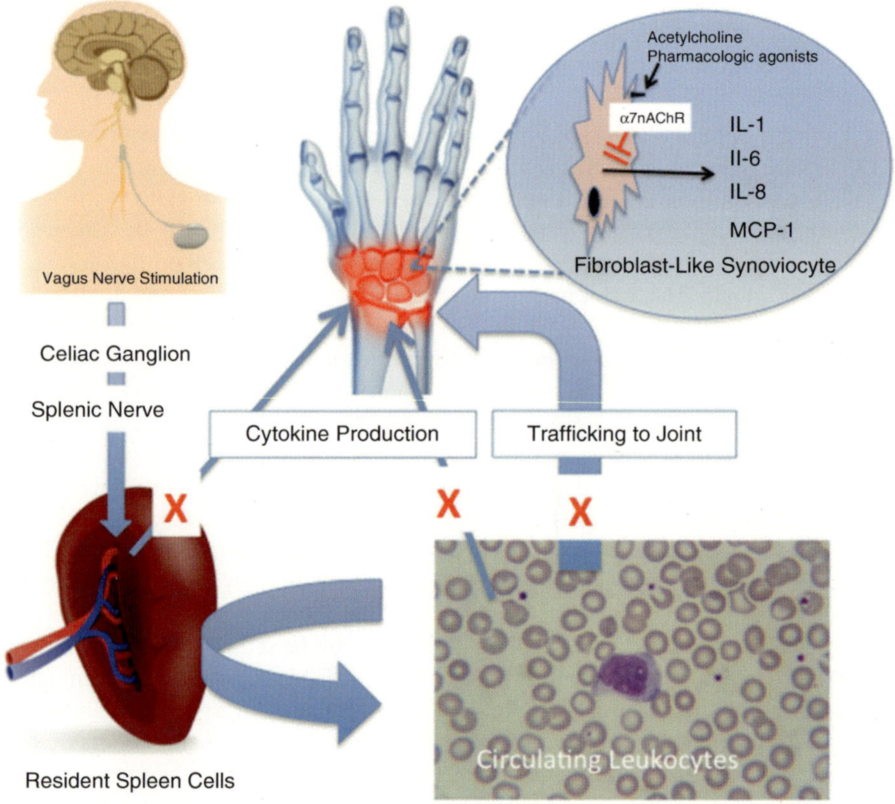

Fig. 2.2 Neurostimulation of the CAP (NCAP) reduces inflammation in rheumatoid arthritis (RA) by three major mechanisms. NCAP induces reduction in cytokine production within the spleen by the mechanism shown in Fig. 2.1. In addition, NCAP causes reduction in cell surface adhesion molecules and thereby reduces trafficking of activated leukocytes to the diseased joint. Further, peripheral blood monocytes that pass through the spleen undergo phenotypic changes after exposure to splenic acetylcholine, and they then secrete lower levels of inflammatory mediators in response to pro-inflammatory signals in the tissue. An inset shows acetylcholine or pharmacologic agonists binding to the fibroblast like synoviocyte (FLS) a7nAChR, in the synovial lining, thereby reducing FLS cytokine production

as Freund's adjuvant. Animals rapidly develop joint inflammation that can be assessed either by direct visualization or caliper measurement of joint swelling. The pathological findings in the rodent joint during CIA exhibit a reasonable degree of similarity to those seen in RA patients, including infiltration of the synovium with immune effector cells, formation of an inflammatory synovial outgrowth termed a "pannus", damage to articular cartilage, and peri-articular erosions of the bone.

Because of the critical role of the α7nAChR in mediating the CAP effect, CIA was induced in mice with targeted disruption of the α7nAChR receptor gene [39]. When compared to wild type littermates, α7NAChR knockout animals had a greater cumulative incidence of disease onset, worsened clinical disease severity and radiographic evidence of bone destruction, increased histological joint inflammation, increased systemic monocyte chemotactic peptide (MCP)-1 and TNF levels, and increased in vitro release of Th1 cytokines from cultured splenocytes. Conversely, the course and severity of CIA was ameliorated by systemic treatment with nicotine or with the selective α7nAChR agonists AR-R17779 [43], PMP-311 and PMP-072 [40].

Directly activating signaling through the vagus nerve itself can improve CIA as evidenced in a rodent study using surgical suspension of the cervical portion of the nerve against the sternocleidomastoid muscle. This surgical apposition of muscle and nerve induced chronic mechanical stimulation, and measurable vagal activation [44]. CIA was induced in sham-operated animals and animals that underwent full surgical suspension of the nerve. When compared with the sham-operated group, animals with surgical suspension had statistically significant improvements in paw swelling, clinical arthritis score, semi-quantitative radiographic assessment of bone erosions, histological evidence of peri-articular bone erosions and inflammation, and reduced serum TNF levels.

Finally, we extended these observations, establishing the practicality and effectiveness of traditional electrical VNS in the CIA model using a chronic implantable rodent system we developed. This system had a cuff lead analogous to those used in humans treated with implantable VNS devices, and was performed as a unique collaboration between an engineering research group experienced in lead design and implantation and a laboratory with extensive experience in the CIA model [38]. In these studies animals were immunized on days 0 and 6, and treatment was initiated after the disease had become semi-established on day 9. When compared to implanted but unstimulated animals, VNS stimulation reduced clinical manifestations as assessed by ankle diameter, and reduced the histological severity of inflammation, pannus formation, cartilage damage and bone resorption, accompanied by a reduction in circulating pro-inflammatory mediators (Fig. 2.3).

Neurostimulation of the CAP in Patients with Rheumatoid Arthritis

On the basis of the compelling biology and evidence in the CIA model cited above, a clinical study was initiated in order to test the hypothesis that NCAP delivered by a standard VNS device can improve the signs and symptoms of RA. The investigational study devices being used are standard, commercially purchased VNS systems, treated as investigational study devices due to their off-label use in patients with RA, but implanted in the recommended manner, as described below (Fig. 2.4).

The study recruited 2 separate patient cohorts: An early stage cohort of patients who have only failed the standard first-line oral drug methotrexate (cohort I, N = 7), and a second cohort including patients who have not responded adequately to at least 2 different biologic RA drugs of the kind typically used sequentially, subsequent to methotrexate in standard RA treatment (cohort II, N = 10).

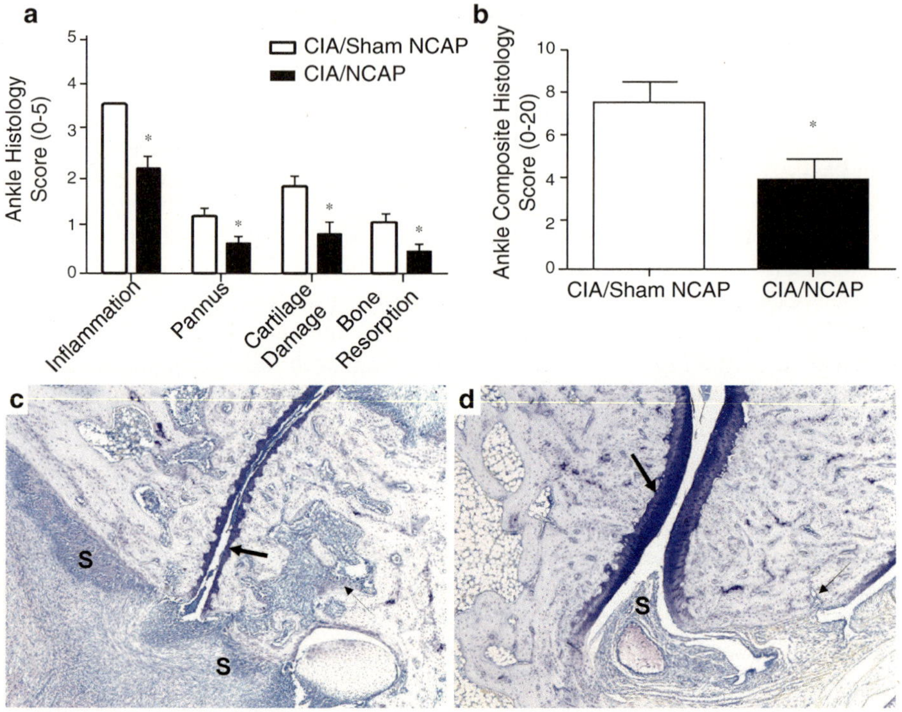

Fig. 2.3 NCAP ameliorates disease in the rodent collagen-induced arthritis (CIA) model. (**a**) Ankle swelling is significantly reduced in animals receiving NCAP. (**b**) NCAP improved histological manifestations of disease with significant reductions in inflammation, pannus formation, cartilage damage, and bone resorption, as assessed by blinded reading on a semi-quantitative scoring scale. (**c**, **d**) Representative toluidine blue stained synovial tissue from NCAP (**c**), and sham (**d**) treated animals. Reductions in synovial inflammation (S), cartilage damage (*thick arrow*), and bone erosions (*thin arrow*) are seen (Figure was taken from [38] under open access policy https://creativecommons.org/licenses/by/4.0/)

This proof-of-concept study has been recently published (Fig. 2.5) [45]. Patients had screening assessments and baseline clinical and biomarker assessments at the day -21 visit, and were implanted under general endotracheal anesthesia at the day -14 visit (Fig. 2.5). The device was then inactivated and the patient allowed recovery from surgery for at least 14 days. On the day 0 visit, patients had postoperative clinical assessments, and were given a single active stimulation. The patients had no stimulation between the day 0 and day 7 visits. On the day 7, 14, and 21 visits patients had clinical and biomarker assessments, and the stimulation output current to be delivered by the device was increased as tolerated. During each of these visits and on the intervening days patients received daily stimulations. At the day 28 visit, if the patient had not achieved a moderate or good clinical response according to EULAR classification [46], the stimulation frequency was increased from once daily to four times daily with other stimulation parameters remaining the same. The primary endpoint of the study was the day 42 visit. On day 42, all subjects had their

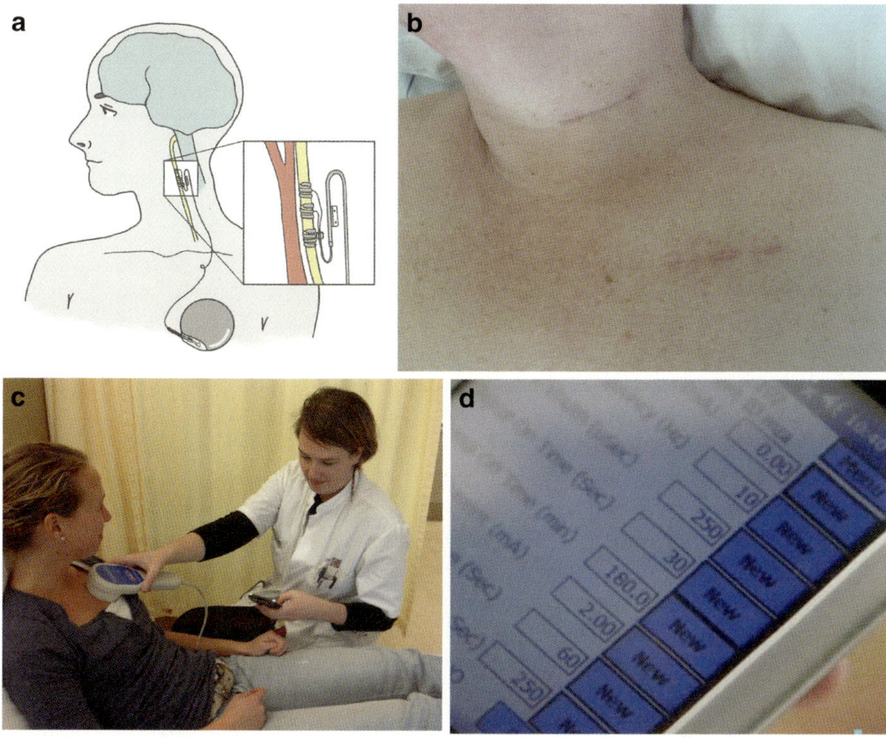

Fig. 2.4 VNS System used in RA proof-of-concept study (**a**) The implantable pulse generator (IPG) placed subcutaneously on the chest wall, and triple helical coiled cuff leads placed within the carotid sheath on the left vagus nerve are shown schematically. (**b**) Typical incision scars on left neck and chest wall from implants are shown. (**c**) In-clinic programming is performed using a handheld controller and a telemetry wand cabled to the controller that is placed over the position of the IPG on the chest wall for programming the implant. (**d**) A close-up view of the stimulation parameter screen of the handheld controller (Reproduced with permission from [45])

device switched off and entered a 14-day treatment withdrawal period. On the day 56 visit, the device was turned on again, and patients received stimulation at the same level and on the same schedule as they were receiving at the day 42 visit, and this was continued through the final study visit at day 84. The primary study endpoint is the mean change in a standard composite RA study endpoint termed the Disease Activity Score (DAS) between baseline and day 42 visit [46].

The DAS was reduced by VNS in both cohorts and when the treatment was paused, the DAS increased, and again was then reduced during retreatment (Fig. 2.5c). The inducible TNF production in whole blood monocytes was measured during the VNS stimulation as a biomarker, similar to the effect we observed in dogs and rodents (Fig. 2.5b). The reduction in TNF production was compared to DAS reductions by linear regression showing a high correlation (Fig. 2.5d), and there was a temporal relationship between the changes in DAS and TNF reductions (Fig. 2.5e). This study provides proof that VNS can cause reduction in a standard rheumatoid arthritis endpoint in association with reductions in a cytokine that drives disease severity.

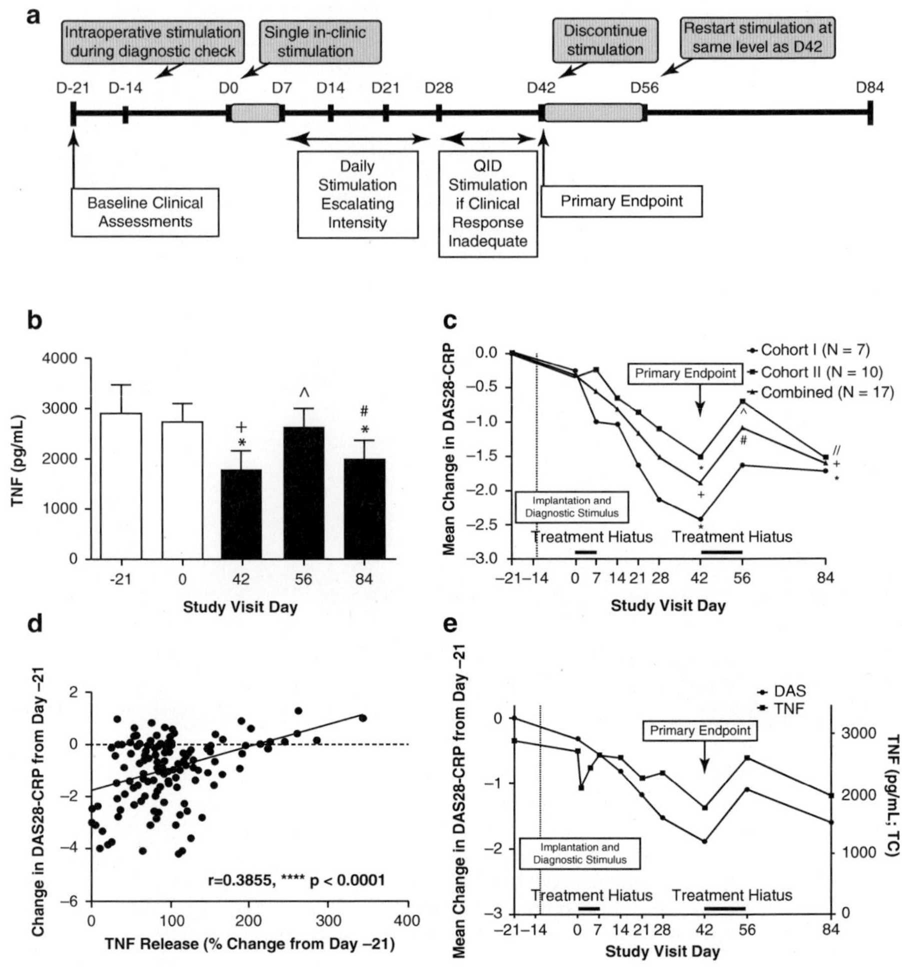

Fig. 2.5 The Effects of VNS on Rheumatoid Arthritis Severity and TNF production (**a**) A schematic of the study design. (**b**) The effect of VNS in reducing in vitro TNF production in whole blood. (**c**) The reduction over time in the Disease Activity Score (DAS), a standard rheumatoid arthritis endpoint. (**d**) The reductions in DAS compared with reductions in TNF production in a regression analysis. (**e**) The temporal association between changes in TNF production and DAS reduction (Reproduced with permission from [45])

Development of an Application-Specific Investigational VNS System for RA

The VNS system used in our present RA study has a standard implanted pulse generator (IPG) containing a non-rechargeable battery, an application-specific integrated circuit (ASIC) that controls system function, and other components necessary for generation and control of electrical pulses and for telemetric communication with a wand-like external device controller (Fig. 2.4c). The IPG is typically placed in a subcutaneous pocket on the anterior chest wall through either an axillary or pectoral incision and connected to the nerve via a lead that is tunneled caudally from a neck incision through the skin, over the clavicle, and into the IPG chest wall pocket [47–49]. The lead is implanted on the nerve through a 2–3 cm left paramedian neck incision to expose the carotid sheath. The left vagus is then isolated within the carotid sheath between the carotid artery and internal jugular vein, and a short segment of perineurium is dissected. The lead has an IPG plug at its proximal end and three helical coiled nerve cuffs having a "corkscrew" appearance at its distal end. The distal and middle coils each have a platinum-iridium electrode to deliver stimulus. The proximal coil has no electrode and serves as an anchor to stabilize the lead on the nerve. The coils have very small suture-like threads at each end that are grasped and used to spread the coil and manually wind it around the nerve. The more proximal part of the lead body is then anchored with a clip to surrounding tissue and a strain relief loop is created, prior to tunneling the lead and closure of the two surgical sites (Fig. 2.4a, b).

The elasticity of the coiled cuffs on the lead serves to facilitate their expansion and contraction, thus minimizing pressure being applied by the cuff to the nerve itself. This is important for the prevention of pressure-induced nerve damage. However, with time, these coils become fibrosed around the nerve, often in an anatomically complex way. While an experienced surgeon can safely remove the lead coils, it is at best a tedious and time-consuming process, and in inexperienced hands, vagus nerve damage can occur during removal attempts [50–53]. When the device is being removed or replaced for reasons other than infection, oftentimes the lead is cut within the neck near the most proximal cuff coil and the distal part of the lead is left in place on the nerve rather than dissecting it free. While this procedure generally works well, implant infection can occur in around 3% of patients, and in such patients full removal of the infected implant is sometimes necessary for infection resolution [52]. The approach also leaves a "bare end" wire, which essentially functions as an antenna, and can overheat and create a tissue damage hazard if the patient is exposed to the radiofrequency energy used during MRI procedures, despite the fact that safe MRI is possible under some conditions if the device is left intact [54].

The investigational VNS system that will be used in future RA studies is fundamentally different from existing systems in that it is implanted directly on the vagus nerve as a single unit that contains a rechargeable battery, pulse generator, as well as a self-contained nerve cuff and electrodes that function without a typical lead wire. The system has four major components (Fig. 2.6): First, a surgically implanted MicroRegulator (MR) functions as both a pulse generator and a leadless cuff electrode. The vagus nerve fits into a groove in the saddle-like base of the unit, and the electrodes in the groove are thereby brought into close apposition to the nerve for efficient stimulation. An onboard ASIC controls the MR. An antenna mounted on the hybrid assembly board allows for radio frequency (RF) telemetry and inductive battery recharging. Second, a surgically implanted Positioning and Orientation Device (POD) is a flexible silicone enclosure that surrounds the MicroRegulator, and holds it against the nerve. The nerve is held in the POD in a cradled position

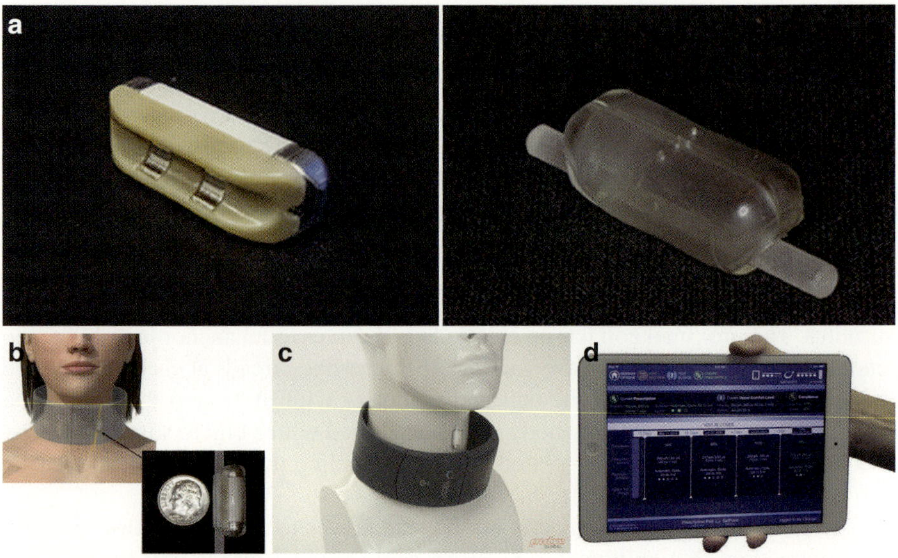

Fig. 2.6 Investigational application-specific VNS system for RA studies (**a**) The MicroRegulator (MR) functions as both and IPG and a "leadless" electrode cuff, and has a groove on the bottom which allows it to cradle the nerve and bring it into close apposition opt the platinum-iridium electrodes in the groove. The MR is secured to the nerve with the Positioning and Orientation Device (POD), a soft enclosure which also isolates the implant electrically from surrounding tissue. (**b**) The position of the MR and POD implanted on the left vagus, and the Energizer collar, used for intermittent telemetry and battery charging are shown. (**c**) The Energizer closes with a magnetic clasp, and is worn intermittently for charging and programming. The Energizer communicates with the MR and charges the onboard MR battery through a radio frequency (RF) interface. The Energizer has a limited number of patient-accessible controls. (**d**) The Prescription Pad is a standard iPad loaded with system-specific software that communicates by Bluetooth with the Energizer and allows the clinician to program the implant

within the electrode groove, allowing for efficient application of electrical charge directly to the nerve, and inducing depolarization. The POD also serves to electrically insulate the device from surrounding tissues other than the target nerve itself. Third, a non-implanted, intermittently worn collar is termed an Energizer. The Energizer collar is positioned on the patient's neck to charge the battery and program the implanted device. Integrated into the collar is a coil running circumferentially, serving to transmit and receive telemetry information, and also to transmit RF energy to the MR antenna for inductive battery recharging. The collar generates an RF field with sufficient range to charge or communicate with the MR, regardless of implantation depth, with the collar placed anywhere on the neck.

The open Energizer collar is positioned on the patient's neck and gently closed with a magnetic clasp. The outward face of the collar has a series of indicator LEDs, control buttons, and a vibrating motor that serve as an interface for patient use to control certain patient-enabled Energizer and MR functions. Finally, the "Prescription Pad" is a system-specific control application for use by caregivers, which is loaded on to a standard

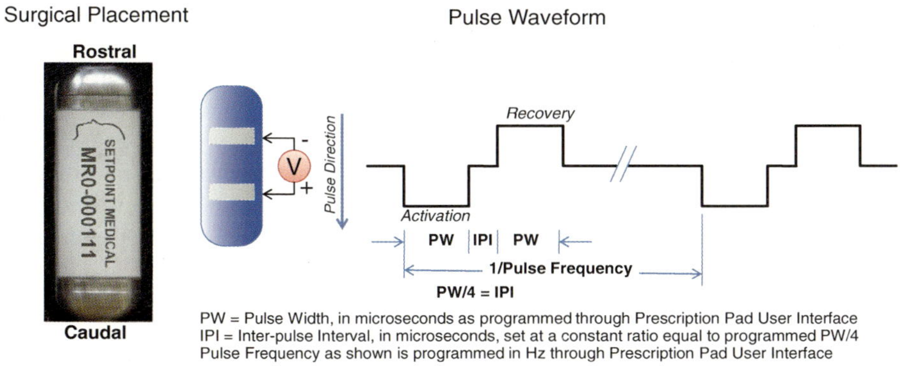

Fig. 2.7 Waveform produced by MR. The MR is placed in the rostral-caudal orientation shown, with a schematic illustration of the anode-cathode orientation, and pulse direction. The pulse waveform produced is charge limited, balanced and biphasic

iPad. The application works through a typical iOS graphic user interface. After programming with the Prescription Pad, the MR delivers bipolar, current-limited, symmetrically biphasic charge-balanced pulses with characteristics as shown in Fig. 2.7.

During the first ambulatory visit, the clinical caregiver will use the Energizer collar and Prescription Pad to program parameters for delivery of stimulation, on a clinician-specified schedule, as the patient's therapy "prescription". The patient will wear the Energizer intermittently to re-charge the MR battery. The Energizer's patient-controllable functions do not require the clinician's Prescription Pad, and include an emergency shut off and a manual dosing function. The use of this novel, application-specific system for delivery of therapy in upcoming clinical studies in RA may prove to offer greater ease of use and patient acceptability than standard VNS systems.

The Future: Potential Steps Toward a Closed Loop "Bioelectronic Medicine"

An effort to increase the therapeutic armamentarium in systemic diseases typically treated with systemically administered drugs has resulted in the concept of "bioelectronic medicines" [55]. As a goal these therapies would have characteristics of both classical medicines and classical medical devices. They would be embedded within the body, and would deliver electrical or other kinds of physical stimulation in a precise and targeted manner that would directly affect the disease pathophysiology.

An inherent part of the definition of an ideal bioelectronic medicine is that the therapeutic entity would be able to continuously monitor the function of the tissue or organ system being treated, adjusting its therapeutic effect in a precise and disease-responsive way that would maximize safety and efficacy. Development of an optimal bioelectronic medicine that can sense activity of individual afferent and efferent nerve fibers communicating with a visceral organ will require a great deal of work in engineering and biology. However, there are a few examples of present day implantable devices that already function in a truly closed loop manner. One such device approved and being marketed in the US alleviates the upper airway anatomic obstruction during sleep apnea by activating the hypoglossal nerve to open the airway, resolving the resultant apneic event. Interestingly, the device has a second lead placed in an intercostal muscle that senses the over-activation of the muscle as the patient struggles to inspire against a closed airway, and instructs the device to fire at that precise moment and open the airway, thus creating a functional closed loop [56]. Several other devices with similar, very simple closed loop designs are in clinical development.

With respect to the treatment of RA and inflammatory disorders, it may be possible to create a device that can "read" the level of systemic inflammation and adjust treatment accordingly. One way to accomplish this would be to build sensors that can directly detect inflammatory mediators and respond to changes by modulating stimulation parameters. However, developing robust closed loop systems that detect and respond to tissue levels of complex proteins will be exceedingly challenging, as evidenced by the lack of a truly closed loop insulin pump system, despite many years of effort to develop one. Alternatively, a device that measures and responds to a neurophysiological or cardiac "proxy" of inflammation may be more immediately feasible.

Epidemiological studies have demonstrated an inverse relationship between vagal tone and disease severity in several inflammatory disorders. Autonomic nervous system activity can be measured indirectly by recording cardiac R-R interval variability and subjecting the data to power spectral analysis. Such heart rate variability (HRV) measurements are influenced by the levels of vagus nerve activity and by balance in cardiac sympathetic-parasympathetic tone. Reduced HRV is indicative of decreased vagal tone, and HRV has a strong inverse correlation with serum levels of c-reactive protein (CRP), an indicator of systemic inflammation, progression of atherosclerosis, and risk of sudden death [57, 58]. HRV is also reduced relative to normals in patients with RA, systemic lupus erythematosus and Sjogren's syndrome, and the extent of reduction in HRV within the patient groups correlates strongly with disease severity [59–62].

Interestingly, a recent study in healthy human volunteers demonstrated that short infusion of very low doses of LPS caused small but measurable dose-dependent changes in body temperature, systemic inflammatory mediator release, and changes in HRV parameters including standard deviation of the average length of interval between each successive heartbeat over a 5-min period (SDNN), the percentage of interval differences of successive intervals between heartbeats greater than 50 milliseconds (pNN50), and high-frequency variability (HF) that correlates with vagal tone. Physiologic measures, mediator levels and HRV indices moved together dynamically during peri-infusion worsening and post infusion recovery [63], demonstrating the potential for HRV parameters to be used as a dynamic surrogate marker of systemic inflammation. Although the above-referenced correlative cross-sectional clinical studies show that HRV and inflammation correlate in RA and other similar diseases, it will be necessary to understand the shorter term variability of HRV indices as the patient's inflammatory disorder moves through its typical clinical cycles of waxing and waning severity. Real-time HRV data from observational studies of RA patients might then be correlated with systemic mediator levels and clinical disease activity assessments to understand the relationship between

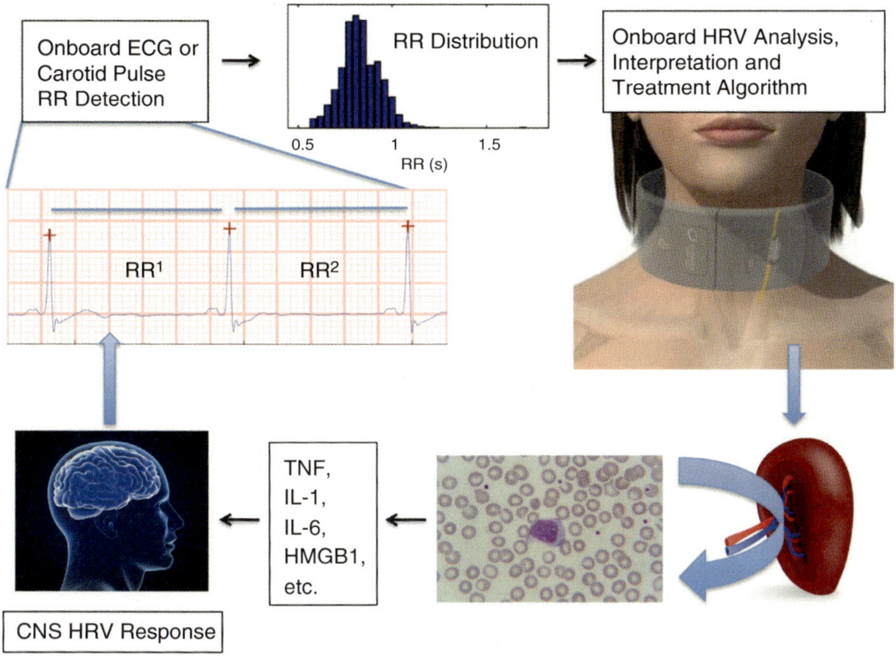

Fig. 2.8 Concept for potential future modifications to create a closed loop system. The central nervous system responds to varying levels of systemic inflammation by causing alterations in heart rate variability (HRV). If the relationship between HRV parameters, inflammation, and disease activity can be understood and modeled, onboard sensors could measure the R wave to R wave (RR) interval, calculate HRV, and adjust stimulation settings using a pre-defined algorithm. This approach might allow a device to automatically tailor the delivered treatment to the patient's changing level of disease activity

HRV and disease, and these data used to model a responsive treatment algorithm that would increase or decrease the delivered VNS stimulation at levels appropriate to the patient's current level of disease activity. The application-specific RA VNS system described above could be modified to sense an ECG signal or carotid pulse movement in order to read the R-R interval, then calculate HRV parameters and algorithmically adjust stimulation output using onboard firmware. A schematic summary of this concept is shown in Fig. 2.8. This research approach may facilitate development of a closed loop VNS system for inflammation therapy in the not-too-distant future.

Summary

The cholinergic anti-inflammatory pathway can be harnessed to reduce systemic and organ-specific inflammation, by virtue of its effects in down-regulating B cell function, reducing T cell, neutrophil, and monocyte inflammatory mediator release, increasing regulatory T cell number and function, and reducing trafficking of leukocytes to inflamed tissue. These pleiotropic effects underlie the improvement in disease activity in several animal models, including the standard rodent collagen-induced arthritis model of human RA. A proof-of-concept study in patients with RA has shown promising preliminary results. Future trials in RA will test a novel nerve stimulation system developed specifically for this application, which will be studied to confirm whether its design offers advantages over existing systems. In the future, this system is capable of being modified to detect and respond to inflammation-induced changes in heart rate variability, allowing the device to respond to changes in the patient's disease status, and thereby offering the potential to become a closed loop, bioelectronic medicine.

References

1. Scott DL, Wolfe F, Huizinga TW. Rheumatoid arthritis. Lancet. 2010;376(9746):1094–108.
2. Avina-Zubieta JA, Thomas J, Sadatsafavi M, Lehman AJ, Lacaille D. Risk of incident cardiovascular events in patients swith rheumatoid arthritis: a meta-analysis of observational studies. Ann Rheum Dis. 2012;71(9):1524–9.
3. Bisoendial RJ, Stroes ES, Tak PP. Critical determinants of cardiovascular risk in rheumatoid arthritis. Curr Pharm Des. 2011;17(1):21–6.
4. Roubille C, Richer V, Starnino T, McCourt C, McFarlane A, Fleming P, et al. The effects of tumour necrosis factor inhibitors, methotrexate, non-steroidal anti-inflammatory drugs and corticosteroids on cardiovascular events in rheumatoid arthritis, psoriasis and psoriatic arthritis: a systematic review and meta-analysis. Ann Rheum Dis. 2015;74(3):480–9.
5. Tak PP, Kalden JR. Advances in rheumatology: new targeted therapeutics. Arthritis Res Ther. 2011;13 Suppl 1:S5.
6. Tracey KJ. The inflammatory reflex. Nature. 2002;420(6917):853–9.
7. Sun J, Singh V, Kajino-Sakamoto R, Aballay A. Neuronal GPCR controls innate immunity by regulating noncanonical unfolded protein response genes. Science. 2011;332(6030):729–32.
8. Tracey KJ. Cell biology. Ancient neurons regulate immunity. Science. 2011;332(6030):673–4.
9. Andersson U, Tracey KJ. Neural reflexes in inflammation and immunity. J Exp Med. 2012;209(6):1057–68.
10. Andersson U, Tracey KJ. Reflex principles of immunological homeostasis. Annu Rev Immunol. 2012;30:313–35.
11. Tracey KJ. Reflex control of immunity. Nat Rev Immunol. 2009;9(6):418–28.
12. Van Maanen M, Vervoordeldonk M, Tak P. The cholinergic anti-inflammatory pathway: towards innovative treatment of rheumatoid arthritis. Nat Rev Rheumatol. 2009;5:229–32.
13. Borovikova L, Ivanova S, Zhang M, Yang H, Botchkina G, Watkins L, et al. Vagus nerve stimulation attenuates the systemic inflammatory response to endotoxin. Nature. 2000;405:458–62.
14. Huston JM, Ochani M, Rosas-Ballina M, Liao H, Ochani K, Pavlov VA, et al. Splenectomy inactivates the cholinergic antiinflammatory pathway during lethal endotoxemia and polymicrobial sepsis. J Exp Med. 2006;203(7):1623–8.
15. Rosas-Ballina M, Ochani M, Parrish WR, Ochani K, Harris YT, Huston JM, et al. Splenic nerve is required for cholinergic antiinflammatory pathway control of TNF in endotoxemia. Proc Natl Acad Sci USA. 2008;105(31):11008–13.
16. Rosas-Ballina M, Olofsson PS, Ochani M, Valdes-Ferrer SI, Levine YA, Reardon C, et al. Acetylcholine-synthesizing T cells relay neural signals in a vagus nerve circuit. Science. 2011;334(6052):98–101.

17. de Jonge WJ, van der Zanden EP, The FO, Bijlsma MF, van Westerloo DJ, Bennink RJ, et al. Stimulation of the vagus nerve attenuates macrophage activation by activating the Jak2-STAT3 signaling pathway. Nat Immunol. 2005;6(8):844–51.
18. Wang H, Yu M, Ochani M, Amella C, Tanovic M, Susarla S, et al. Nicotinic acetylcholine receptor alpha7 subunit is an essential regulator of inflammation. Nature. 2003;421: 384–8.
19. Lu B, Kwan K, Levine YA, Olofsson PS, Yang H, Li J, et al. Alpha7 nicotinic acetylcholine receptor signaling inhibits inflammasome activation by preventing mitochondrial DNA release. Mol Med. 2014;20:350–8.
20. Bottini N, Firestein GS. Duality of fibroblast-like synoviocytes in RA: passive responders and imprinted aggressors. Nat Rev Rheumatol. 2013;9(1):24–33.
21. Bruchfeld A, Goldstein RS, Chavan S, Patel NB, Rosas-Ballina M, Kohn N, et al. Whole blood cytokine attenuation by cholinergic agonists ex vivo and relationship to vagus nerve activity in rheumatoid arthritis. J Intern Med. 2010;268(1):94–101.
22. Olofsson PS, Levine YA, Caravaca A, Chavan SS, Pavlov VA, Faltys M, et al. Single pulse and unidirectional activation of the cervical vagus nerve reduces TNF in endotoxemia. Bioelectronic Med. 2015;2:37–42.
23. van Westerloo DJ, Giebelen IA, Florquin S, Bruno MJ, Larosa GJ, Ulloa L, et al. The vagus nerve and nicotinic receptors modulate experimental pancreatitis severity in mice. Gastroenterology. 2006;130(6):1822–30.
24. Krzyzaniak MJ, Peterson CY, Cheadle G, Loomis W, Wolf P, Kennedy V, et al. Efferent vagal nerve stimulation attenuates acute lung injury following burn: the importance of the gut-lung axis. Surgery. 2011;150(3):379–89.
25. Borovikova LV, Ivanova S, Nardi D, Zhang M, Yang H, Ombrellino M, et al. Role of vagus nerve signaling in CNI-1493-mediated suppression of acute inflammation. Auton Neurosc: basic & clinical. 2000;85(1–3):141–7.
26. Huston JM, Rosas-Ballina M, Xue X, Dowling O, Ochani K, Ochani M, et al. Cholinergic neural signals to the spleen down-regulate leukocyte trafficking via CD11b. J Immunol. 2009;183(1):552–9.
27. Mina-Osorio P, Rosas-Ballina M, Valdes-Ferrer SI, Al-Abed Y, Tracey KJ, Diamond B. Neural signaling in the spleen controls B-cell responses to blood-borne antigen. Mol Med. 2012;18:618–27.
28. Grant CR, Liberal R, Mieli-Vergani G, Vergani D, Longhi MS. Regulatory T-cells in autoimmune diseases: challenges, controversies and-yet-unanswered questions. Autoimmun Rev. 2015;14(2):105–16.
29. Wang DW, Zhou RB, Yao YM, Zhu XM, Yin YM, Zhao GJ, et al. Stimulation of alpha7 nicotinic acetylcholine receptor by nicotine increases suppressive capacity of naturally occurring CD4+CD25+ regulatory T cells in mice in vitro. J Pharmacol Exp Ther. 2010;335(3):553–61.
30. Galitovskiy V, Qian J, Chernyavsky AI, Marchenko S, Gindi V, Edwards RA, et al. Cytokine-induced alterations of alpha7 nicotinic receptor in colonic CD4 T cells mediate dichotomous response to nicotine in murine models of Th1/Th17- versus Th2-mediated colitis. J Immunol. 2011;187(5):2677–87.
31. Ghia JE, Blennerhassett P, Collins SM. Vagus nerve integrity and experimental colitis. Am J Physiol Gastrointest Liver Physiol. 2007;293(3):G560–7.
32. Ghia JE, Blennerhassett P, El-Sharkawy RT, Collins SM. The protective effect of the vagus nerve in a murine model of chronic relapsing colitis. Am J Physiol Gastrointest Liver Physiol. 2007;293(4):G711–8.
33. Morishita K, Costantini TW, Eliceiri B, Bansal V, Coimbra R. Vagal nerve stimulation modulates the dendritic cell profile in posthemorrhagic shock mesenteric lymph. J Trauma Acute Care Surg. 2014;76(3):610–7.
34. O'Mahony C, van der Kleij H, Bienenstock J, Shanahan F, O'Mahony L. Loss of vagal anti-inflammatory effect: in vivo visualization and adoptive transfer. Am J Physiol Regul Integr Comp Physiol. 2009;297(4):R1118–26.

35. Karimi K, Bienenstock J, Wang L, Forsythe P. The vagus nerve modulates CD4+ T cell activity. Brain Behav Immun. 2010;24(2):316–23.
36. van Maanen MA, Stoof SP, van der Zanden EP, de Jonge WJ, Janssen RA, Fischer DF, et al. The alpha7 nicotinic acetylcholine receptor on fibroblast-like synoviocytes and in synovial tissue from rheumatoid arthritis patients: a possible role for a key neurotransmitter in synovial inflammation. Arthritis Rheum. 2009;60(5):1272–81.
37. Waldburger JM, Boyle DL, Pavlov VA, Tracey KJ, Firestein GS. Acetylcholine regulation of synoviocyte cytokine expression by the alpha7 nicotinic receptor. Arthritis Rheum. 2008;58(11):3439–49.
38. Levine YA, Koopman FA, Faltys M, Caravaca A, Bendele A, Zitnik R, et al. Neurostimulation of the cholinergic anti-inflammatory pathway ameliorates disease in rat collagen-induced arthritis. PLoS One. 2014;9(8):e104530.
39. van Maanen M, Stoof S, Larosa G, Vervoordeldonk M, Tak P. Role of the cholinergic nervous system in rheumatoid arthritis: aggravation of arthritis in nicotinic acetylcholine receptor alpha7 subunit gene knockout mice. Ann Rheum Dis. 2010;69:1717–23.
40. van Maanen MA, Papke RL, Koopman FA, Koepke J, Bevaart L, Clark R, et al. Two novel alpha7 nicotinic acetylcholine receptor ligands: in vitro properties and their efficacy in collagen-induced arthritis in mice. PLoS One. 2015;10(1):e0116227.
41. Bevaart L, Vervoordeldonk MJ, Tak PP. Evaluation of therapeutic targets in animal models of arthritis: how does it relate to rheumatoid arthritis? Arthritis Rheum. 2010;62(8):2192–205.
42. Levine YA, Koopman F, Faltys M, Zitnik R, Tak PP. Neurostimulation of the cholinergic anti-inflammatory pathway in rheumatoid arthritis and inflammatory bowel disease. Bioelectron Med. 2014;1(1):34–43.
43. van Maanen M, Lebre M, van der Poll T, LaRosa G, Elbaum D, Vervoordeldonk M, et al. Stimulation of nicotinic acetylcholine receptors attenuates collagen-induced arthritis in mice. Arthritis Rheum. 2009;60:114–22.
44. Zhang P, Han D, Tang T, Zhang X, Dai K. Inhibition of the development of collagen-induced arthritis in Wistar rats through vagus nerve suspension: a 3-month observation. Inflamm Res. 2008;57(7):322–8.
45. Koopman FA, Chavan SS, Miljko S, Grazio S, Sokolovic S, Schuurman PR, Mehta AD, Levine YA, Faltys M, Zitnik R, Tracey KJ, Tak PP. Vagus nerve stimulation inhibits cytokine production and attenuates disease severity in rheumatoid arthritis. Proc Natl Acad Sci. 2016;113(29):8284–9.
46. Fransen J, van Riel PL. The Disease Activity Score and the EULAR response criteria. Clin Exp Rheumatol. 2005;23(5 Suppl 39):S93–9.
47. Felson DT, Anderson JJ, Boers M, Bombardier C, Furst D, Goldsmith C, et al.; American College of Rheumatology. Preliminary definition of improvement in rheumatoid arthritis. Arthritis Rheum 1995;38(6):727–735.
48. Beekwilder JP, Beems T. Overview of the clinical applications of vagus nerve stimulation. J Clin Neurophysiol: official publication of the American Electroencephalographic Society. 2010;27(2):130–8.
49. Ben-Menachem E, Revesz D, Simon BJ, Silberstein S. Surgically implanted and non-invasive vagus nerve stimulation: a review of efficacy, safety and tolerability. Eur J Neurol. 2015;22(9):1260–8.
50. Agarwal G, Wilfong AA, Edmonds Jr JL. Surgical revision of vagus nerve stimulation electrodes in children. Otolaryngol Head Neck Surg. 2011;144(1):123–4.
51. Air EL, Ghomri YM, Tyagi R, Grande AW, Crone K, Mangano FT. Management of vagal nerve stimulator infections: do they need to be removed? J Neurosurg Pediatr. 2009;3(1): 73–8.
52. Horowitz G, Amit M, Fried I, Neufeld MY, Sharf L, Kramer U, et al. Vagal nerve stimulation for refractory epilepsy: the surgical procedure and complications in 100 implantations by a single medical center. Eur Arch Otorhinolaryngol: official journal of the European Federation of Oto-Rhino-Laryngological Societies (EUFOS) : affiliated with the German Society for Oto-Rhino-Laryngology - Head and Neck Surgery. 2013;270(1):355–8.

53. Ng WH, Donner E, Go C, Abou-Hamden A, Rutka JT. Revision of vagal nerve stimulation (VNS) electrodes: review and report on use of ultra-sharp monopolar tip. Childs Nerv Syst. 2010;26(8):1081–4.
54. Gorny KR, Bernstein MA, Watson Jr RE. 3 Tesla MRI of patients with a vagus nerve stimulator: initial experience using a T/R head coil under controlled conditions. J Magn Reson Imaging. 2010;31(2):475–81.
55. Birmingham K, Gradinaru V, Anikeeva P, Grill WM, Pikov V, McLaughlin B, et al. Bioelectronic medicines: a research roadmap. Nat Rev Drug Discov. 2014;13(6):399–400.
56. Strollo Jr PJ, Soose RJ, Maurer JT, de Vries N, Cornelius J, Froymovich O, et al. Upper-airway stimulation for obstructive sleep apnea. N Engl J Med. 2014;370(2):139–49.
57. Huikuri HV, Jokinen V, Syvanne M, Nieminen MS, Airaksinen KE, Ikaheimo MJ, et al. Heart rate variability and progression of coronary atherosclerosis. Arterioscler Thromb Vasc Biol. 1999;19(8):1979–85.
58. Sajadieh A, Nielsen OW, Rasmussen V, Hein HO, Abedini S, Hansen JF. Increased heart rate and reduced heart-rate variability are associated with subclinical inflammation in middle-aged and elderly subjects with no apparent heart disease. Eur Heart J. 2004;25(5):363–70.
59. Evrengul H, Dursunoglu D, Cobankara V, Polat B, Seleci D, Kabukcu S, et al. Heart rate variability in patients with rheumatoid arthritis. Rheumatol Int. 2004;24(4):198–202.
60. Janse van Rensburg DC, Ker JA, Grant CC, Fletcher L. Autonomic impairment in rheumatoid arthritis. Int J Rheum Dis. 2012;15(4):419–26.
61. Louthrenoo W, Ruttanaumpawan P, Aramrattana A, Sukitawut W. Cardiovascular autonomic nervous system dysfunction in patients with rheumatoid arthritis and systemic lupus erythematosus. QJM. 1999;92(2):97–102.
62. Stojanovich L, Milovanovich B, de Luka SR, Popovich-Kuzmanovich D, Bisenich V, Djukanovich B, et al. Cardiovascular autonomic dysfunction in systemic lupus, rheumatoid arthritis, primary Sjogren syndrome and other autoimmune diseases. Lupus. 2007;16(3):181–5.
63. Herlitz GN, Arlow RL, Cheung NH, Coyle SM, Griffel B, Macor MA, et al. Physiologic variability at the verge of systemic inflammation: multiscale entropy of heart rate variability is affected by very low doses of endotoxin. Shock. 2015;43(2):133–9.

Chapter 3
Electroceutical Approaches for the Treatment of Traumatic Brain Injury

Harvey Leung, Ali Ali, Christopher Heath, Arshad Majid, and Jessica Redgrave

Abstract Existing treatments for traumatic brain injury (TBI) include surgical intervention for the acute phase and rehabilitative therapies for the chronic/recovery phase. There is a brief time period after TBI has occurred when surgical intervention can reduce cerebral ischemia, limiting the damage this would otherwise cause. For example, decompressive craniectomy, can treat intracranial hypertension following TBI and may also improve regional cerebral blood flow. Surgical evacuation of haematomas may also help return cerebral blood flow regulation to normal. Various forms of therapy are used in the rehabilitation process for humans following TBI. For example, speech therapy, occupational therapy and physiotherapy all play a key role in helping patients to return to as normal a level of functioning as possible. Cognitive therapies may focus on specific areas such as working memory or attention deficits. Psychotherapy can help patients to adapt to their disability, and lead to improvements in mood and self-esteem.

Keywords Electroceuticals • Traumatic brain injury • Vagus nerve stimulation • Deep brain stimulation • Transcranial magnetic stimulation • Transcranial direct current stimulation

Introduction

Traumatic brain injury (TBI) is generally defined as any brain injury caused by trauma inflicted on the brain by an outside source [1]. It is difficult to quantify the overall prevalence of TBI as minor cases may not always receive medical treatment. TBI also often occurs in combination with other injuries, leading to possible

H. Leung, MSc • A. Ali, MSc • C. Heath, MSc • A. Majid, MBChB • J. Redgrave, D Phil (✉)
Sheffield Institute of Translational Neuroscience, University of Sheffield,
385a Glossop Road, Sheffield S10 2HQ, UK
e-mail: Jessica.Redgrave@sth.nhs.uk

A. Majid (ed.), *Electroceuticals*, DOI 10.1007/978-3-319-28612-9_3

under-reporting. However, the number of TBI serious enough to cause hospitalisation or death have been estimated to be over 10 million per year worldwide [1–3]. The most common causes of TBI are incidents such as falls, traffic accidents, struck by/against events and assaults. In terms of demographics, people below 19 and over 75 show the highest incidences of TBI, and males have a higher incidence than females [4].

As TBI encompasses a wide range of potential severities and injury locations within the brain, it can present with a wide range of symptoms. Adults with mild TBI have reported posttraumatic cognitive symptoms such as headaches, fatigue, forgetfulness, and sleep difficulties [5], as well as problems with balance and concentration [6]. In more severe cases, many different brain functions may be compromised, and secondary effects may include movement and sleep disorders, visual deficits, and long-term cognitive and behavioural problems [1]. Studies have also highlighted an increased prevalence of seizures, epilepsy, depression and neurodegenerative diseases such as Alzheimer's disease [2, 6] in those who have experienced TBI.

The damage caused by TBI can generally be separated into two parts. Initially, the trauma causes specific areas of tissue damage and may impair cerebral blood flow regulation. Secondary, more diffuse damage may then occur to the brain through a variety of mechanisms. For example, the reduced regulation of cerebral blood flow may result in ischaemia or hyperaemia, and metabolic failure. Oedema and inflammation may lead to further brain damage.

Existing treatments for TBI include surgical intervention for the acute phase and rehabilitative therapies for the chronic/recovery phase. There is a brief time period after TBI has occurred when surgical intervention can reduce cerebral ischemia, limiting the damage this would otherwise cause [7]. For example, decompressive craniectomy, can treat intracranial hypertension following TBI [8] and may also improve regional cerebral blood flow [9]. Surgical evacuation of haematomas may also help return cerebral blood flow regulation to normal [10].

Various forms of therapy are used in the rehabilitation process for humans following TBI. For example, speech therapy, occupational therapy and physiotherapy all play a key role in helping patients to return to as normal a level of functioning as possible. Cognitive therapies may focus on specific areas such as working memory or attention deficits [11]. Psychotherapy can help patients to adapt to their disability, and lead to improvements in mood and self-esteem [1].

Electroceutical Therapies in TBI

Electroceutical treatments such as vagus nerve stimulation (VNS), deep brain stimulation (DBS), transcranial magnetic stimulation (TMS) and direct cortical stimulation (DCS) may play a role in the treatment and recovery from TBI in the future.

However, owing to the diversity of types, locations, size and symptoms arising from TBI, evaluation of these potential treatments within standardised human trials is difficult. Human trials rely on volunteers or consent from third parties and it can be difficult to find large enough samples of participants with comparable brain injuries undergoing the same form of treatment. The frequency with which TBI occurs in conjunction with other injuries and illnesses also make it difficult to isolate the effects of TBI specifically. Therefore, we mostly rely on controlled animal studies when exploring the potential for electroceutical treatments in the context of TBI.

Animal Models of TBI

Various methods have been used to induce TBI in animals to study the effects of VNS. These include: fluid percussion injury (FPI) [12–15], weight drop [16, 17], controlled cortical impact (CCI) [18], and explosive injury [19]. In all cases, craniotomy is performed to expose the brain with the dura mater intact prior to inducing TBI.

In fluid percussion injury (FPI), an injury cap is fitted over an exposed area of the brain then sealed and filled with saline to create a closed system. A fluid-filled cylinder is attached to the cap and a weight pushes a piston to create a fluid pressure pulse directly onto the dura mater and underlying brain. This creates a pressure pulse lasting approximately 23 milliseconds and a pressure of 1.82 atmospheres (SD = 0.09). Following injury, the injury cap is removed and the craniotomy is covered with sterile gel foam [12–15].

In the "weight drop" model of TBI, a weight is dropped directly onto the brain. Bansal et al. [16] and Lopez et al. [17] deployed this technique in mice and exposed the brain first by creating a burr hole with a diameter of 4 mm, and a 250 g metal rod was dropped from a high of 2 cm onto the intact dura mater. Following this, the incision was closed using Vetbond [16, 17].

Pruitt et al. used controlled cortical impact (CCI), in which they deployed a spring-loaded device, to induce TBI in a consistent manner [18]. The motor cortex of rats was exposed, and the 3 mm diameter impactor tip was lowered onto the surface of the brain. The impactor tip was then lowered 2 mm below the surface of the brain at a velocity of 3 m/s and remained in place for 5 s before being removed. The craniotomy was then covered with a silicone polymer and sealed with acrylic [18].

Another model of TBI is so-called "explosive injury" as used by Zhou et al. in their studies on rabbits [19]. Following craniotomy to expose the brain, an incision was made in the dura mater to expose the parietal cortex. A firecracker wrapped in fine iron wire was then placed 0.5 cm from the exposed brain tissue. Five pieces of metal debris were placed on the right parietal cortex directly and then the firecrackers were lit from a distance to induce TBI. Following this, the bone window was filled with bone wax and a whole-layer suture was performed [19].

Evidence for Electroceutical Therapies in TBI

Vagus Nerve Stimulation

The vagus nerve is the tenth cranial nerve and takes a long meandering course through the body, connecting to centres within the brain as well as several other organs. Vagus nerve stimulation (VNS) historically has involved implanting an electrode directly onto the vagus nerve in the neck. This electrode is then connected to a stimulator unit implanted into the chest wall [20]. Whilst already in widespread use to treat epilepsy and depression in humans, VNS is currently being explored as a treatment for a number of other disorders, including TBI [21].

The vagus nerve is composed of 80% afferent fibres and 20% efferent fibres [22]. The afferent fibres receive innervation primarily from visceral organs of the thorax and abdomen and project to the nucleus tractus solitarius (NTS) in the medulla, which then relays information to the forebrain, thalamic region, and the orbitofrontal and prefrontal cortices. Whilst the neuroprotective effects of vagus nerve stimulation are not well understood, several potential mechanisms have been proposed. For example, the NTS connects to several structures in the brain, including the locus ceruleus (LC) [22]. The LC releases large amounts of norepinephrine, which leads to neurogenesis, release of serotonin from the dorsal raphe nucleus (DRN), and acetylcholine secretion [23, 24]. Both norepinephrine and serotonin have been found to stimulate neurogenesis [25], inhibit excitotoxicity [26], and suppress seizures [27] indicating possible mechanisms underlying therapeutic effects of VNS. Furthermore, acetylcholine, another neurotransmitter released by VNS, blocks glutamate excite-toxicity and the synthesis of inflammatory cytokines, thereby reducing the production of reactive oxygen species and disruption of the blood-brain barrier [28–30].

Experimental Models of Vagus Nerve Stimulation in Traumatic Brain Injury

To date, animal models have been used to investigate the effects of VNS on motor recovery [12, 13, 15, 18], brain swelling [15, 19], ischaemia [12–14, 17–19], blood brain barrier permeability [17], and inflammatory changes [16, 19] following TBI. These studies are summarised in Table 3.1. Changes in the level of cytokines such as TNF-α, IL-1β, and IL-10, or hormones like ghrelin after VNS may contribute to the attenuation of inflammation and oedema formation following TBI [15–17, 19] to limit the size of the final injury [14].

Table 3.1 Summary of VNS studies on TBI.

Reference	TBI model/ type	Species, group (n)	Stimulation side	Stimulation parameters					Tested measures	Results
				VNS switched on	Intensity (mA or V)	Frequency (Hz)	Pulse width (ms)	Duty cycle % (on/off time)		
Smith et al. [12]	Fluid percussion injury	**Male rats (n = 49[a]):** Sham- surgery only; TBI only; TBI + VNS	Left	2 h post-TBI	0.5 mA	20	0.5	1.64% (30s/30min)	Behavioural assessments: limb mobility, cognition. Histology	No sig. Differences in histology in VNS+FPI compared to FPI alone. Improved rate of recovery of mobility and cognitive outcomes after 14 days of VNS.
Smith et al. [13]	Fluid percussion injury	**Rats[b]:** Sham-craniotomy without TBI (n = 16); TBI only (n = 16); TBI + VNS (n = 16)	Left	24 h post-TBI	0.5 mA	20	0.5	1.64% (30s/30min)	Behavioural assessments: limb mobility, cognition. Histology	No sig. Differences in histology in VNS+FPI compared to FPI alone. Improved rate of recovery of mobility and cognitive outcomes after 14 days of VNS. Despite VNS being administered later, recovery rate was similar to VNS administered at 2 h and similar outcomes at 14 days post-TBI.
Neese et al. [14]	Fluid percussion injury	**Male rats:** Sham-craniotomy without TBI (n = 8); TBI only (n = 8); TBI + VNS (n = 8)	Left	24 h post-TBI	0.5 mA	20	0.5	1.67% (30s/29.5 min)	Histology	VNS reduces loss of GABA neurons following FPI

(continued)

Table 3.1 (continued)

Reference	TBI model/ type	Species, group (n)	Stimulation side	Stimulation parameters: VNS switched on	Intensity (mA or V)	Frequency (Hz)	Pulse width (ms)	Duty cycle % (on/off time)	Tested measures	Results
Clough et al. [15]	Fluid percussion injury	**Male rats:** Sham-Craniotomy without TBI (n = 5) TBI only (n = 6) TBI + VNS (n = 8)	Left	2 h post-TBI	0.5 mA	20	0.5	1.67% (30s/29.5 min)	Motility, brain water content	VNS significantly recovered motility and attenuated oedema formation 48 h post-TBI.
Pruitt et al. [18]	Spring-loaded controlled cortical impact device	**Female rats:** TBI + Rehab (n = 14) TBI + VNS + Rehab (n = 14)	Left	Post-TBI. Within 45 ms of forelimb pulling response force > 120 g.	0.8 mA	30	0.1	Paired to successful forelimb pulling response	Conditioned forelimb pulling responses, Histology	VNS paired to rehabilitation in rats significantly increased forelimb recovery at 3–6 weeks post-TBI. Lesion size from TBI did not differ between VNS + rehabilitation vs. rehabilitation only.
Bansal et al. [16]	Weight drop	**Male mice:** Sham- no TBI (n = 8) TBI only (n = 8) TBI + Ghrelin (n = 8) TBI + VNS (n = 8) TBI + VNS + Ghrelin antagonist (n = 8)	Right	10 mins pre-TBI	2 mA	Not reported	Not reported	100% (10 min continuous)	Serum levels of TNF-α and Ghrelin, tissue levels of Ghrelin	VNS attenuated secondary inflammation. Ghrelin is important in VNS-mediated anti-inflammatory response

Lopez et al. [17]	Weight drop	**Male mice:** Sham surgery (no TBI or VNS) (n = 4) TBI only (n = 4) TBI + VNS (n = 4)	Right	10 mins pre-TBI	2 mA	Not reported	Not reported	100% (10 min continuous)	Histology, blood brain barrier permeability	VNS reduces expression of AQP-4 and attenuates blood brain barrier breakdown following TBI.
Zhou et al. [19]	Explosive injury	**Male rabbits:** Control- No TBI or VNS (n = 4) Sham surgery with no TBI or VNS (n = 6) TBI (n = 10) TBI + VNS (n = 8)	Right	1 h post-TBI	10 V	5	5	100% (20 mins continuous)	Serum and brain tissue levels of TNF-a, IL-1b, and IL-10. Brain water content. Histology	Reduction in oedema in VNS treated TBI group. Reduction in inflammatory cytokine levels (TNF-a and IL-1b) and increased anti-inflammatory cytokine levels (Il-10) in serum and brain tissue following VNS.
Englot et al. [31]	Post-traumatic epilepsy	**Humans:** Posttraumatic epilepsy (n = 317) Non posttraumatic epilepsy (n = 1763)	Left	Not reported	Not reported	Not reported	Not reported	Not reported	Seizure frequency and types, Engel outcome class	PTE patients respond better to VNS than non-PTE patients with a greater reduction in seizure frequency and overall more positive outcomes

TBI traumatic brain injury, *VNS* vagus nerve stimulation, *PTE* post-traumatic epilepsy, *IL* interleukin, *TNF* tumor necrosis factor, *FPI* fluid percussion injury

[a]Group n not reported (all groups underwent vagus nerve implant surgery)

[b]Gender not reported

Effects of VNS on Motor and Cognitive Recovery Post TBI in Rats

The potential for VNS to enhance motor recovery following TBI have been reported in studies in rats [12, 13] (Table 3.1). For example, electrical stimulation of the left cervical vagus nerve at 30 min intervals for 2 weeks initiated at 2 h [12] or 24 h [13] after FPI both significantly improved the rate and degree of recovery of forelimb motor function by the end of the treatment period [12, 13]. Furthermore, "reference memory" as assessed by a Morris water maze task had improved in mice that received VNS at 2 h post-FPI but not in those who received VNS at 24 h post FPI [13]. Performance of VNS-treated animals in both motor and memory tasks was the same as that in the uninjured controls (craniotomy without injury) at 2 weeks post-TBI [12].

In another study by Pruitt et al., 28 female rats were trained to perform a "pull" task prior to TBI [18]. A successful trial in pulling the handle with a force greater than 120 g resulted in a single pellet reward and the rats achieved a >85% success rate in surpassing the 120 g threshold. A spring-loaded device was then used to induce controlled cortical impact (CCI) at the left motor cortex. The rats were divided into 2 groups, one group received rehabilitative training alone (n = 14) and the other group received rehabilitative training paired with VNS (n = 14) (VNS delivered within 45 ms of each successful pull trial). In the VNS group, there was pairing of electrical stimulation with the forelimb pulling task initiated at 3–4 weeks following TBI but stimulation was turned off during the 6th week in order to assess whether the effects of stimulation were sustained. By week 4 post-TBI, the forelimb maximal force strength and percentage of successful pull attempts in the VNS group were significantly increased in VNS treated rats compared to unstimulated rats. These differences were maintained at the end of week 6 ($p < 0.05$) leading the authors to conclude that the beneficial effects of VNS may persist after actual stimulation has ceased [18]. Interestingly, upon sacrifice of the animals at the end of week 6, there were no differences in final lesion size between stimulated and unstimulated rats [18]. Other studies have confirmed no effects of VNS on the severity of tissue injury or cell death in the cortex or hippocampus following stimulation at either 2 or 24 h post TBI [12, 13]. The beneficial effects of VNS on motor recovery therefore do not appear to be mediated through alterations in in size or extent of initial brain damage.

Effects of VNS on Neuronal Survival Post TBI

A study by Neese et al. administered VNS in rats at 30 minute intervals for 2 weeks starting at 24 h following FPI in the left hemisphere. Here, 24 rats were implanted with a VNS device and 8 rats received FPI only, 8 received FPI followed by VNS, and 8 received sham FPI (craniotomy without injury) without VNS [14]. The VNS-treated rats had a significantly higher number of GABAergic neurons compared to FPI-only group in the cortex at the end of the 2 weeks treatment ($p < 0.05$) [14]. The study also found a 32% increase in GABAergic-like cells in the hippocampus following VNS. The authors hypothesised that this could be due to an increase in neurogenesis triggered by VNS or an increased number of newly divided neurons acquiring a GABAergic phenotype [14].

Effects of VNS on Oedema Post TBI in Rats

One mechanism whereby VNS may reduce neuronal cell death following TBI is by attenuating cerebral oedema. In a study by Clough et al., 19 rats implanted with VNS and were divided into three groups: FPI with VNS ($n = 8$), FPI without VNS ($n = 6$), and sham (craniotomy without FPI) without stimulation ($n = 5$). All rats were tethered via their skulls to a stimulation device, but the devices for the sham and FPI minus VNS groups were inactive, ensuring the assessors were blind to the treatment group allocation. VNS was then initiated at either 2 h or 24 h post-FPI and given at 30-min intervals for 48 h. The rats underwent a beam walk test and were then sacrificed so that sections of brain tissues could be weighed before and after dehydration to determine water content as a measure of oedema [15]. A reduced level of oedema at the cerebral cortex ipsilateral to FPI was found in the VNS group compared to the FPI-only group ($p < 0.04$). Reductions in brain oedema were significantly correlated with improved beam walk performance at 2 days post-FPI ($p < 0.039$). Taking these two observations together, the authors hypothesised that oedema reduction is one mechanism by which VNS may improve motor recovery post TBI.

Additional evidence for anti-oedema effects of VNS comes from a study by Zhou et al. in 28 rabbits following explosion-induced TBI [19]. The animals were divided into four groups: blank control ($n = 4$), sham surgery (craniotomy and vagus nerve implantation but no TBI) ($n = 6$), explosive injury without VNS ($n = 10$) and explosive injury with VNS ($n = 8$). In that study, VNS was administered 1 h post-TBI and serum and brain tissue were collected 24 h later to assess oedema and cytokine levels. Histological examination of brain tissue demonstrated that oedema was reduced in rabbits that received VNS post TBI compared to TBI alone [19].

Biochemical Changes Following VNS Post TBI

In the same study by Zhou et al., pro- and anti-inflammatory cytokines in serum and brain tissue were measured using enzyme-linked immunosorbent assays (ELISA). Pro-inflammatory TNF-α and IL-1β levels were significantly lower in the VNS group than in the TBI-only group in both serum and brain tissue ($p < 0.01$). Furthermore, VNS increased the levels of the anti-inflammatory cytokine IL-10 in serum and brain tissue compared to the TBI-only group ($p < 0.01$). On further analysis, both TNF-α and IL-1β levels in the brain were strongly associated with brain water content at 24 h post-TBI. This suggests that VNS may attenuate oedema formation through lowering levels of TNF-α and IL-1β and increasing levels of IL-10 (19).

Another study also measured serum and tissue levels of TNF-α post-TBI [16]. Bansal et al. divided 40 mice into Five groups: Sham surgery (right cervical neck incision and vagus nerve exposure only) (n = 8), TBI without VNS (n = 8), TBI with VNS (n = 8), TBI with ghrelin injections and no VNS (n = 8), and TBI with ghrelin injections and VNS. In mice stimulated with VNS prior to weight drop TBI attenuated oedema formation was seen [16]. These "pre-conditioned" animals also demonstrated no increase in brain TNF-α following TBI unlike those that received TBI without prior VNS [16].

Ghrelin, a hormone with anti-inflammatory properties has also been studied as a possible mechanism behind beneficial effects of VNS post TBI. Ghrelin is responsible for multiple physiological and biological functions to maintain homeostasis (e.g. appetite, gut motility, gastric acid balance) [32]. In one study ghrelin was elevated in plasma 2 h following TBI in mice who had received VNS immediately prior to TBI and levels returned to those in TBI-only mice by 6 h post-TBI [16]. Vagotomy performed prior to preconditioning with VNS abolished the increased levels of ghrelin, providing further evidence that VNS up-regulates ghrelin [16].

Effects of VNS on Blood Brain Barrier

A study by Lopez et al. investigated the effects of "preconditioning" with VNS on blood brain barrier breakdown following TBI [17]. In their study of 12 mice, 4 mice underwent weight drop-induced TBI alone, 4 mice received VNS for 10-minutes prior to TBI, and 4 mice underwent sham injury without VNS. Vascular permeability was measured using a fluorescent permeability tracer and mice preconditioned with VNS had significantly reduced vascular permeability compared to those who received TBI-only ($p < 0.05$) Upon histological examination of brain tissue 200 μm medial to the injury site, the preconditioned mice had a decrease in vacuolization (an indicator of oedema) compared to those who had not received VNS [17]. Aquaphorins (AQP) are water channel proteins with AQP-4 being the predominant subtype found in brain [33]. Following TBI, AQP-4 upregulation is found at the site of injury, leading to oedema formation [34]. AQP-4 levels in mice who were preconditioned with VNS prior to TBI remained similar to those in mice who received sham injury [17]. Taken together, these findings raise the hypothesis that VNS initiate biochemical changes, possibly involving AQP-4 to alter vascular permeability which may improve outcomes following TBI.

Challenges with Translating VNS Studies to Humans Post-TBI

Whilst there is evidence from the aforementioned studies that VNS may be both neuro-protective and boost neuroplasticity in animal models of TBI, the optimum VNS stimulation settings to achieve these beneficial effects e.g. pulse width, frequency, intensity, duty cycle, duration of stimulation or number of doses per day, are still unknown. Another area of uncertainty is the therapeutic window for VNS post TBI. Although VNS has been given both before and after TBI in animal models, this may not accurately represent the timescale for treating TBI in humans. Another potential barrier to translation is that some animal studies stimulated the right vagus nerve [16, 17, 19], which is generally avoided in humans as the right vagus nerve carries efferent fibres to the heart. Transient changes in heart rate, blood pressure, and cerebral blood flow have been found in response to stimulation of the right vagus nerve in rodent models of stroke [35, 36] further contributing to fears that right sided stimulation in humans might induce cardiac side effects and potentially be unsafe. Whilst such concerns remain, it is likely that human trials of VNS will need to stimulate on the left side. To our knowledge, no studies have compared efficacy of left versus right sided VNS in either humans or animals.

A further consideration is that studies in animals have tended to observe effects of VNS for up to 3 weeks following TBI i.e. persistence of beneficial effects of VNS in the longer term is unclear. Additionally, VNS was generally administered up to 24 h after injury in the animal studies such that the effects of more delayed VNS are unknown. Since brain injuries in humans can go unrecognised for days or even longer, this is an important question to be addressed. Other unanswered questions include the influence of age and gender on the effects of VNS post TBI. It is known, for example, that oestrogen has neuro-protective properties and in humans treated with VNS for epilepsy, seizure reduction is greater in younger age groups [37]. Nevertheless, age and gender influences on the effects of VNS have not been rigorously studied in animals with TBI.

Human Studies of VNS Post TBI

It is not ethically possible to test the effects of VNS "preconditioning" on TBI outcomes in humans, and studies involving delivery of VNS within 2 h of TBI might be difficult to recruit due to the narrow time intervals involved. However, several human studies have determined the effects of VNS on modification of symptoms and long term complications of TBI. One study, for example, investigated the effects of VNS on post-traumatic epilepsy (PTE) from the VNS Therapy Patient Outcome Registry [31]. Amongst 317 PTE patients and 1763 non-posttraumatic epilepsy (non-PTE) patients, those with PTE patients responded better to VNS [31]. Specifically, the median reduction in seizure frequency was higher in PTE than non-PTE patients following 24 months of VNS treatment (PTE = 73%, non-PTE = 57% reduction, $p = 0.15$). Furthermore, 78% of PTE patients had a ≥50% reduction in seizure frequency after 24 months of treatment, whereas only 61% of non-PTE patients achieved this target ($p = 0.02$).

Interestingly, the vagus nerve can now be stimulated noninvasively –either via the auricular branch, which supplies the concha of the outer ear, or via the cervical branch stimulated transcutaneously at the neck. Several commercially available devices are now available to treat patients in this way and trials have shown beneficial effects in treatment of conditions such as: epilepsy [38–41], migraine [42–45], depression [46, 47], and tinnitus [48–51], all of which are common complications of TBI. Non-invasive VNS activates similar regions of the brain to invasive VNS [52, 53] and may therefore provide an alternative to invasive VNS in the future.

Review of Other Electroceuticals Traumatic Brain Injury (TBI)

Other brain stimulation techniques have shown promise in the treatment of traumatic brain injury. For example, Transcranial magnetic stimulation (TMS), Transcranial direct cortical stimulation (tDCS) and Deep Brain Stimulation (DBS) have been evaluated in animal models and in human case series. Each of these three electroceutical techniques will be discussed in the next section along with a summary of available evidence supporting their role in TBI.

Transcranial Magnetic Stimulation (TMS)

In TMS, an electrical current is passed through a copper coil, inducing a small magnetic field. The coil is passed over the scalp and the current depolarizes neurons at the axon hillock or indirectly via inter-neurons. When applied as single pulses, TMS can be used to measure parameters which reflect cortical excitability such as motor threshold (MT), motor evoked potential (MEP), and silent period (SP) duration [54]. These parameters change in the months following TBI in conjunction with clinical recovery [55] and therefore "single-pulse" TMS be useful to record surrogate outcomes in future trials of potential TBI therapies.

When TMS is used repeatedly over weeks or months, it can also have therapeutic effects [56]. For example, so-called "repetitive TMS (rTMS) was used in a trial of 24 veterans with headache persisting for more than 3 months following TBI. In that trial, 12 veterans were given 2000 pulses of TMS at 10 Hz frequency (3 study treatments within 1 week) and 12 were given sham TMS. At one-week follow-up, 58% of those in the TMS treated group achieved a >50% reduction in headache frequency compared to only 17% of those given sham TMS ($P = 0.04$) [57]. In another study in rats, the delivery of 10 Hz repetitive TMS (rTMS) per day for 14 days post TBI resulted in increased success in a pellet-reaching task compared to sham stimulation and this was accompanied by an increase c-fos protein expression (a marker of neuronal activity) in the cerebral cortex [58]. However the "optimum" stimulation settings for rTMS remain unclear as dose finding studies have not yet been performed [59].

There are several case reports of rTMS having been used to treat sequelae of TBI such as auditory hallucinations, tinnitus and visuo-spatial inattention. [60–64] There has also been one sham-controlled treatment trial of rTMS in depression post TBI in which ex-military personnel were given either 3 days of high dose, high frequency rTMS over the left DLPFC or sham rTMS. Although small in size, that trial showed a rapid "anti-suicide" effect in those given rTMS [65].

Another potentially useful property of rTMS is that the generated electric field can either increase or decrease cortical excitability depending on the frequency of stimulation used. For example, high frequencies tend to increase cortical excitability whereas low frequencies decrease it. This is particularly relevant in the context of TBI where the unaffected hemisphere may become "hyper-excitable" due to a lack of inhibition by the damaged hemisphere [66]. A commonly used regime is low frequency (1 Hz) TMS to the dorsolateral prefrontal cortex (DLPFC) followed by high frequency (10 Hz) TMS to the contralateral DLPFC [67]. Such "sequential bilateral" rTMS has been found to be superior to standard unilateral high-frequency left sided rTMS in the treatment of patients with major depression [67] and may in future be shown to be useful in patients with depression secondary to TBI [68].

A further advantage is that rTMS may lead to changes in the cortex and a "pro-plasticity state". A meta-analysis of 18 studies (392 patients) of rTMS given to patients with limb weakness who were at various time intervals post stroke found an effect size 0.55 for the motor outcome (95% CI, 0.37–0.72) in favour of treatment with VNS [69]. However, only seven studies in that meta-analysis performed follow-up assessments and no study followed up for more than 1 year [69]. Thus it remains unclear whether the effects of rTMS on motor recovery are sustained in the longer term. Whilst similar studies in motor recovery have not yet been performed in humans with deficit post TBI, the cortical reorganisation which occurs following recovery from TBI is similar to that following stroke, and so rTMS may similarly be helpful in post TBI recovery.

The most serious side effect of TMS is inducement epileptic seizures. To minimise this risk, patients with focal frontal lesions, subdural haematomas, previous surgery for clot evacuation, TBI within 3 months or a history of seizures are often excluded from human trials of rTMS. However, whilst likely leading to improved safety outcomes in trials, such exclusions will inevitably limit the clinical application of rTMS post TBI.

Deep Brain Stimulation

Deep brain stimulation (DBS) was introduced in 1987 as a therapy for a number of neurological disorders. DBS involves implantation of a stimulator unit into the chest wall which is then connected by a wire to electrodes which are strategically placed into specific regions of the brain depending on the symptom/disease being treated. For example, electrodes may be implanted into the ventromedial thalamus to treat essential tremor, into the globus pallidus to treat symptoms of Parkinson's disease, or into the nucleus accumbens to treat depression/obsessive compulsive disorder. The mechanisms of action are considered to be a combination of depolarisation blockade and synaptic inhibition [70].

In the context of TBI, studies have shown increased arousal in minimally conscious patients e.g. 8/21 emerged from persistent vegetative state when DBS was applied [71]. There have also been reports of DBS having been used to treat tremor, hemi-dystonia [72, 73] (commonly found in patients with injuries to the basal ganglia and thalamus) and parkinsonism [74] post TBI. However, randomised controlled trials are lacking and are hampered by heterogeneity of functional and anatomical deficits and ethical boundaries of undertaking such studies.

Direct Cortical Stimulation

Transcranial direct current stimulation (tDCS) involves attaching one electrode to a specific place on the scalp which then transmits a weak but direct current to an electrode placed on the contralateral side of the head or on the chin. Cortex excitability is either increased or decreased depending on the distance from each electrode. For example, the cortex near the "cathode" experiences reduced excitability and the area near the "anode" experiences increased excitability (a shift of neuro-membrane potentials towards depolarisation) [75, 76]. Thus depending on the positioning of the electrodes in relation to the precise site of brain injury, either of these cortical effects can be harnessed at appropriate time-points after TBI for therapeutic gain [77]. For example, "cathodal" stimulation may be useful in the acute phase to suppress glutamate whereas "anodal" stimulation may be useful in the sub-acute phase to counteract the GABA-ergic effects.

There is evidence from studies in other neurological diseases e.g. Parkinson's disease and stroke, that tDCS can boost neuroplasticity thereby enabling improvements in motor function [78–80]. There is also evidence that tDCS can be used to treat symptoms that commonly occur post TBI e.g. pain [81], gait disorder [82], aphasia [80], depression [76], and attention/working memory deficits [83, 84] although studies in patients following TBI specifically, are lacking.

There have been no reports of seizures following administration of tDCS [85] and it is therefore considered safer than rTMS in the context of TBI. Indeed tDCS may have anti-seizure effects as cathodal DCS has been used to successfully treat refractory epilepsy in a paediatric patient [86].

Summary

There is mounting evidence from animal models and from smaller studies and from case series in humans to suggest a role for VNS, TMS, tDCS, and DBS in the recovery from TBI, e.g. for the relief of symptoms such as headache, and memory deficits, for improving consciousness and for the promotion of neuroplasticity to assist in recovery of neurological function. However, large randomised placebo controlled studies in humans are lacking. There are also significant challenges in translating results from animal studies to humans with TBI. Further research is required to understand how variations in individual stimulation settings (such as frequency and intensity), and the timings and frequency of delivery post TBI may influence the effects of electroceutical treatments. Furthermore, the effects of age and sex on the effects of electromodulation post TBI requires further study.

References

1. NIH Consensus Development Panel on Rehabilitation of Persons With Traumatic Brain Injury. Consensus conference. Rehabilitation of persons with traumatic brain injury. JAMA. 1999;282(10):974–83.
2. Langlois JA, Rutland-Brown W, Wald MM. The epidemiology and impact of traumatic brain injury: a brief overview. J Head Trauma Rehabil. 2006;21(5):375–8.
3. Hyder AA, Wunderlich CA, Puvanachandra P, Gururaj G, Kobusingye OC. The impact of traumatic brain injuries: a global perspective. NeuroRehabilitation. 2007;22(5):341–53.
4. Faul M, Xu L, Wald MM CV. Traumatic brain injury in the United States: emergency department visits, hospitalizations, and deaths. Centers for Disease Control and Prevention, National Center for Injury Prevention and Control. 2010. p. 891–904.
5. Carroll L, Cassidy JD, Peloso P, Borg J, von Holst H, Holm L, et al. Prognosis for mild traumatic brain injury: results of the who collaborating centre task force on mild traumatic brain injury. J Rehabil Med. 2004;36(0):84–105.
6. Bazarian JJ, Cernak I, Noble-Haeusslein L, Potolicchio S, Temkin N. Long-term neurologic outcomes after traumatic brain injury. J Head Trauma Rehabil. 2009;24(6):439–51.
7. Irimia A, Goh S-YM, Torgerson CM, Stein NR, Chambers MC, Vespa PM, et al. Electroencephalographic inverse localization of brain activity in acute traumatic brain injury as a guide to surgery, monitoring and treatment. Clin Neurol Neurosurg. 2013;115(10): 2159–65.
8. Taylor A, Butt W, Rosenfeld J, Shann F, Ditchfield M, Lewis E, et al. A randomized trial of very early decompressive craniectomy in children with traumatic brain injury and sustained intracranial hypertension. Childs Nerv Syst. 2001;17(3):154–62.
9. Huang AP-H, Tu Y-K, Tsai Y-H, Chen Y-S, Hong W-C, Yang C-C, et al. Decompressive craniectomy as the primary surgical intervention for hemorrhagic contusion. J Neurotrauma. 2008;25(11):1347–54.
10. Chauhan NB, Gatto R, Chauhan MB. Neuroanatomical correlation of behavioral deficits in the CCI model of TBI. J Neurosci Methods. 2010;190(1):1–9.
11. Elliott M, Parente F. Efficacy of memory rehabilitation therapy: a meta-analysis of TBI and stroke cognitive rehabilitation literature. Brain Inj. 2014;9052(12):1–7.
12. Smith DC, Modglin AA, Roosevelt RW, Neese SL, Jensen RA, Browning RA, et al. Electrical stimulation of the vagus nerve enhances cognitive and motor recovery following moderate fluid percussion injury in the rat. J Neurotrauma. 2005;22(12):1485–502.
13. Smith DC, Tan AA, Duke A, Neese SL, Clough RW, Browning RA, et al. Recovery of function after vagus nerve stimulation initiated 24 hours after fluid percussion brain injury. J Neurotrauma. 2006;23(10):1549–60.
14. Neese SL, Sherill LK, Tan AA, Roosevelt RW, Browning RA, Smith DC, et al. Vagus nerve stimulation may protect GABAergic neurons following traumatic brain injury in rats: An immunocytochemical study. Brain Res. 2007;1128(1):157–63.
15. Clough RW, Neese SL, Sherill LK, Tan AA, Duke A, Roosevelt RW, et al. Cortical edema in moderate fluid percussion brain injury is attenuated by vagus nerve stimulation. Neuroscience. 2007;147(2):286–93.
16. Bansal V, Ryu SY, Lopez N, Allexan S, Krzyzaniak M, Eliceiri B, et al. Vagal stimulation modulates inflammation through a ghrelin mediated mechanism in traumatic brain injury. Inflammation. 2012;35(1):214–20.
17. Lopez NE, Krzyzaniak MJ, Costantini TW, Putnam J, Hageny A-M, Eliceiri B, et al. Vagal nerve stimulation decreases blood-brain barrier disruption after traumatic brain injury. J Trauma Acute Care Surg. 2012;72(6):1562–6.
18. Pruitt DT, Schmid AN, Kim LJ, Abe CM, Trieu JL, Choua C, et al. Vagus nerve stimulation delivered with motor training enhances recovery of function after traumatic brain injury. J Neurotrauma. 2016;33(9):871–9.

19. Zhou L, Lin J, Lin J, Kui G, Zhang J, Yu Y. Neuroprotective effects of vagus nerve stimulation on traumatic brain injury. Neural Regen Res. 2014;9(17):1585–91.
20. Chambers A, Bowen JM. Electrical stimulation for drug-resistant epilepsy: an evidence-based analysis. Ont Health Technol Assess Ser. 2013;13(18):1–37.
21. Shi C, Flanagan SR, Samadani U. Vagus nerve stimulation to augment recovery from severe traumatic brain injury impeding consciousness: a prospective pilot clinical trial. Neurol Res. 2013;35(3):263–76.
22. Cheyuo C, Jacob A, Wu R, Zhou M, Coppa GF, Wang P. The parasympathetic nervous system in the quest for stroke therapeutics. J Cereb Blood Flow Metab. 2011;31(5):1187–95.
23. Fornai F, Ruffoli R, Giorgi FS, Paparelli A. The role of locus coeruleus in the antiepileptic activity induced by vagus nerve stimulation. Eur J Neurosci. 2011;33(12):2169–78.
24. Masuda T, Nakagawa S, Boku S, Nishikawa H, Takamura N, Kato A, et al. Noradrenaline increases neural precursor cells derived from adult rat dentate gyrus through β2 receptor. Prog Neuropsychopharmacol Biol Psychiatry. 2012;36(1):44–51.
25. Young SZ, Taylor MM, Bordey A. Neurotransmitters couple brain activity to subventricular zone neurogenesis. Eur J Neurosci. 2011;33(6):1123–32.
26. Kamei J, Igarashi H, Kasuya Y. Modulation by serotonin of glutamate-induced lethality in mice. Res Commun Chem Pathol Pharmacol. 1991;74(2):167–84.
27. Neuman RS, Thompson PM. Serotonin mediates suppression of focal epileptiform activity induced by noxious stimulation. Epilepsia. 1989;30(3):307–13.
28. Wehrwein E, Thompson SA, Coulibaly SF, Linn DM, Linn CL. Acetylcholine protection of adult pig retinal ganglion cells from glutamate-induced excitotoxicity. Invest Ophthalmol Vis Sci. 2004;45(5):1531–43.
29. Giuliani D, Ottani A, Altavilla D, Bazzani C, Squadrito F, Guarini S. Melanocortins and the cholinergic anti-inflammatory pathway. Adv Exp Med Biol. 2010;681:71–87.
30. Fraser PA. The role of free radical generation in increasing cerebrovascular permeability. Free Radic Biol Med. 2011;51(5):967–77.
31. Englot DJ, Rolston JD, Wang DD, Hassnain KH, Gordon CM, Chang EF. Efficacy of vagus nerve stimulation in posttraumatic versus nontraumatic epilepsy. J Neurosurg. 2012; 117(5):970–7.
32. Eissa N, Ghia JE. Immunomodulatory effect of ghrelin in the intestinal mucosa. Neurogastroenterol Motil. 2015;27(11):1519–27.
33. Neely JD, Christensen BM, Nielsen S, Agre P. Heterotetrameric composition of aquaporin-4 water channels. Biochemistry. 1999;38(34):11156–63.
34. Sun M-C, Honey CR, Berk C, Wong NLM, Tsui JKC. Regulation of aquaporin-4 in a traumatic brain injury model in rats. J Neurosurg. 2003;98(3):565–9.
35. Ay I, Lu J, Ay H, Gregory SA. Vagus nerve stimulation reduces infarct size in rat focal cerebral ischemia. Neurosci Lett. 2009;459(3):147–51.
36. Ay I, Sorensen AG, Ay H. Vagus nerve stimulation reduces infarct size in rat focal cerebral ischemia: an unlikely role for cerebral blood flow. Brain Res. 2011;1392:110–5.
37. Englot DJ, Chang EF, Auguste KI. Efficacy of vagus nerve stimulation for epilepsy by patient age, epilepsy duration, and seizure type. Neurosurg Clin N Am. 2011;22(4):443–8. v
38. Stefan H, Kreiselmeyer G, Kerling F, Kurzbuch K, Rauch C, Heers M, et al. Transcutaneous vagus nerve stimulation (t-VNS) in pharmacoresistant epilepsies: a proof of concept trial. Epilepsia. 2012;53(7):e115–8.
39. He W, Jing X, Wang X, Rong P, Li L, Shi H, et al. Transcutaneous auricular vagus nerve stimulation as a complementary therapy for pediatric epilepsy: a pilot trial. Epilepsy Behav. 2013;28(3):343–6.
40. Rong P, Liu A, Zhang J, Wang Y, Yang A, Li L, et al. An alternative therapy for drug-resistant epilepsy: transcutaneous auricular vagus nerve stimulation. Chin Med J (Engl). 2014;127(2):300–4.
41. Aihua L, Lu S, Liping L, Xiuru W, Hua L, Yuping W. A controlled trial of transcutaneous vagus nerve stimulation for the treatment of pharmacoresistant epilepsy. Epilepsy Behav. 2014;39:105–10.

42. Goadsby PJ, Grosberg BM, Mauskop A, Cady R, Simmons KA. Effect of noninvasive vagus nerve stimulation on acute migraine: an open-label pilot study. Cephalalgia. 2014;34(12):986–93.
43. Grazzi L, Padovan A, Barbanti P. Role of neurostimulation in migraine. Neurol Sci. 2015;36 Suppl 1(S1):121–3.
44. Barbanti P, Grazzi L, Egeo G, Padovan AM, Liebler E, Bussone G. Non-invasive vagus nerve stimulation for acute treatment of high-frequency and chronic migraine: an open-label study. J Headache Pain. 2015;16(1):61.
45. Straube A, Ellrich J, Eren O, Blum B, Ruscheweyh R. Treatment of chronic migraine with transcutaneous stimulation of the auricular branch of the vagal nerve (auricular t-VNS): a randomized, monocentric clinical trial. J Headache Pain. 2015;16(1):543.
46. Hein E, Nowak M, Kiess O, Biermann T, Bayerlein K, Kornhuber J, et al. Auricular transcutaneous electrical nerve stimulation in depressed patients: a randomized controlled pilot study. J Neural Transm. 2013;120(5):821–7.
47. Fang J, Rong P, Hong Y, Fan Y, Liu J, Wang H, et al. Transcutaneous vagus nerve stimulation modulates default mode network in major depressive disorder. Biol Psychiatry. 2016;79(4):266–73.
48. Kreuzer PM, Landgrebe M, Husser O, Resch M, Schecklmann M, Geisreiter F, et al. Transcutaneous vagus nerve stimulation: retrospective assessment of cardiac safety in a pilot study. Front Psych. 2012;3:70.
49. Kreuzer PM, Landgrebe M, Resch M, Husser O, Schecklmann M, Geisreiter F, et al. Feasibility, safety and efficacy of transcutaneous vagus nerve stimulation in chronic tinnitus: an open pilot study. Brain Stimul. 2014;7(5):740–7.
50. Lehtimäki J, Hyvärinen P, Ylikoski M, Bergholm M, Mäkelä JP, Aarnisalo A, et al. Transcutaneous vagus nerve stimulation in tinnitus: a pilot study. Acta Otolaryngol. 2013;133(4):378–82.
51. Hyvärinen P, Yrttiaho S, Lehtimäki J, Ilmoniemi RJ, Mäkitie A, Ylikoski J, et al. Transcutaneous vagus nerve stimulation modulates tinnitus-related beta- and gamma-band activity. Ear Hear. 2014;36(3):e76–85.
52. Dietrich S, Smith J, Scherzinger C, Hofmann-Preiss K, Freitag T, Eisenkolb A, et al. A novel transcutaneous vagus nerve stimulation leads to brainstem and cerebral activations measured by functional MRI. Biomed Tech (Berl). 2008;53(3):104–111.
53. Frangos E, Ellrich J, Komisaruk BR. Non-invasive access to the vagus nerve central projections via electrical stimulation of the external ear: fMRI evidence in humans. Brain Stimul. 2015;8(3):624–36.
54. Kobayashi M, Pascual-Leone A. Transcranial magnetic stimulation in neurology. Lancet Neurol. 2003;2(3):145–56.
55. Chistyakov AV, Soustiel JF, Hafner H, Elron M, Feinsod M. Altered excitability of the motor cortex after minor head injury revealed by transcranial magnetic stimulation. Acta Neurochir. 1998;140(5):467–72.
56. Lefaucheur J. Methods of therapeutic cortical stimulation. Neurophysiol Clin. 2009;39(1):1–14.
57. Leung A, Shukla S, Fallah A, Song D, Lin L, Golshan S, et al. Repetitive transcranial magnetic stimulation in managing mild traumatic brain injury-related headaches. Neuromodulation. 2016;19(2):133–41.
58. Yoon MS, Han J, Tse WW, Rogers R. Effects of vagal stimulation, atropine, and propranolol on fibrillation threshold of normal and ischemic ventricles. Am Heart J. 1977;93(1):60–5.
59. Hiscock A, Miller S, Rothwell J, Tallis RC, Pomeroy VM. Informing dose-finding studies of repetitive transcranial magnetic stimulation to enhance motor function: a qualitative systematic review. Neurorehabil Neural Repair. 2008;22(3):228–49.
60. Cosentino G, Giglia G, Palermo A, Panetta ML, Lo Baido R, Brighina F, et al. A case of post-traumatic complex auditory hallucinosis treated with rTMS. Neurocase. 2010;16(3):267–72.
61. Cavinato M, Iaia V, Piccione F. Repeated sessions of sub-threshold 20-Hz rTMS. Potential cumulative effects in a brain-injured patient. Clin Neurophysiol. 2012;123(9):1893–5.

62. Bonni S, Mastropasqua C, Bozzali M, Caltagirone C, Koch G. Theta burst stimulation improves visuo-spatial attention in a patient with traumatic brain injury. Neurol Sci. 2013;34(11):2053–6.
63. Kreuzer PM, Landgrebe M, Frank E, Langguth B. Repetitive transcranial magnetic stimulation for the treatment of chronic tinnitus after traumatic brain injury: a case study. J Head Trauma Rehabil. 2013;28(5):386–9.
64. Louise-Bender Pape T, Rosenow J, Lewis G, Ahmed G, Walker M, Guernon A, et al. Repetitive transcranial magnetic stimulation-associated neurobehavioral gains during coma recovery. Brain Stimul. 2009;2(1):22–35.
65. George MS, Raman R, Benedek DM, Pelic CG, Grammer GG, Stokes KT, et al. A two-site pilot randomized 3 day trial of high dose left prefrontal repetitive transcranial magnetic stimulation (rTMS) for suicidal inpatients. Brain Stimul. 2014;7(3):421–31.
66. Mori F, Koch G, Foti C, Bernardi G, Centonze D. The use of repetitive transcranial magnetic stimulation (rTMS) for the treatment of spasticity. Prog Brain Res. 2009;175:429–39.
67. Fitzgerald PB, Hoy KE, Herring SE, McQueen S, Peachey AVJ, Segrave RA, et al. A double blind randomized trial of unilateral left and bilateral prefrontal cortex transcranial magnetic stimulation in treatment resistant major depression. J Affect Disord. 2012;139(2):193–8.
68. Fitzgerald PB, Hoy KE, Maller JJ, Herring S, Segrave R, McQueen S, et al. Transcranial magnetic stimulation for depression after a traumatic brain injury: a case study. J ECT. 2011;27(1):38–40.
69. Hsu W-Y, Cheng C-H, Liao K-K, Lee I-H, Lin Y-Y. Effects of repetitive transcranial magnetic stimulation on motor functions in patients with stroke: a meta-analysis. Stroke. 2012;43(7):1849–57.
70. McIntyre CC, Savasta M, Kerkerian-Le Goff L, Vitek JL. Uncovering the mechanism(s) of action of deep brain stimulation: activation, inhibition, or both. Clin Neurophysiol. 2004;115(6):1239–48.
71. Yamamoto T, Katayama Y, Kobayashi K, Oshima H, Fukaya C, Tsubokawa T. Deep brain stimulation for the treatment of vegetative state. Eur J Neurosci. 2010;32(7):1145–51.
72. Sellal F, Hirsch E, Barth P, Blond S, Marescaux C. A case of symptomatic hemidystonia improved by ventroposterolateral thalamic electrostimulation. Mov Disord. 1993;8(4):515–8.
73. Kim JP, Chang WS, Chang JW. The long-term surgical outcomes of secondary hemidystonia associated with post-traumatic brain injury. Acta Neurochir. 2012;154(5):823–30.
74. Shahaduzzaman M, Acosta S, Bickford PC, Borlongan CV. α-Synuclein is a pathological link and therapeutic target for Parkinson's disease and traumatic brain injury. Med Hypotheses. 2013;81(4):675–80.
75. Nitsche MA, Paulus W. Excitability changes induced in the human motor cortex by weak transcranial direct current stimulation. J Physiol. 2000;527 Pt 3:633–9.
76. Nitsche MA, Boggio PS, Fregni F, Pascual-Leone A. Treatment of depression with transcranial direct current stimulation (tDCS): a review. Exp Neurol. 2009;219(1):14–9.
77. Vahedi K, Hofmeijer J, Juettler E, Vicaut E, George B, Algra A, et al. Early decompressive surgery in malignant infarction of the middle cerebral artery: a pooled analysis of three randomised controlled trials. Lancet Neurol. 2007;6(3):215–22.
78. Fregni F, Boggio PS, Santos MC, Lima M, Vieira AL, Rigonatti SP, et al. Noninvasive cortical stimulation with transcranial direct current stimulation in Parkinson's disease. Mov Disord. 2006;21(10):1693–702.
79. Boggio PS, Nunes A, Rigonatti SP, Nitsche MA, Pascual-Leone A, Fregni F. Repeated sessions of noninvasive brain DC stimulation is associated with motor function improvement in stroke patients. Restor Neurol Neurosci. 2007;25(2):123–9.
80. Monti A, Cogiamanian F, Marceglia S, Ferrucci R, Mameli F, Mrakic-Sposta S, et al. Improved naming after transcranial direct current stimulation in aphasia. J Neurol Neurosurg Psychiatry. 2008;79(4):451–3.
81. Fregni F, Boggio PS, Lima MC, Ferreira MJL, Wagner T, Rigonatti SP, et al. A sham-controlled, phase II trial of transcranial direct current stimulation for the treatment of central pain in traumatic spinal cord injury. Pain. 2006;122(1–2):197–209.

82. Madhavan S, Weber KA, Stinear JW. Non-invasive brain stimulation enhances fine motor control of the hemiparetic ankle: implications for rehabilitation. Exp Brain Res. 2011;209(1): 9–17.
83. Ulam F, Shelton C, Richards L, Davis L, Hunter B, Fregni F, et al. Cumulative effects of transcranial direct current stimulation on EEG oscillations and attention/working memory during subacute neurorehabilitation of traumatic brain injury. Clin Neurophysiol. 2015;126(3): 486–96.
84. Kang E-K, Kim D-Y, Paik N-J. Transcranial direct current stimulation of the left prefrontal cortex improves attention in patients with traumatic brain injury: a pilot study. J Rehabil Med. 2012;44(4):346–50.
85. Iyer MB, Mattu U, Grafman J, Lomarev M, Sato S, Wassermann EM. Safety and cognitive effect of frontal DC brain polarization in healthy individuals. Neurology. 2005;64(5):872–5.
86. Yook S-W, Park S-H, Seo J-H, Kim S-J, Ko M-H. Suppression of seizure by cathodal transcranial direct current stimulation in an epileptic patient – a case report. Ann Rehabil Med. 2011;35(4):579–82.

Chapter 4
Deep Brain Stimulation for Movement Disorders Other than Parkinson's Disease

Monty Silverdale

Abstract As well as being an effective treatment for well selected Parkinson's disease patients, Deep Brain Stimulation (DBS) is also a beneficial treatment for Movement Disorders other than Parkinson's disease. In the treatment of dystonia, the most common target is the internal globus pallidus (GPi). Focal and generalised primary dystonia will often respond extremely well to bilateral GPi DBS. More modest improvements can be seen in the management of secondary dystonia. In the treatment of Essential Tremor, the usual target is either the ventral intermediate nucleus of the thalamus (VIM) or the zona incerta (ZI). Bilateral VIM or ZI DBS is often a very effective treatment for Essential Tremor and other tremor syndromes. DBS is sometimes used to treat Tourette syndrome, chorea, myoclonus and tardive syndromes. Impressive results are often seen in these other conditions, although further research is needed to clarify which patients will benefit. DBS does not improve patients with Parkinson Plus disorders.

Keywords Deep brain stimulation • Dystonia • Chorea • Tremor • Tourette syndrome • Tics • Myoclonus • Tardive dyskinesia

Introduction

Movement Disorders are a group of neurological conditions, which impair the control of movement. Hypokinetic disorders are associated with a pathological reduction in movement whereas hyperkinetic disorders are associated with a pathological increase in movement.

Parkinson's disease is the most common hypokinetic Movement Disorder. The main clinical features of Parkinson's disease are resting tremor, rigidity (stiffness)

M. Silverdale, MD, PhD
Salford Royal NHS Foundation Trust, Department of Neurology,
Stott Lane, Salford, Greater Manchester, UK
e-mail: Monty.silverdale@srft.nhs.uk

A. Majid (ed.), *Electroceuticals*, DOI 10.1007/978-3-319-28612-9_4

and bradykinesia (slowness of movement). Deep Brain Stimulation has been used in the treatment of Parkinson's disease for some years now and can be a very effective treatment for many patients [1].

Parkinson Plus disorders may present in a similar fashion to Parkinson's disease with tremor, rigidity and bradykinesia (although classical parkinsonian resting tremor is rare in Parkinson Plus disorders). However Parkinson Plus disorders do not usually respond well to levodopa or other antiparkinsonian therapies and they tend to progress much more quickly and relentlessly than Parkinson's disease. Parkinson Plus disorders include Progressive Supranuclear Palsy (PSP), Multiple System Atrophy (MSA) and Corticobasal Degeneration (CBD) [2–4].

Hyperkinetic movement disorders are conditions associated with excess involuntary movements that often interfere with normal movements. There are several different types of hyperkinetic movement disorder which can usually be distinguished by clinical assessment: in chorea, the involuntary movements are random in nature; in dystonia the movements are patterned; in tremor, the movements are rhythmic; in myoclonus the movements are very brief; in tics, the movements are suppressible and associated with an underlying urge sensation.

This chapter will discuss the role of Deep Brain Stimulation (DBS) in the management of movement disorders other than Parkinson's disease. The data are summarised in Table 4.1.

The History of DBS

In 1908 Horsley and Clarke developed a device which could make anatomically defined lesions in the brain of a monkey [38]. The device used a 3-dimensional coordinate system and was thus the first stereotactic device. The development of stereotactic surgery in humans did not start until 1947 when Spiegel and Wycis developed a similar device that could be used on humans. Stereotactic surgery gradually became very popular and by 1965 around 25,000 stereotactic operations had been used in the treatment of various neurological conditions including movement disorders, pain and epilepsy as well as in the treatment of psychiatric disorders [39].

Stereotactic surgery most commonly involves the use of a stereotactic frame. The frame initial developed by Spiegel and Wycis has been adapted and modified over the years and other frames, including the Leksell frame are also used [40]. An example of the Leksell frame is shown in Fig. 4.1. The Leksell frame uses an arc system, which allows the carrier to move along the arc to any location and still be able to terminate at the desired target. The centre of the arc indicates the desired target. Thus any part of the brain can be accurately targeted by using a specific (x,y,z) coordinate system. Prior to the surgery itself, an image is taken of the patient with the frame in situ. This image can be x ray, CT or MRI. Part of the frame includes markers, called fiducials, that are visible on the imaging. Different types of markers

Table 4.1 DBS for the treatment of movement disorders other than Parkinson's disease

Movement disorder	Specific conditions	Effects of DBS	References
Parkinson plus disorders	PSP, MSA, CBD	Very little benefit from traditional DBS (bilateral STN or GPi DBS). Some interest in the possibility of PPN DBS for PSP although results show modest benefit at best	[5–7]
Dystonia	Primary torsion dystonia	Very good results with bilateral GPi DBS. 50–90% improvement in generalised dystonia. 50–70% improvements with cervical dystonia. Good results with blepharospasm and Meige's syndrome	[8–15]
	Myoclonus dystonia	Encouraging results with GPi and thalamic VIM DBS	[16, 17]
	Secondary dystonia	Bilateral GPi DBS. Less Effective than in the treatment of primary dystonia. Modest improvements (around 25%) in dystonic cerebral palsy. Similar modest improvements in other secondary dystonia syndromes. Very good results with tardive dystonia (50–90% improvement)	[18–21]
Tremor	Essential tremor	Bilateral VIM or bilateral ZI DBS. Excellent results. 50–90% improvement	[22–26]
	Other tremor syndromes	VIM DBS or ZI DBS. Good results for dystonic tremor. Modest efficacy for Holmes Tremor with unilateral VIM DBS. Variable results with MS tremor. Modest efficacy for orthostatic tremor	[27–31]
Tourette syndrome		Modest efficacy of DBS in small studies. Various targets including GPi, GPe and thalamus (centromedian parafascicular nucleus)	[32–34]
Myoclonus		Good results for myoclonus dystonia (bilateral GPi DBS).	[16, 17]
Chorea		Modest efficacy for Huntington's disease (bilateral GPi DBS). GPi and thalamic DBS have shown modest efficacy for hemiballism / hemichorea	[35, 36]
Tardive dyskinesia	Classical tardive dyskinesia	Bilateral GPi DBS – modest efficacy	[37]
	Tardive dystonia	Bilateral GPi DBS – good response	[19, 20]

PSP progressive supranuclear palsy, *MSA* multiple system atrophy, *CBD* corticobasal degeneration, *DBS* deep brain stimulation, *GPi* internal globus pallidus, *STN* subthalamic nucleus, *PPN* pedunculopontine nucleus, *GPe* external globus pallidus, *VIM* ventral intermediate nucleus of thalamus, *ZI* zona incerta

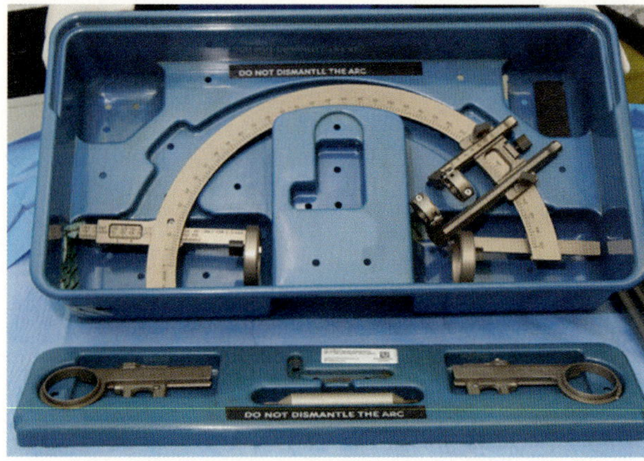

Fig. 4.1 The Leksell frame

are used depending on whether x ray, CT or MRI imaging is to be undertaken. The surgeon can then indicate to the computer software the location of all the fiducials on the image, thus informing the computer software the exact location of the image within the frame. The surgeon then identifies the target on the image and the computer software will calculate the desired (x,y,z) coordinates to use on the frame in order to reach the target [39].

Stereotactic lesioning has been used for many years in the treatment of movement disorders. However a significant drawback of lesioning surgery is that the lesions are irreversible. Thus if a lesion is inaccurately placed or is larger than had been intended then neighbouring structures can be damaged. For example the internal capsule sits very close to both the subthalamic nucleus and the globus pallidus and is potentially damaged during a lesioning procedure leading to hemiparesis. Furthermore the risks of bilateral lesioning procedures are very high such that bilateral lesioning is very rarely undertaken [41].

In the 1950s it was shown that stereotactic high frequency stimulation of the globus pallidus could be used to alleviate tremor when applied to the globus pallidus. Initially this type of high frequency stimulation was used to identify the exact location of the target prior to lesioning surgery [42]. In the 1980s the company Medtronic developed implantable cardiac pacemakers. This led to Benabid and colleagues developing implantable Deep Brain Stimulators as an alternative to lesioning procedures [43, 44]. DBS of a brain region produces a very similar effect to lesioning. However the effect of DBS is reversible such that if side effects are produced, for example due to internal capsule stimulation, then the DBS settings can be altered. DBS is therefore much safer than lesioning and has become the surgical procedure of choice for most movement disorders. Over 100,000 DBS systems have been implanted around the world and lesioning procedures are now fairly rarely performed [45].

Surgical Technique: Getting the Lead to the Target

Initial Surgical Procedure

As detailed in the previous section, most DBS procedures involve the use of a stereotactic frame. All procedures now involve the use of an MRI scan to enable accurate identification of the target structure. Some surgeons perform the MRI during the DBS surgical procedure, using an MRI compatible frame with fiducials that are visible on the MRI scan. Another technique involves performing the MRI scan prior to the surgery. On the day of surgery, after the frame has been attached, a CT scan is performed. The frame has fiducials, which are visible on a CT scanner. The intraoperative CT is then fused with the pre-operative MRI such that the location of the fiducials can now been seen with respect to the MRI image.

Once the computer software has identified the coordinates, the surgeon then drills a hole in the skull and passes the DBS lead to the desired coordinates.

Checking That the Target Location Has Been Reached

There are several different ways in which the surgeon can check that the lead is now lying in the appropriate target structure.

The first method involves microelectrode recording from a lead during the last few millimetres of the approach to target [46]. Signals from the lead are passed to an oscilloscope screen where they can be seen and heard. Typical "firing patterns" have been defined for all the commonly targeted structures, including the "firing patterns" just above the target, the "firing patterns" in the target structure and also the firing patterns just below the target structure. A neurophysiologist is able to therefore determine whether the lead is just above the appropriate target structure, whether the lead is inside the target structure and whether the lead is just below the target structure. Microelectrode recording is an effective way to ensure the correct target structure has been reached, although sometimes involves more than one pass (taking the lead out and putting it back in along a slightly different tract) therefore theoretically may add to the potential risks of the procedure [46].

A second method to determine accurate location of the lead requires waking the patient up during surgery (or performing the whole procedure awake) and testing the lead by switching on the DBS (awake stimulation) [47]. If the operation is being performed for Parkinson's disease or for tremor then one would expect an immediate improvement in symptoms as the lead is switched on. One can also ask the patient about side effects as well as examining the patient looking for the presence of side effects which may indicate that the lead is incorrectly placed or simply that the stimulation parameters are too high. If performing DBS for dystonia one would not expect a beneficial effect during awake stimulation as beneficial effects can take several months, however one can still test for side effects due to inaccurately placed leads. Testing the DBS during surgery is a very effective way to ensure correct lead placement. However some patients find awake surgery very frightening and may be put off the procedure because of worrying about being awake during brain surgery.

A third method to determine accurate location of the lead requires postoperative imaging [48, 49]. There are theoretical concerns regarding the use of MRI imaging in a patient with an implanted DBS system as there are concerns that the lead may heat up in the MRI scanner and cause brain damage at the tip of the lead. Although one or two such cases have been reported [50], a great deal of research has been performed in order to develop guidelines for the safe use of MRI in DBS patients. Fairly strict guidelines are now available, and by following these guidelines several groups have shown that MRI brain scans can be safely undertaken after DBS [48, 51]. Thus a postoperative MRI scan can be used to ensure accuracy of targeting. This method potentially avoids the need for microelectrode recordings or awake stimulation. A similar method involves placing an MRI compatible stylet (cut to the exact dimensions of the DBS lead) down a "guide tube" similar to putting in an IV cannula. The stylet is visible on the MRI scan and therefore can be imaged via MRI entirely safely to check the accuracy of lead location. If the location is accurate the stylet can be removed and the actual lead placed down the guide tube [49].

Once accurate positioning of the lead has been confirmed, the lead is connected to a "pacemaker" battery placed into the chest wall. Subsequently a computer system is able to wirelessly communicate with this pacemaker allowing adjustment of stimulator settings (stimulator programming).

Programming the Deep Brain Stimulator

Timing of Stimulator Programming

Initially placing the DBS lead can sometimes improve symptoms including parkinsonian symptoms and tremor. This "impact effect" is thought to be due to a small lesion caused by the surgery itself. The impact effect often lasts a few weeks and can complicate stimulator programming. Thus most, although not all units, wait a few weeks after surgery before switching on the stimulator so that the effects of stimulation can be assessed without the complicating factor of an impact effect.

The initial programming session takes between about 1 and 3 h depending on the number of parameters the programmer needs to assess. The main aim of the initial programming session is to work out the most effective stimulator settings for that patient.

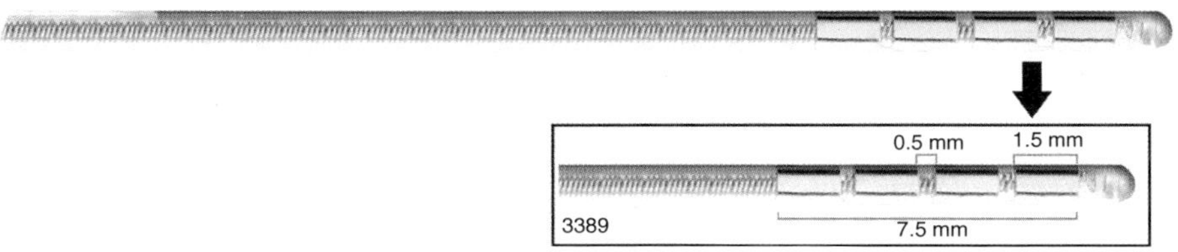

Fig. 4.2 The Medtronic *3389* lead. The lead has four contacts. These contacts are *1.5 mm* long and are spaced a *0.5 mm* intervals. On the left lead, the contacts are labelled from distal to proximal (0, 1, 2, 3) and on the right lead, the contacts are labelled from distal to proximal (8, 9, 10, 11) (© Medtronic Inc.)

Selecting the Best Configuration of Contacts

The most commonly used stimulator system is the Medtronic system, although the Boston and St Jude's system are also frequently used. The Medtronic 3389 lead is commonly used at the time of writing and is shown in Fig. 4.2. The lead has four contacts. These contacts are 1.5 mm long and are spaced a 0.5 mm intervals. On the left lead, the contacts are labelled from distal to proximal (0, 1, 2, 3) and on the right lead, the contacts are labelled from distal to proximal (8, 9, 10, 11). Stimulation is provided through the cathode (i.e. through the negative electrode).

Before programming, the initial step is to check the impedance across all the contacts. Impedance is the term used for resistance to flow of the electric current. The terms resistance and impedance are sometimes used interchangeably. However resistance is not altered by frequency and is the correct term to use for a direct current. Impedance is altered by frequency and is therefore the correct term to use for a varying current. As DBS is a varying current, impedance is the correct term to use.

Usual levels of impedance are between 500 and 2000 Ω. Very low impedance levels may indicate a short circuit somewhere in the DBS system, whereas very high impedance levels may indicate a lead fracture or a problem with one of the contacts.

Following impedance checking, the programmer then checks the stimulator to decide on the best contacts to use. It is important to check all the contacts in a systematic fashion. For example, initially the programmer might start on the left lead and select the case as the positive electrode and contact 0 as the negative electrode. Stimulation is started at a low level and gradually increased observing for any beneficial effects and any side effects. If beneficial effects are seen at a low setting, but side effects do not occur until very high settings then this would represent a "good" contact to use going forwards. Subsequently contacts 1, 2 and 3 would be tried (with case positive) in the same fashion in order to select the best contact. Thus it is possible to move the area of stimulation along the lead, in order to identify the best contact. When assessing certain symptoms such as parkinsonian symptoms and tremor, one expects a beneficial effect a few seconds after a change in settings has been made. However when assessing other symptoms such as dystonia, one would not expect a beneficial effect during stimulator programming as beneficial effects can take many months. Thus when programming a dystonia DBS system, one is reliant on determining which contacts cause side effects and which do not cause side effects to help decide on the best contact to use.

Monopolar stimulation is the term used when using one of the contacts as the negative electrode and the case as the positive electrode. One can also use bipolar stimulation where one of the contacts acts as the negative electrode and one of the other contacts acts as the positive electrode. Bipolar stimulation produces a smaller, more concentrated area of stimulation than monopolar stimulation.

A useful analogy, described by Montgomery, is to think of a round table with a hose pipe connected to a hole in the centre of the table ([52]). The hosepipe is connected from the underneath and projects up onto the table. When the hose is switched on, the whole table becomes covered with water, which pores off the sides. This situation is similar to monopolar stimulation where the cathode sends negatively charged electrons into the tissue and these conduct in all directions through the body and back to the case (anode). If however one drills a fairly large hole in the table separate from the hole that the hose is using, and perhaps applies some suction at this other hole, then the water will come out of the hose, pass towards the other hole, then drain back under the table. There is thus a more concentrated area of water between the hose and the other hole, with the rest of the table remaining fairly dry. This is the situation with bipolar stimulation during which the cathode sends negatively charged electrons into the tissue and these electrons pass directly towards the positive contact, which is acting as the anode. This produces a fairly small intense area of stimulation between the two contacts. Bipolar stimulation can sometimes be a useful technique to reduce side effects in a well-placed lead when the side effects are due to the stimulation conducting too far away from the cathode into a neighbouring brain structure.

Other contact configurations that can be used include using two cathodes (two separate negative contacts producing a fairly large area of stimulation) or tripolar stimulation (a negative contact with a positive contact on either side, producing a very small intense area of stimulation).

Adjusting Stimulator Parameters

In the preceding section I talked about gradually increasing the stimulator parameters, and I will now elaborate on what is meant by that.

Figure 4.3 shows the typical output from a Deep Brain Stimulator. Thus brief pulses of stimulation are applied at a very fast frequency. The pulse width defines the duration of each pulse, the amplitude defines the size of each pulse and the frequency determines how many pulses there are per second. As well as being able to vary the active contacts as detailed in the previous section, it is also possible to vary the pulse width, frequency and amplitude.

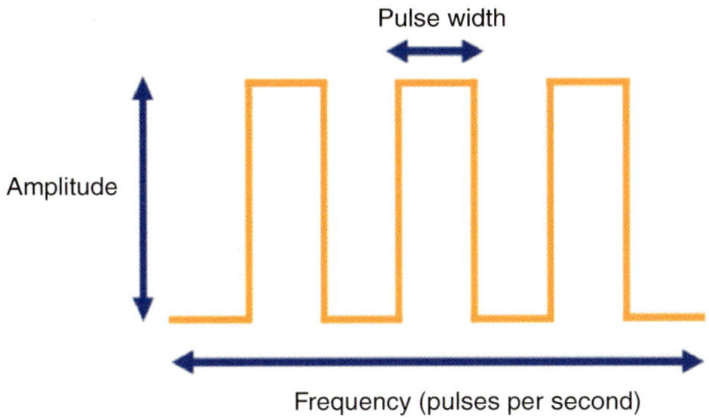

Fig. 4.3 Adjustable stimulator parameters. The pulse width defines the duration of each pulse, the amplitude defines the size of each pulse and the frequency determines how many pulses there are per second

Typical settings for pulse width vary between 60 and 150 μs although higher pulse widths (up to 450 μs) are occasionally used for the treatment of dystonia. The electrical properties of neurons are such that low pulse widths stimulate mainly axons whereas higher pulse widths stimulate cell bodies as well as axons [53]. The low pulse widths typically used for DBS stimulate mainly the axons [54].

The frequency (F), measured in Hertz (Hz) can also be varied. Low frequency stimulation (<50 Hz) is generally not effective for most movement disorders. Typical stimulation parameters would be around 130 Hz.

The voltage (V), measured in volts or the current (I), measured in milliamps can be varied as well. Voltage, current and impedance are related to each other via Ohms law.

$$\text{Impedance} = \frac{V}{I}.$$

Thus as long as the impedance remains stable, increasing either the current or the voltage has the same effect. The Medtronic DBS system is typically programmed by varying the voltage, whereas the Boston and the St. Jude DBS systems are typically programmed by varying the current.

Although rarely noted by the programmer, the most important setting is probably the Total Electrical Energy Delivered to the tissue (TEED) [55]. This is dependent on the pulse width in microseconds, frequency in Hertz, voltage in volts and impedance (Imp) in Ohms of the tissue. The relationship between these parameters is as follows:

$$\text{TEED} = \frac{V^2 + PW + F}{Imp}$$

Although there is a wide range of typical DBS settings used by different units, evidence indicates that in many cases the clinical effect of varying settings such as pulse width is not very great [56]. Usually the Voltage (or Current) will be reduced at the same time and the TEED will therefore be fairly similar despite different pulse widths. It is probably the TEED, which is most important as long as Pulse Width, Frequency and Voltage are kept within reasonable parameters.

In our unit we typically use the Medtronic system with a frequency of 130 Hz and pulse width of 60 μs. We would not alter the frequency or pulse width in most cases. We then start at an amplitude 0.5 V, slowly increasing to 5 or 6 V assessing for beneficial effects and side effects. We try out each contact that way in a monopolar configuration, moving to bipolar stimulation or even tripolar if needed. Once the best contacts have been identified we would usually send the patient home with a stimulator amplitude of around 1 V, gradually increasing to a maintenance amplitude over the next few weeks. A typical maintenance amplitude would often be around 3.5 V.

How Does DBS Work?

The mechanism by which DBS of a target improves movement disorders is not fully understood. The following is a brief summary of some of the current thinking in this area.

What Effect Does DBS Have on the Electrical Properties of the Nerve Cell?

The neuronal cell membrane contains a lipid bilayer, which is impermeable to electric current. In electrical circuit terminology, the neuronal membrane acts as a capacitor. In the resting state, there is a "potential difference" between the outside of the cell and the inside of the cell, whereby the inside of the cell is negatively charged compared to the outside of the cell [57].

As detailed in the previous section, DBS is usually applied to the target via the cathode (negative electrode). Thus a strong negative stimulation is applied to the outside of the nerve cells and nerve axons within the target structure. Since the neuronal membrane does not conduct electricity, the strong negative charge is stored outside the membrane. This external negative charge creates a potential difference across the neuronal membrane whereby the inside of the cell is now positive with respect to the outside. The potential difference changes the conformation of sodium permeable pores (sodium channels) in the membrane causing them to open. The opening of these sodium channels can lead to an Action Potential [58].

As the effects of DBS are very similar to the effects of a lesion, initial theories regarding the mechanism of DBS assumed that DBS caused overstimulation of the target structure leading to a "depolarising block" whereby the over-stimulated neurones switched off, perhaps due to inactivation of sodium channels [59]. A similar mechanism is known to underlie the action at the neuromuscular junction of a group of paralysing agents called depolarising muscle blockers. However DBS is no longer thought to work in this way [45, 60].

What Part of the Neuron Does DBS Effect?

In principle, stimulation of three possible structures could be involved in the action of DBS: the stimulation could be primarily affecting the cell body; the stimulation could predominantly be affecting axons terminating or starting within the target structure; or the stimulation could predominantly be affecting axons which are simply passing through the target structure.

However, as detailed in the previous section, due to the electrical properties of nerve cells and nerve axons, the pulse widths that are used in DBS have been shown to predominantly stimulate nerve axons rather than cell bodies [54]. Thus the effects of DBS are not felt to be due to an action on the cell body. Having said that, the effects of DBS may well be on the axon just as it is leaving the cell body and thus have an effect very similar to stimulation of the cell body itself. A combination of effects is currently thought to occur including stimulation of axons terminating in the target neurons, stimulation of the axon projections from the target neurons and stimulation of the axon projections through the target neurons.

Effects of DBS on Brain Oscillatory Activity

It is now being increasingly recognised that the effects of DBS cannot simply be considered as those of stimulating or inhibiting a brain structure. All the areas of the basal ganglia are connected in a complex fashion and these interconnected areas produce rhythmic oscillatory activity. Recording the rhythmical activity within the basal ganglia has led to the concept of normal and pathological brain rhythms. This concept has been best studied in Parkinson's disease but almost certainly applies to other conditions such as dystonia and tremor. Thus in Parkinson's disease it is found that bradykinesia (slowness of movement) is related to an increase in rhythmic activity within the basal ganglia at a rate of 13–30 Hz. This abnormal rhythmic activity is called beta oscillations and is thought to signal a "don't move" message to the brain. In the non-Parkinsonian brain, beta activity reduces before voluntary movement allowing the brain to move. Thus abnormal synchronised rhythmic beta activity in Parkinson's disease is thought to be important in the production of bradykinesia. Using intracranial recording it has been shown that DBS reduces beta activity, probably in a similar fashion to a radar jamming signal. Thus it is unlikely that the DBS itself contains any "information" for the basal ganglia. Most likely the DBS simply gets in the way of the ability of the Parkinsonian basal ganglia to generate a beta rhythm. Reduction in beta activity will then allow movement to proceed [61, 62].

Why Do Some Effects of DBS Take So Long?

It is well recognised that DBS can improve parkinsonian symptoms very quickly (within seconds) and this may well be due to reduction in beta activity. However the beneficial effects of DBS on dystonia take much longer, often many months. This more prolonged effect is thought to be due to synaptic plasticity within the brain, whereby synapses gradually change their strength over time [59]. Some evidence that synaptic strength gradually changes over time when DBS is used for dystonia has been demonstrated in experiments using transcranial magnetic stimulation (TMS) of the cortex [63].

Parkinson Plus Disorders

The parkinson plus disorders are a group of conditions which can sometimes be misdiagnosed as Parkinson's disease. They cause Parkinsonian features including tremor, rigidity and bradykinesia, although a typical Parkinsonian resting tremor is rare in Parkinson plus disorders. These disorders tend to respond poorly if at all to levodopa and other anti-Parkinsonian treatments. They usually progress relentlessly towards severe disability and subsequently death. Median survival times are much lower than in Parkinson's disease. Pathologically the Parkinson plus disorders are associated with much more widespread neurodegeneration in the basal ganglia than would typically be seen in Parkinson's disease which may be the main reason why they do not respond well to levodopa or to DBS [64].

The three main Parkinson plus disorders are Multiple System Atrophy (MSA), Progressive Supranuclear Palsy (PSP) and Corticobasal Degeneration (CBD). As well as Parkinsonian features responding poorly to levodopa treatment Parkinson plus disorders are associated with other clinical features. Thus in MSA, autonomic symptoms and cerebellar symptoms are common; in PSP patients develop impairment of volitional eye movements (supranuclear gaze palsy); in CBD patients often present with apraxia (a disorder of higher motor control) and myoclonus in a limb as well as Parkinsonism [2–4].

There have been a small number of case reports using subthalamic nucleus (STN) DBS in patients with parkinson plus disorders and in general there has been very little benefit [5, 6]. STN and Globus Pallidus Internus (GPi) DBS are not recommended in patients with Parkinson plus disorders Indeed standard recommendations for assessing Parkinson's disease patients for DBS suitability usually stipulate that the patient should have had PD for at least 5 years [65]. One of the main reasons for this timing is that Parkinson plus disorders can look like PD in the first few years, however in the vast majority of cases a Parkinson plus disorder would have "declared" itself within 5 years of onset.

There have been attempts to treat the gait disorder in PSP using pedunculopontine (PPN) nucleus DBS with some reports showing modest improvements [7]. However PPN DBS is very much an experimental treatment at present.

Dystonia

Phenomenology of Dystonia

Dystonia is a hyperkinetic movement disorder whereby the increased involuntary movement is patterned. The word patterned means that the same movement(s) are performed repeatedly. Dystonia causes sustained muscle contractions leading to abnormal postures and repetitive movements [66].

Tremor is often associated with dystonia. When tremor occurs in a body affected by dystonia it is termed "dystonic tremor", whereas when tremor occurs in a separate body part from dystonia it is termed "tremor associated with dystonia". Some patients with dystonia have a "sensory trick" whereby gently touching the dystonic area will lead to an improvement in dystonia [67].

Classification of Dystonia: Classification by Body Part Affected

Dystonia can be classified according to the body part(s) affected: in generalised dystonia, the legs, trunk and another body part are affected; in hemidystonia the limbs down one side of the body are affected; in segmental dystonia two neighbouring body parts are affected; whereas in focal dystonia only one body part is affected [66].

Virtually any body part can be affected by dystonia, either as a focal dystonia or as part of a more widespread dystonic syndrome. Dystonia can affect the neck (cervical dystonia) causing the neck to develop abnormal postures. When dystonia affects the eyelids (blepharospasm) they tend to forcefully close and when severe the patient can be functionally blind. Dystonia can also affect the limbs (limb dystonia), including the lower limbs which may develop unusual postures on walking, or the upper limbs which may develop unusual postures for example when writing. When dystonia affects the mouth and jaw (oromandibular dystonia) the mouth can tend to opening or closing when eating or speaking. Sometimes the larynx is affected by dystonia (laryngeal dystonia) often causing a strained "dystonic" speech.

When dystonia presents in childhood, it often presents in the lower limbs and gradually becomes generalised. However when dystonia presents in adulthood it is usually focal or segmental dystonia.

Classification of Dystonia: Classification by Method of Activation

Dystonia can be classified according to the method of activation. Thus when dystonia first presents it often occurs only when doing a specific task (task-specific dystonia). For example some people find that when they write, their hand and/or arm develops an abnormal posture, which can make normal writing difficult or impossible. This is called writers cramp and is a form of task-specific dystonia. Other task-specific dystonias include those associated with playing musical instruments. Often dystonia remains as a task specific phenomenon and does not progress past this. However in some people the dystonia can start to affect any movement of limb (action dystonia). Further progression in the condition can lead to dystonia even at rest (rest dystonia) and occasionally the limb may develop a fixed immobile posture (fixed dystonia).

Classification of Dystonia: Classification by Cause

Dystonia can be classified as primary dystonia, dystonia plus syndromes or secondary dystonia [68, 69].

Primary Dystonia: Primary Torsion Dystonia (PTD)

Primary torsion dystonia (PTD) is the term given to the development of dystonia in the absence of any other movement disorder (except tremor), any other neurological problem, any causative abnormality on imaging or anything in the history to suggest a secondary cause. Primary dystonia accounts for about 75% of dystonia cases and many forms have a genetic cause. Childhood onset PTD typically starts in the lower limbs and then becomes generalised. Childhood onset PTD is often due to a mutation in the DYT1 gene. Adult onset PTD is usually focal dystonia. Many cases of adult onset focal PTD have a family history suggesting genetic factors, although the majority of genes have not yet been identified.

Dystonia Plus Conditions

The dystonia plus conditions are a group of conditions where dystonia is associated with another movement disorder (other than tremor). The main dystonia plus disorders are Dopa Responsive Dystonia (DRD), Myoclonus Dystonia Syndrome (MDS) and Rapid Onset Dystonia Parkinsonism (RODP).

DRD is a rare form of generalised dystonia, which usually presents in childhood. It presents with lower limb dystonia that may mimic PTD or dystonic cerebral palsy. Diurnal fluctuations are common whereby the condition is improved in the morning and worsens through the day. Parkinsonian features can occur later. Most cases of DRD are due to a mutation in the GTP cyclohydrolase 1 gene, which codes for a protein that is important in dopamine synthesis. DRD usually responds dramatically to low doses of levodopa which are almost curative therefore this condition should not be missed and anyone with this phenotype should have a trial of levodopa.

MDS causes a combination of dystonia and myoclonus. Myoclonic jerks typically affect the face and upper limbs and are often the most troublesome feature of the condition. Patients also often have dystonia including cervical dystonia or writers cramp. MDS is a genetic condition often due to a mutation in the epsilon sarcoglycans gene. Drug therapy is often unsatisfactory. Psychiatric problems including obsessive compulsive disorder are common. The myoclonic jerks often respond to alcohol and many patients therefore develop alcoholism.

RODP is a rare condition that usually starts in childhood or early adolescence. Dystonia, which often affects the cranio-cervical region as well as generalised Parkinsonism, often develops over hours-to-weeks. The condition is caused by a mutation in the ATP1A3 gene.

Secondary Dystonia

Dystonia can be caused by a vast number of secondary causes often associated with brain and in particular basal ganglia injury. Dystonic cerebral palsy is usually a generalised dystonia. Although classically associated with ABO incompatibility leading to haemolysis and jaundice (kernicterus) dystonic cerebral palsy can occur due to any cause of perinatal injury. Hypoxic injury or vascular injury to the brain can be complicated by dystonia. When a basal ganglia stroke leads to dystonia it is often contralateral hemidystonia. A large number of metabolic and hereditary conditions can lead to basal ganglia injury and dystonia, including glutaric aciduria, neuroacanthocytosis, pantothenate-kinase associated neurodegeneration, Wilson's disease, Lesch-Nyhan Syndrome and Huntington's disease. Dystonia can also be a feature of neurodegenerative conditions including Parkinson's disease and PSP. Finally dystonia can be caused by medication: levodopa treatment in PD can be associated with dystonic dyskinesia and neuroleptic treatment of psychiatric disorders can cause a persistent dystonic syndrome termed tardive dystonia.

Pathophysiology of Dystonia

The pathophysiology of dystonia is not well understood and is discussed in detail elsewhere [68]. Neurophysiological studies have demonstrated a reduction in inhibition affecting various levels of the nervous system in patients with dystonia [70]. Sensory deficits have been demonstrated in dystonia including impaired temporal discrimination (the ability to perceive two successive stimuli as being separate) [71]. Most current theories of dystonia pathophysiology suggest that heightened synaptic plasticity (i.e. pathological strengthening of synaptic connections) in motor areas leads to the generation of pathological dystonic movements. The impaired inhibition may well lead to over-excitation thus driving this synaptic plasticity [68].

Treatment of Dystonia

Various drugs have been used in the treatment of dystonia. Antidopaminergic drugs are often used. These include dopamine blocking drugs (neuroleptics including haloperidol and risperidone) and dopamine depleting drugs (in particular tetrabenazine). Antidopaminergic drugs have modest efficacy against dystonic symptoms and are often associated with side effects. Anticholinergic drugs such as trihexyphenidyl can be somewhat effective treatments for dystonia but again side effects are common. Benzodiazepines such as clonazepam can give modest benefit as can the GABA-B agonist baclofen. In general however, drug treatment of dystonia has modest efficacy at best [72].

Botulinum toxin is a very effective treatment for focal dystonia. The toxin weakens the muscle by impairing acetyl choline release at the neuromuscular junction. The effect usually lasts about 3 months after which the injections need to be repeated. Dramatic beneficial effects can be seen in many forms of focal dystonia if the appropriate muscles are targeted with the appropriate dose. In particular cervical dystonia, blepharospasm and laryngeal dystonia often respond well to botulinum toxin treatment. Treatment of limb dystonia such as writer's cramp is more difficult. The dystonia can often be improved but sometimes only at the expense of weakness which itself can cause disability. Generalised dystonia is difficult to treat with botulinum toxin as so many muscles would need targeted and there is a limit to how much toxin can be injected before side effects such as respiratory muscle weakness become a problem [72].

Rating Scales for Dystonia

Several rating scales exist for the assessment of dystonia, allowing fairly unified assessment between units. The Burke Fahn Marsden Dystonia Rating Scale (BFMDRS) is a rating scale for dystonia affecting any part of the body and is most useful in patients with generalised dystonia. Dystonia is assessed in several body parts and each part is rated between 0 (normal/none) and 4 (severe dystonia). The final score is between 0 and 120. The Toronto Western Spasmodic Torticollis Rating Scale (TWSTRS) is a similar scale focussing only on cervical dystonia.

DBS for Dystonia

DBS in Primary Torsion Dystonia (PTD)

In some patients medical treatment of dystonia is unsatisfactory. Some patients are very disabled by the condition hence the requirement for alternative treatments. In the 1950s the first attempts were made to treat dystonia surgically with lesions in various sites including the GPi, the thalamus, the zona incerta and the subthalamic nucleus. DBS for dystonia was developed in the 1980s in parallel with the development of DBS for PD. The majority of DBS operations for dystonia have targeted the internal globus pallidus bilaterally (bilateral GPi DBS). As mentioned previously, the beneficial effects of DBS on dystonia can take several months to occur, probably due to the gradual alterations in synaptic plasticity within motor areas of the brain [18].

Most DBS operations for dystonia have been on patients with primary torsion dystonia (PTD). A large number of case reports, case series and large multi-centre clinical trials have demonstrated the efficacy and safety of DBS in the treatment of PTD [8–10]. The benefit in generalised PTD can very dramatic. Most cases show improvements of 50–60% in the BFMDRS with some patients achieving improvement of as much as 90%. The beneficial effects of bilateral GPi DBS on cervical dystonia are also well established, with improvements in TWSTRS of between 50 and 70% in most studies [11–13].

Although there is a large body of evidence regarding the efficacy of GPi DBS in the treatment of cervical dystonia, the data on the treatment of other forms of focal dystonia are more limited. Nonetheless good results have been reported in blepharospasm and Meige's syndrome (Meige's syndrome is the term given to the combination of blepharospasm and oromandibular dystonia) [14, 15]. A small number of case reports have successfully used DBS to treat writers cramp, although the ventral oral nucleus of the thalamus was chosen as the target rather than the GPi based on encouraging results with lesioning studies [18].

DBS in Dystonia Plus Conditions

DBS has been used to treat myoclonus dystonia. The two main targets used have been the GPi and the ventral intermediate nucleus of the thalamus (VIM). Encouraging results have been demonstrated with improvements in both myoclonus and dystonia [16, 17]. I am not aware of any cases of DRD or RODP treated with DBS.

DBS in the Treatment of Secondary Dystonia

GPi DBS is much less effective in the treatment of secondary dystonia than in the treatment of PTD. Nonetheless improvements can be seen. A number of studies have investigated DBS in the treatment of dystonic cerebral palsy with modest improvements (around 25%) seen in many patients [19]. It is important to distinguish dystonia (which may be improved by DBS) from spasticity (which will not be improved by DBS, although may be improved by intrathecal baclofen). Dystonia and spasticity often co-exist in patients with secondary dystonia such as cerebral palsy. Similar modest improvements, mainly in case reports, have been demonstrated in the treatment of other secondary dystonia syndromes including pantothenate kinase associated neurodegeneration, neurodegeneration with brain iron accumulation and Lesch-Nyhan disease [18].

Although most cases of secondary dystonia respond only modestly to GPi DBS, many case reports and case series have demonstrated that tardive dystonia can respond extremely well to bilateral GPi DBS with improvements seen between about 50 and 90% in most patients [20, 21].

A small number of patients with generalised dystonia can present with a severe exacerbation of their dystonia called dystonic storm. This condition can lead to rhabdomyolysis, renal failure, respiratory compromise and even death. Dystonic storm can be provoked by infections or medication, although a provoking factor is not always found. Urgent bilateral GPi DBS has been used in the treatment of dystonic storm with generally positive results [73].

Tremor

Tremor is an oscillatory, rhythmic, usually regular movement affecting one or more body parts such as the limbs, neck, tongue, face or larynx. When examining a patient with tremor it is useful to determine whether the tremor is present at rest (resting tremor), with posture holding such as extending out the arms (postural tremor), with action such as writing or pouring water between cups (action tremor) or with intention such as when bringing the finger to a target (intention tremor).

Classification of Tremor

There are many different causes of tremor including parkinsonian tremor, essential tremor, dystonic tremor, orthostatic tremor and secondary tremors [67, 74].

Physiological Tremor

We all have a low amplitude physiological tremor, which can be demonstrated on electromyography (EMG). In certain conditions the physiological tremor can be enhanced such as with anxiety and hyperthyroidism. Enhanced physiological tremor is never severe enough to consider DBS.

Parkinsonian Tremor

Most although not all patients with Parkinson's disease have a tremor. Parkinsonian tremor is usually a resting tremor. Occasionally Parkinsonian tremor can be a postural tremor (with or without resting tremor) that often takes a few seconds to develop after the arms are held outstretched (postural re-emergent tremor). Most patients with Parkinsonian tremor have other Parkinsonian features including rigidity and bradykinesia. Resting tremor in PD can be a nuisance and can be embarrassing but is rarely disabling as the tremor improves on action. Postural re-emergent tremor on the other hand can be very disabling as it can affect activities such as using cutlery and holding a cup. Parkinsonian tremor is usually asymmetrical. Jaw tremor is common. Head tremor and vocal tremor are fairly rare in PD.

Essential Tremor

Essential tremor is a common condition that causes a predominantly postural and action tremor. Thus various actions such as writing, pouring and holding a cup will bring out the tremor. Essential tremor can present at almost any age. In patients with a large amplitude tremor, essential tremor can be very disabling and in severe cases simple tasks such as drinking from a cup or using cutlery become almost impossible. Essential tremor often runs in families and is therefore felt to be genetic however most genes have not yet been found. Essential tremor often affects the upper limbs however can also affect the head, the face, the speech, the trunk and the lower limbs.

Dystonic Tremor

Dystonic tremor is a fairly poorly-characterised condition. As detailed in the section of dystonia, when tremor occurs in a body part affected by dystonia it is termed "dystonic tremor", whereas when tremor occurs in a separate body part it is called "tremor associated with dystonia". Similar to essential tremor, dystonic tremor causes a predominantly postural and action tremor. It can affect the limbs, head, trunk, face and speech and in many cases is very disabling. The presence or absence of subtle dystonic features in a patient can be the only difference between whether they are diagnosed with essential tremor or dystonic tremor and there is some debate regarding the correct diagnosis in many patients.

Orthostatic Tremor

Orthostatic tremor is a tremor that mainly affects the anti-gravity muscles and thus is most commonly demonstrated in the lower limbs. Orthostatic tremor tends to be at a much higher frequency (13–18 Hz) than essential tremor (4–10 Hz). Orthostatic tremor tends to be worse on standing than on walking. Patients may therefore report the unusual symptom that they are unsteady while standing but not while walking. When examining a patient while standing, the orthostatic tremor can sometimes be seen as a high frequency rhythmic movement in the quadriceps muscles. Sometimes the tremor can be palpated. The tremor can sometimes be heard by placing the bell of the stethoscope over the quadriceps and listening for a noise similar to that of rotating helicopter blades. Orthostatic tremor can be demonstrated in the upper limbs if they act as anti-gravity muscles such as when the patient stands and leans on a table with straight arms, allowing the table to take their weight.

Cerebellar Tremor

Lesions and diseases affecting the cerebellum can cause a variety of "cerebellar signs" including an intention tremor. Cerebellar or intention tremor tends to affect the limb while moving and tends to get larger in amplitude as the limb approaches the target.

Holmes Tremor

Holmes tremor, sometimes called rubral tremor or midbrain tremor is due to a lesion affecting the midbrain or its connections. The tremor tends to be fairly large amplitude and disabling. It predominantly affects the upper limb and is a unilateral tremor, contralateral to the causative lesion. Holmes tremor is present at rest and on posture but becomes much more exaggerated as the limb approaches the target (intention tremor). The resting tremor component may be due to the lesion affecting the substantia nigra and its pathways whereas the intention component of the tremor may be due to the lesion affecting the cerebellum or its pathways. Various lesions including stroke, tumour and vascular malformations can cause a Holmes tremor.

Multiple Sclerosis (MS) Tremor

Tremor is common in MS and an important cause of disability. The prevalence of tremor in MS is around 25% in the community and over 50% in specialist clinics. MS tremor is often an upper extremity postural and intention tremor although rest tremors and rubral tremors have been rarely reported [75].

Treatment of Tremor

Various drugs are used in the treatment of tremor [76]. The most commonly used medication for tremor is beta blockers. In particular propranolol has been shown to have modest efficacy in the treatment of most tremors. Although most beta blockers may well be efficacious for tremor, the enhanced lipid solubility of propranolol (enabling good brain penetration) as well as the pharmacological profile of propranolol (blocks beta 2 adrenergic receptors as well as beta 1) may potentially indicate that propranolol is more effective than other beta blockers. Nonetheless propranolol has only modest efficacy against tremor and rarely provides satisfactory relief of severe essential tremor. It is contraindicated in patients with asthma.

Primidone is another anti-tremor drug with reasonable efficacy although often associated with side effects such as sedation. Other medications occasionally used include topiramate, gabapentin, benzodiazepines (such as clonazepam) and pregabalin. Occasionally botulinum toxin injections can improve tremor. Resting tremor in PD will often improve with levodopa and other antiparkinsonian medications. Occasionally levodopa can improve the resting tremor component of a Holmes tremor. Treatment options for orthostatic tremor include gabapentin and clonazepam.

Although there are quite a few drugs available for the treatment of tremor, the effects of these drugs is modest at best and most patients with severe tremor syndromes will not achieve satisfactory control of their tremor with medication.

Tremor Rating Scales

The most commonly used tremor rating scale is the Fahn Tolosa Marin Tremor Rating Scale (FTMTRS). This scale assesses tremor in various body parts as well as asking about activities of daily living and assessing actions including pouring and writing. Each assessment is graded from 0 (normal or none) to 4 (severely impaired). The FTMTRS enables fairly unified assessment of tremor between different units.

DBS for Tremor

In the 1950s stereotactic lesioning of the thalamus was widely used in the treatment of tremor. During some of these operations, high frequency stimulation of the thalamus was used to suppress tremor intra-operatively enabling the surgeon to know that they were at the correct target before the permanent lesioning was performed. In parallel with the development of DBS for PD in the 1990s, DBS was also developed for tremor [22].

The majority of DBS operations for tremor have targeted the thalamus. Thalamic anatomy is very complicated with many different nomenclature methods used for classifying over 120 thalamic nuclei. This has made it very difficult to compare targets between centres. Over time, an evolving consensus has been reached indicating that bilateral DBS of the ventral intermediate thalamic nucleus (VIM) is an appropriate thalamic target for the treatment of tremor.

The efficacy of DBS in the treatment of essential tremor has been demonstrated in many studies [22–24]. When assessed using the FTMTRS, improvements in tremor range from 50 to 90%. Improvement in tremor usually occurs within seconds of switching on the stimulator at the appropriate settings. Another region that has received attention is the Zona Incerta lying dorsal to the STN. Bilateral Zona Incerta

DBS can also produce very impressive improvements in essential tremor and other tremor syndromes [25, 26].

Dystonic tremor is also improved with bilateral VIM DBS although is a less well investigated and less well defined condition ([27]). A small number of case reports have demonstrated modest efficacy when treating Holmes tremor with either unilateral VIM or GPi DBS [28]. DBS management of MS tremor is difficult, partly due to the problems distinguishing tremor (which may be improved by DBS) from ataxia (which will not be improved by DBS). Most studies indicate fairly disappointing results when using VIM stimulation for MS tremor, but some fairly encouraging results have been demonstrated [29, 30]. A small number of case reports have demonstrated efficacy of bilateral thalamic DBS for the treatment of orthostatic tremor [31].

Tics and Tourette's Syndrome

A tic can take a wide variety of forms including eye blinking, shoulder rotation, facial movements, limb movements and vocalisations [77]. The cardinal feature of a tic is that the patient will describe an uncomfortable sensation in the body part and an urge to make the movement, similar to an itch that you have to scratch. The patient makes the movement voluntarily in response to the urge/uncomfortable sensation leading to a transient improvement in the urge and sensory component. The movement can be suppressed via a force of will on behalf of the patient, however during this time the urge and uncomfortable sensation get stronger and stronger until a rebound increase in tics is seen. Although there are formal diagnostic criteria, Tourette disorder can basically be considered a severe form of tic disorder. There is a spectrum with mild tic disorder at one end and severe Tourette syndrome at the other end. Tics affect around 5% of school children being more common in boys than in girls. Tics usually present in early adolescence and will often reduce as the child moves into adulthood. Occasionally tics continue into adulthood, and adult onset tic disorder is described. As well as motor tics, vocalisations are common in tic disorder and Tourette syndrome. Vocalisations usually include grunting, throat clearing and other vocal noises. Coprolalia (swearing) occurs in less than 50% of patients with Tourette syndrome. Many patients with Tourette syndrome have obsessive compulsive disorder (OCD) and attention deficit hyperactivity disorder (ADHD).

Treatment of Tic Disorder and Tourette Syndrome

The main drugs used to treat tics include dopamine blockers (such as haloperidol, risperidone and sulpiride), dopamine depleting medication (tetrabenazine), baclofen and alpha 2 agonists (clonidine). These drugs are often not very effective and may well cause side effects. In most cases of simple tic disorder and in some cases of Tourette syndrome, treatment is not helpful, causing side effects and not improving the tics to any great degree. Therefore often it is best to avoid medication. However some patients will achieve meaningful benefit from medication without side effects. Botulinum toxin injections can sometimes be helpful for focal tics. Psychological strategies are available to try and reduce tics and can sometimes be helpful. However in most patients with severe Tourette syndrome, drug treatment and psychological treatment is unsatisfactory [77].

Rating Scales for Tourette Syndrome

The main rating scale for Tourette syndrome is the Yale Global Tic Severity Scale (YGTSS). The scale documents number, frequency, intensity, complexity and interference of both motor and vocal tics grading each question from 0 (none) to 5 (severe). The scale also documents how much the tics interfere with normal activities of daily living. Total scores range from 0 to 100. The YGTSS enables Tourette syndrome severity to be compared between different units.

DBS for Tourette Syndrome

Thalamic lesioning as a treatment for Tourette syndrome was first reported in the 1970s and the first case report of thalamic DBS for Tourette syndrome was in 1999. Since then there have been many case reports, case series and a small number of trials investigating the use of DBS for Tourette syndrome. The main targets have been the medial thalamus (in particular the centromedian parafascicular nuceleus), the GPi, the external Globus Pallidus (GPe) and the internal capsule/nucleus accumbens. Most of the studies have shown fairly significant improvements in YGTSS in the range of 50%, sometimes more [32]. A randomised double-blind crossover trial of GPi DBS for medically-refractory Tourette's syndrome has been recently reported. GPi DBS led to a significant improvement in tic severity, with an overall acceptable safety profile [78].

Myoclonus

Myoclonus describes sudden involuntary jerking movements of the muscles. Myoclonic movements are very brief, typically <100 ms if measured by EMG. A large number of conditions can cause myoclonus and are reviewed in detail elsewhere [33, 34, 79]. As mentioned in the section on dystonia, myoclonus dystonia is a genetic condition causing myoclonus and dystonia. Bilateral GPi DBS has been used in the management of myoclonus dystonia in several case reports and case series. Thalamic DBS has also been reported. Fairly impressive reductions in both myoclonus and dystonia have been demonstrated [16, 17]. With the exception of one study demonstrating efficacy of thalamic DBS for myoclonus associated with perinatal hypoxia [80], I am not aware of studies investigating DBS for other forms of myoclonus.

Chorea

Chorea is a hyperkinetic movement disorder in which the movements are completely random. The most well recognised cause of chorea is Huntington's disease (HD), which is caused by a mutation in the Huntington gene. HD is an autosomal dominant condition causing chorea, dystonia, parkinsonism, dementia, behavioural problems and psychiatric issues [81]. A small number of case reports have demonstrated useful reduction in chorea in HD using bilateral GPi DBS [35]. However chorea is one of a large number of problems that HD patients face therefore DBS should be reserved only for those with very disabling chorea. Hemiballism / hermichorea usually results from a vascular or metabolic insult to the basal ganglia, often near the subthalamic nucleus. The condition causes severe chorea down one side of the body contralateral to the lesion. Usually the condition will gradually settle over a few months although not in all cases [82]. GPi and thalamic DBS have been shown to be an effective treatment for refractory hemiballism / hemichorea [36]. There are a large number of other causes of chorea, reviewed elsewhere, but I am not aware of DBS being used for any these other causes of chorea [83].

Tardive Dyskinesia

Long term treatment with dopamine blocking drugs can cause involuntary movements termed tardive dyskinesia [84]. The most common clinical scenario is the use of neuroleptic drugs to treat psychiatric disorders such as schizophrenia. Tardive dyskinesia is a hyperkinetic movement disorder. The involuntary movements often affect the orolingual region and are stereotyped in nature. The movements will often settle when the patient tries to eat or speak, only to recur again afterwards. The term stereotypy is sometimes used to define this type of hyperkinetic movement disorder and tardive dyskinesia is therefore sometimes called tardive stereotypy. Tardive dyskinesia sometimes affects other body parts as well including the limbs. A few case reports and case series have documented beneficial effects of bilateral GPi DBS in the treatment of Tardive Dyskinesia [37].

A more disabling complication of long-term dopamine blocking treatment is that of tardive dystonia where the involuntary movements tend to be dystonic rather than stereotypic. Classically tardive dystonia affects the neck and axial muscles causing dystonic spasms, which tend to throw the neck and body backwards into an extensor posture. However many other forms of dystonia can be seen. Tardive dystonia usually responds well to bilateral GPi DBS as detailed in the section on dystonia [20, 21].

Adverse Effects of DBS

I will split the adverse effects of DBS into surgical complications, stimulation related adverse effects and cognitive/neuropsychiatric adverse effects.

Surgical Complications of DBS

DBS involves placing a small wire deep into the brain. It will never be possible to perform such a procedure without any risk, however modern surgical techniques have minimised the risk. The most feared complication is haemorrhage. Sometimes intracranial haemorrhage complicating DBS can be asymptomatic however intracranial haemorrhage can be complicated by hemiparesis and even death. A fairly recent meta-analysis has indicated a haemorrhage rate of around 1.57% (95% confidence intervals 1.26–1.95%) [85].

Another surgical complications of DBS is infection. Minor infections of the battery site are not uncommon and usually respond to antibiotic treatment, occasionally requiring removal of the battery. More major infections tracking down the lead itself are uncommon however will require prolonged antibiotic treatment as well as removal of the whole DBS system including the intracranial lead.

Occasionally the leads can become damaged leading to fracture or short circuit. These type of problems will declare themselves when the stimulator impedance is measured and this should therefore be done regularly. Although not a complication as such, the stimulator battery will usually need replaced every 5 years or so unless a rechargeable battery is used.

Stimulation Related Adverse Effects of DBS

No matter which target is being used, many important structures pass close to the DBS target. Thus the conduction of electrical DBS activity to neighbouring structures can cause side effects depending on the normal function of the structure involved [52].

With STN DBS the electrical activity can stimulate the nearby internal capsule causing muscle spasms. Other structures that can be stimulated include the oculomotor region causing double vision, the sensory pathways causing paraesthesia and the brachium conjunctivum causing ataxia. Stimulation induced dysarthria is also common, probably due to capsular stimulation

With GPi DBS nearby structure include the visual pathways, stimulation of which can cause flashing lights and the internal capsule, stimulation of which can cause muscle spasms.

With VIM DBS, stimulation induced side effects include paraesthesia (due to stimulating the sensory thalamus), tonic muscle spasms due to capsular stimulation and dysarthria.

The main advantage of DBS over lesioning is that these stimulation-induced side effects are not permanent and can be treated by changing stimulator parameters as detailed in the section on stimulator programming.

Neuropsychiatric and Cognitive Effects of DBS

A large body of literature has investigated the cognitive effects of DBS in the treatment of Parkinson's disease. There is fairly good evidence for mild cognitive side effects in particular "frontal lobe" problems including verbal fluency. Similarly there are many case reports and case series detailing neuropsychiatric complications of DBS in PD including depression, apathy, mania and impulsivity [86–88].

However there are several potential causes for cognitive and neuropsychiatric complications of DBS in PD including: effects of the disease itself (cognitive impairment and neuropsychiatric symptoms are common in PD); effects of the medication (medication reduction may be the main cause of apathy) [86]; effects of the surgery itself (the lead usually passes through the frontal lobe on its way to target); and the effects of the stimulation. Thus both disease related and DBS-related factors may be implicated [87].

Neuropsychiatric and cognitive effects of DBS in the treatment of other movement disorders, in particular dystonia have been much less investigated. However current evidence suggests very little in the way of cognitive or neuropsychiatric complications when DBS is used to treat dystonia [89]. Nonetheless careful monitoring is still recommended.

Future Directions

Although DBS is now a well-established treatment for dystonia and tremor, there is still work to be done in order to clarify the role of DBS in the management of Tourette syndrome, chorea, myoclonus and other movement disorders. We also need to clarify the best target for each condition. Clinical trials, ideally double blind are required.

Improved stereotactic MRI-guided techniques are starting to improve the accuracy and safety of targeting and there will probably come a time when microelectrode recording and/or awake stimulation are not necessary.

Improved battery technology including rechargeable batteries and much smaller batteries will make the whole process easier for the patient. Rechargeable batteries are already in common use.

Improved lead technology will allow many more contacts as well as being able to stimulate in a certain direction from a contact. The ability to fuse the patient's MRI image with an image of their lead placement as well as using computer algorithms will enable the programmer to visualise anatomically the effects of specific stimulator settings on the area stimulated. This will vastly speed up the time taken to programme and potentially allow the programmer to choose the appropriate settings without resorting to trial and error.

One of the more exciting developments is so called adaptive DBS. So far this has mainly been used in Parkinson's disease where beta activity is known to be associated with a Parkinsonian state (see previous section). Using adaptive stimulation, the stimulator can assess for beta activity and switch itself on only when required rather than all the time. Early studies using adaptive stimulation suggest that it may be more effective than continuous stimulation [90]. In the future it is likely that similar techniques may enable the DBS system to programme itself without the requirement for a programmer.

The ability to safely implant a lead into the brain in order to record, analyse and modify activity within a discrete neuronal area is an extremely exciting development. The future of DBS opens up possibilities, which at this present moment would be considered farfetched even in a science fiction movie.

References

1. Deuschl G, Paschen S, Witt K. Clinical outcome of deep brain stimulation for Parkinson's disease. Handb Clin Neurol. 2013;116:107–28.
2. Armstrong MJ, Litvan I, Lang AE, Bak TH, Bhatia KP, Borroni B, et al. Criteria for the diagnosis of corticobasal degeneration. Neurology. 2013;80(5):496–503.
3. Esper CD, Weiner WJ, Factor SA. Progressive supranuclear palsy. Rev Neurol Dis. 2007;4(4):209–16.
4. Quinn N. Multiple system atrophy–the nature of the beast. J Neurol Neurosurg Psychiatry. 1989;52(Suppl):78–89.
5. Shih LC, Tarsy D. Deep brain stimulation for the treatment of atypical parkinsonism. Mov Disord Off J Mov Disord Soc. 2007;22(15):2149–55.
6. Thavanesan N, Gillies M, Farrell M, Green AL, Aziz T. Deep brain stimulation in multiple system atrophy mimicking idiopathic Parkinson's disease. Case Rep Neurol. 2014;6(3):232–7.
7. Hazrati LN, Wong JC, Hamani C, Lozano AM, Poon YY, Dostrovsky JO, et al. Clinicopathological study in progressive supranuclear palsy with pedunculopontine stimulation. Mov Disord Off J Mov Disord Soc. 2012;27(10):1304–7.

8. Kupsch A, Benecke R, Muller J, Trottenberg T, Schneider GH, Poewe W, et al. Pallidal deep-brain stimulation in primary generalized or segmental dystonia. N Engl J Med. 2006;355(19):1978–90.
9. Vidailhet M, Vercueil L, Houeto JL, Krystkowiak P, Benabid AL, Cornu P, et al. Bilateral deep-brain stimulation of the globus pallidus in primary generalized dystonia. N Engl J Med. 2005;352(5):459–67.
10. Air EL, Ostrem JL, Sanger TD, Starr PA. Deep brain stimulation in children: experience and technical pearls. J Neurosurg Pediatr. 2011;8(6):566–74.
11. Cacciola F, Farah JO, Eldridge PR, Byrne P, Varma TK. Bilateral deep brain stimulation for cervical dystonia: long-term outcome in a series of 10 patients. Neurosurgery. 2010;67(4):957–63.
12. Skogseid IM, Ramm-Pettersen J, Volkmann J, Kerty E, Dietrichs E, Roste GK. Good long-term efficacy of pallidal stimulation in cervical dystonia: a prospective, observer-blinded study. Eur J Neurol Off J Eur Federation Neurol Soc. 2012;19(4):610–5.
13. Volkmann J, Mueller J, Deuschl G, Kuhn AA, Krauss JK, Poewe W, et al. Pallidal neurostimulation in patients with medication-refractory cervical dystonia: a randomised, sham-controlled trial. Lancet Neurol. 2014;13(9):875–84.
14. Limotai N, Go C, Oyama G, Hwynn N, Zesiewicz T, Foote K, et al. Mixed results for GPi-DBS in the treatment of cranio-facial and cranio-cervical dystonia symptoms. J Neurol. 2011;258(11):2069–74.
15. Reese R, Gruber D, Schoenecker T, Bazner H, Blahak C, Capelle HH, et al. Long-term clinical outcome in meige syndrome treated with internal pallidum deep brain stimulation. Mov Disord Off J Mov Disord Soc. 2011;26(4):691–8.
16. Azoulay-Zyss J, Roze E, Welter ML, Navarro S, Yelnik J, Clot F, et al. Bilateral deep brain stimulation of the pallidum for myoclonus-dystonia due to epsilon-sarcoglycan mutations: a pilot study. Arch Neurol. 2011;68(1):94–8.
17. Cif L, Valente EM, Hemm S, Coubes C, Vayssiere N, Serrat S, et al. Deep brain stimulation in myoclonus-dystonia syndrome. Mov Disord Off J Mov Disord Soc. 2004;19(6):724–7.
18. Vidailhet M, Jutras MF, Roze E, Grabli D. Deep brain stimulation for dystonia. Handb Clin Neurol. 2013;116:167–87.
19. Vidailhet M, Yelnik J, Lagrange C, Fraix V, Grabli D, Thobois S, et al. Bilateral pallidal deep brain stimulation for the treatment of patients with dystonia-choreoathetosis cerebral palsy: a prospective pilot study. Lancet Neurol. 2009;8(8):709–17.
20. Chang EF, Schrock LE, Starr PA, Ostrem JL. Long-term benefit sustained after bilateral pallidal deep brain stimulation in patients with refractory tardive dystonia. Stereotact Funct Neurosurg. 2010;88(5):304–10.
21. Gruber D, Trottenberg T, Kivi A, Schoenecker T, Kopp UA, Hoffmann KT, et al. Long-term effects of pallidal deep brain stimulation in tardive dystonia. Neurology. 2009;73(1):53–8.
22. Nazzaro JM, Lyons KE, Pahwa R. Deep brain stimulation for essential tremor. Handb Clin Neurol. 2013;116:155–66.
23. Benabid AL, Pollak P, Gao D, Hoffmann D, Limousin P, Gay E, et al. Chronic electrical stimulation of the ventralis intermedius nucleus of the thalamus as a treatment of movement disorders. J Neurosurg. 1996;84(2):203–14.
24. Limousin P, Speelman JD, Gielen F, Janssens M. Multicentre European study of thalamic stimulation in parkinsonian and essential tremor. J Neurol Neurosurg Psychiatry. 1999;66(3):289–96.
25. Plaha P, Javed S, Agombar D, O' Farrell G, Khan S, Whone A, et al. Bilateral caudal zona incerta nucleus stimulation for essential tremor: outcome and quality of life. J Neurol Neurosurg Psychiatry. 2011;82(8):899–904.
26. Plaha P, Khan S, Gill SS. Bilateral stimulation of the caudal zona incerta nucleus for tremor control. J Neurol Neurosurg Psychiatry. 2008;79(5):504–13.

27. Hedera P, Phibbs FT, Dolhun R, Charles PD, Konrad PE, Neimat JS, et al. Surgical targets for dystonic tremor: considerations between the globus pallidus and ventral intermediate thalamic nucleus. Parkinsonism Relat Disord. 2013;19(7):684–6.
28. Diederich NJ, Verhagen Metman L, Bakay RA, Alesch F. Ventral intermediate thalamic stimulation in complex tremor syndromes. Stereotact Funct Neurosurg. 2008;86(3):167–72.
29. Alusi SH, Aziz TZ, Glickman S, Jahanshahi M, Stein JF, Bain PG. Stereotactic lesional surgery for the treatment of tremor in multiple sclerosis: a prospective case-controlled study. Brain (A Journal of neurology). 2001;124(Pt 8):1576–89.
30. Starr PA. Deep brain stimulation for other tremors, myoclonus, and chorea. Handb Clin Neurol. 2013;116:209–15.
31. Espay AJ, Duker AP, Chen R, Okun MS, Barrett ET, Devoto J, et al. Deep brain stimulation of the ventral intermediate nucleus of the thalamus in medically refractory orthostatic tremor: preliminary observations. Mov Disord Off J Mov Disord Soc. 2008;23(16):2357–62.
32. Muller-Vahl KR, Cath DC, Cavanna AE, Dehning S, Porta M, Robertson MM, et al. European clinical guidelines for Tourette syndrome and other tic disorders. Part IV: deep brain stimulation. Eur Child Adolesc Psychiatry. 2011;20(4):209–17.
33. Huasen B, McCreary R, Evans J, Potter G, Silverdale M. Cervical myelopathy secondary to Tourette's syndrome managed by urgent deep brain stimulation. Mov Disord Off J Mov Disord Soc. 2014;29(4):452–3.
34. Martinez-Fernandez R, Zrinzo L, Aviles-Olmos I, Hariz M, Martinez-Torres I, Joyce E, et al. Deep brain stimulation for Gilles de la Tourette syndrome: a case series targeting subregions of the globus pallidus internus. Mov Disord Off J Mov Disord Soc. 2011;26(10):1922–30.
35. Cubo E, Shannon KM, Penn RD, Kroin JS. Internal globus pallidotomy in dystonia secondary to Huntington's disease. Mov Disord Off J Mov Disord Soc. 2000;15(6):1248–51.
36. Hasegawa H, Mundil N, Samuel M, Jarosz J, Ashkan K. The treatment of persistent vascular hemidystonia-hemiballismus with unilateral GPi deep brain stimulation. Mov Disord Off J Mov Disord Soc. 2009;24(11):1697–8.
37. Damier P, Thobois S, Witjas T, Cuny E, Derost P, Raoul S, et al. Bilateral deep brain stimulation of the globus pallidus to treat tardive dyskinesia. Arch Gen Psychiatry. 2007;64(2):170–6.
38. Clarke RH, Horsley V. THE CLASSIC: on a method of investigating the deep ganglia and tracts of the central nervous system (cerebellum). Br Med J 1906:1799–1800. Clin Orthop Relat Res. 2007;463:3–6.
39. Khan FR, Henderson JM. Deep brain stimulation surgical techniques. Handb Clin Neurol. 2013;116:27–37.
40. Leksell L. The stereotaxic method and radiosurgery of the brain. Acta Chir Scand. 1951;102(4):316–9.
41. Hariz MI, Hariz GM. Therapeutic stimulation versus ablation. Handb Clin Neurol. 2013;116:63–71.
42. Hassler R, Riechert T, Mundinger F, Umbach W, Ganglberger JA. Physiological observations in stereotaxic operations in extrapyramidal motor disturbances. Brain (Journal of Neurology). 1960;83:337–50.
43. Benabid AL, Pollak P, Louveau A, Henry S, de Rougemont J. Combined (thalamotomy and stimulation) stereotactic surgery of the VIM thalamic nucleus for bilateral Parkinson disease. Appl Neurophysiol. 1987,50(1–6):344–6.
44. Olanow CW, Obeso J. Profile of Mahlon DeLong and Alim Benabid, 2014 Lasker-DeBakey Medical Research awardees. Proc Natl Acad Sci U S A. 2014;111(50):17693–5.
45. Agnesi F, Johnson MD, Vitek JL. Deep brain stimulation: how does it work? Handb Clin Neurol. 2013;116:39–54.
46. Kinfe TM, Vesper J. The impact of multichannel microelectrode recording (MER) in deep brain stimulation of the basal ganglia. Acta Neurochir Suppl. 2013;117:27–33.

47. Machado A, Rezai AR, Kopell BH, Gross RE, Sharan AD, Benabid AL. Deep brain stimulation for Parkinson's disease: surgical technique and perioperative management. Mov Disord Off J Mov Disord Soc. 2006;21(Suppl 14):S247–58.
48. Aviles-Olmos I, Kefalopoulou Z, Tripoliti E, Candelario J, Akram H, Martinez-Torres I, et al. Long-term outcome of subthalamic nucleus deep brain stimulation for Parkinson's disease using an MRI-guided and MRI-verified approach. J Neurol Neurosurg Psychiatry. 2014;85(12):1419–25.
49. Patel NK, Plaha P, O'Sullivan K, McCarter R, Heywood P, Gill SS. MRI directed bilateral stimulation of the subthalamic nucleus in patients with Parkinson's disease. J Neurol Neurosurg Psychiatry. 2003;74(12):1631–7.
50. Henderson JM, Tkach J, Phillips M, Baker K, Shellock FG, Rezai AR. Permanent neurological deficit related to magnetic resonance imaging in a patient with implanted deep brain stimulation electrodes for Parkinson's disease: case report. Neurosurgery. 2005;57(5):E1063. discussion E.
51. Oluigbo CO, Rezai AR. Magnetic resonance imaging safety of deep brain stimulator devices. Handb Clin Neurol. 2013;116:73–6.
52. Montgomery EB. Deep brain stimulation programming. Oxford: Oxford University Press; 2010.
53. Ranck Jr JB. Which elements are excited in electrical stimulation of mammalian central nervous system: a review. Brain Res. 1975;98(3):417–40.
54. Holsheimer J, Demeulemeester H, Nuttin B, de Sutter P. Identification of the target neuronal elements in electrical deep brain stimulation. Eur J Neurosci. 2000;12(12):4573–7.
55. Koss AM, Alterman RL, Tagliati M, Shils JL. Calculating total electrical energy delivered by deep brain stimulation systems. Ann Neurol. 2005;58(1):168. author reply -9.
56. Vercueil L, Houeto JL, Krystkowiak P, Lagrange C, Cassim F, Benazzouz A, et al. Effects of pulse width variations in pallidal stimulation for primary generalized dystonia. J Neurol. 2007;254(11):1533–7.
57. Hodgkin AL, Huxley AF. Resting and action potentials in single nerve fibres. J Physiol. 1945;104(2):176–95.
58. Brocker DT, Grill WM. Principles of electrical stimulation of neural tissue. Handb Clin Neurol. 2013;116:3–18.
59. Shin DS, Samoilova M, Cotic M, Zhang L, Brotchie JM, Carlen PL. High frequency stimulation or elevated K+ depresses neuronal activity in the rat entopeduncular nucleus. Neuroscience. 2007;149(1):68–86.
60. Benabid AL, Benazzous A, Pollak P. Mechanisms of deep brain stimulation. Mov Disord Off J Mov Disord Soc. 2002;17(Suppl 3):S73–4.
61. Brittain JS, Sharott A, Brown P. The highs and lows of beta activity in cortico-basal ganglia loops. Eur J Neurosci. 2014;39(11):1951–9.
62. Little S, Brown P. The functional role of beta oscillations in Parkinson's disease. Parkinsonism Relat Disord. 2014;20(Suppl 1):S44–8.
63. Tisch S, Rothwell JC, Bhatia KP, Quinn N, Zrinzo L, Jahanshahi M, et al. Pallidal stimulation modifies after-effects of paired associative stimulation on motor cortex excitability in primary generalised dystonia. Exp Neurol. 2007;206(1):80–5.
64. Dickson DW. Parkinson's disease and parkinsonism: neuropathology. Cold Spring Harb Perspect Med. 2012;2(8).
65. Pollak P. Deep brain stimulation for Parkinson's disease – patient selection. Handb Clin Neurol. 2013;116:97–105.
66. Albanese A, Bhatia K, Bressman SB, Delong MR, Fahn S, Fung VS, et al. Phenomenology and classification of dystonia: a consensus update. Mov Disord Off J Mov Disord Soc. 2013;28(7):863–73.
67. Deuschl G, Bain P, Brin M. Consensus statement of the Movement Disorder Society on Tremor. Ad Hoc Scientific Committee. Mov Disord Off J Mov Disord Soc. 1998;13(Suppl 3):2–23.

68. Phukan J, Albanese A, Gasser T, Warner T. Primary dystonia and dystonia-plus syndromes: clinical characteristics, diagnosis, and pathogenesis. Lancet Neurol. 2011;10(12):1074–85.
69. Balint B, Bhatia KP. Dystonia: an update on phenomenology, classification, pathogenesis and treatment. Curr Opin Neurol. 2014;27(4):468–76.
70. Hallett M. Neurophysiology of dystonia: the role of inhibition. Neurobiol Dis. 2011;42(2):177–84.
71. Sanger TD, Tarsy D, Pascual-Leone A. Abnormalities of spatial and temporal sensory discrimination in writer's cramp. Mov Disord Off J Mov Disord Soc. 2001;16(1):94–9.
72. Jankovic J. Medical treatment of dystonia. Mov Disord Off J Mov Disord Soc. 2013;28(7):1001–12.
73. Walcott BP, Nahed BV, Kahle KT, Duhaime AC, Sharma N, Eskandar EN. Deep brain stimulation for medically refractory life-threatening status dystonicus in children. J Neurosurg Pediatr. 2012;9(1):99–102.
74. Alty JE, Kempster PA. A practical guide to the differential diagnosis of tremor. Postgrad Med J. 2011;87(1031):623–9.
75. Alusi SH, Worthington J, Glickman S, Bain PG. A study of tremor in multiple sclerosis. Brain (A Journal of neurology). 2001;124(Pt 4):720–30.
76. Schneider SA, Deuschl G. Medical and surgical treatment of tremors. Neurol Clin. 2015;33(1):57–75.
77. McNaught KS, Mink JW. Advances in understanding and treatment of Tourette syndrome. Nat Rev Neurol. 2011;7(12):667–76.
78. Kefalopoulou Z, Zrinzo L, Jahanshahi M, Candelario J, Milabo C, Beigi M, et al. Bilateral globus pallidus stimulation for severe Tourette's syndrome: a double-blind, randomised crossover trial. Lancet Neurol. 2015;14(6):595–605.
79. Kojovic M, Cordivari C, Bhatia K. Myoclonic disorders: a practical approach for diagnosis and treatment. Ther Adv Neurol Disord. 2011;4(1):47–62.
80. Kobayashi K, Katayama Y, Otaka T, Obuchi T, Kano T, Nagaoka T, et al. Thalamic deep brain stimulation for the treatment of action myoclonus caused by perinatal anoxia. Stereotact Funct Neurosurg. 2010;88(4):259–63.
81. Novak MJ, Tabrizi SJ. Huntington's disease. BMJ. 2010;340:c3109.
82. Hawley JS, Weiner WJ. Hemiballismus: current concepts and review. Parkinsonism Relat Disord. 2012;18(2):125–9.
83. Walker RH. Differential diagnosis of chorea. Curr Neurol Neurosci Rep. 2011;11(4):385–95.
84. Bhidayasiri R, Boonyawairoj S. Spectrum of tardive syndromes: clinical recognition and management. Postgrad Med J. 2011;87(1024):132–41.
85. Kimmelman J, Duckworth K, Ramsay T, Voss T, Ravina B, Emborg ME. Risk of surgical delivery to deep nuclei: a meta-analysis. Mov Disord Off J Mov Dis Soc. 2011;26(8):1415–21.
86. Thobois S, Ardouin C, Lhommee E, Klinger H, Lagrange C, Xie J, et al. Non-motor dopamine withdrawal syndrome after surgery for Parkinson's disease: predictors and underlying mesolimbic denervation. Brain (A Journal of neurology). 2010;133(Pt 4):1111–27.
87. Volkmann J, Daniels C, Witt K. Neuropsychiatric effects of subthalamic neurostimulation in Parkinson disease. Nat Rev Neurol. 2010;6(9):487–98.
88. Witt K, Daniels C, Reiff J, Krack P, Volkmann J, Pinsker MO, et al. Neuropsychological and psychiatric changes after deep brain stimulation for Parkinson's disease: a randomised, multicentre study. Lancet Neurol. 2008;7(7):605–14.
89. Jahanshahi M, Czernecki V, Zurowski AM. Neuropsychological, neuropsychiatric, and quality of life issues in DBS for dystonia. Mov Disord Off J Mov Disord Soc. 2011;26(Suppl 1):S63–78.
90. Little S, Pogosyan A, Neal S, Zavala B, Zrinzo L, Hariz M, et al. Adaptive deep brain stimulation in advanced Parkinson disease. Ann Neurol. 2013;74(3):449–57.

Chapter 5
Deep Brain Stimulation for Parkinson Disease

Kelvin L. Chou, Emily L. Levin, Parag G. Patil, and Daniel Leventhal

Abstract Deep brain stimulation (DBS) therapy is now considered one of the most important advances in the treatment of Parkinson disease (PD), a progressive neurodegenerative disorder. DBS improves the cardinal motor symptoms of PD (rest tremor, bradykinesia, rigidity), markedly reduces motor complications (dyskinesias and wearing off), and dramatically improves quality of life. In this chapter, we review how DBS came to be and present the current science behind how DBS works. Clinical indications and up-to-date evidence on clinical outcomes of DBS are presented. Finally, the risks and side effects of DBS, and advances in DBS technology are discussed.

Keywords Parkinson disease • Deep brain stimulation • Basal ganglia • Surgery • Tremor • Bradykinesia • Rigidity • Dyskinesias • Motor fluctuations

K.L. Chou, MD (✉)
University of Michigan Medical School,
2301 Commonwealth Blvd., Michigan House Room 1032B,
Ann Arbor, MI 48105-2945, USA
e-mail: klchou@med.umich.edu

E.L. Levin, MD
University of Michigan Health Systems/VA Ann Arbor Healthcare System,
Department of Neurosurgery, Ann Arbor, MI, USA
e-mail: emilyleh@med.umich.edu

P.G. Patil, MD, PhD
University of Michigan, Department of Neurosurgery, Ann Arbor, MI, USA
e-mail: pgpatil@umich.edu

D. Leventhal, MD, PhD
University of Michigan Health Systems/VA Ann Arbor Healthcare System,
Department of Neurology, Ann Arbor, MI, USA
e-mail: dleventh@med.umich.edu

A. Majid (ed.), *Electroceuticals*, DOI 10.1007/978-3-319-28612-9_5

Overview

Deep brain stimulation (DBS) therapy involves the surgical placement of electrodes in precise areas of the brain. These electrodes are then connected by extension wires to a pacemaker-like device in the chest called an implantable pulse generator. The tip of the electrode has four metal rings at the end of it, called "contacts" (see Fig. 5.1). When the stimulator is turned on, electrical impulses travel from the pulse generator, through the extension wires and out the contacts (see Fig. 5.2). The resulting electrical stimulation of the brain can improve the symptoms of many medical conditions.

DBS is currently an established treatment for many movement disorders, including Parkinson disease (PD). PD affects approximately 1% of the population greater than 65 years of age and 2.5% of the population greater than 80 years of age [1]. Between 4.1 and 4.6 million individuals over the age of 50 are affected worldwide and this number is expected to double by the year 2030 [2]. The cardinal features of rest tremor, bradykinesia, rigidity and postural instability progressively worsen over time, and the disease is associated with increased morbidity and a high economic burden. The symptoms of PD respond very well to medications such as levodopa and other dopaminergic agents. These medications can be increased as the motor symptoms of tremor, bradykinesia and rigidity worsen. At some point, however, most patients with PD develop

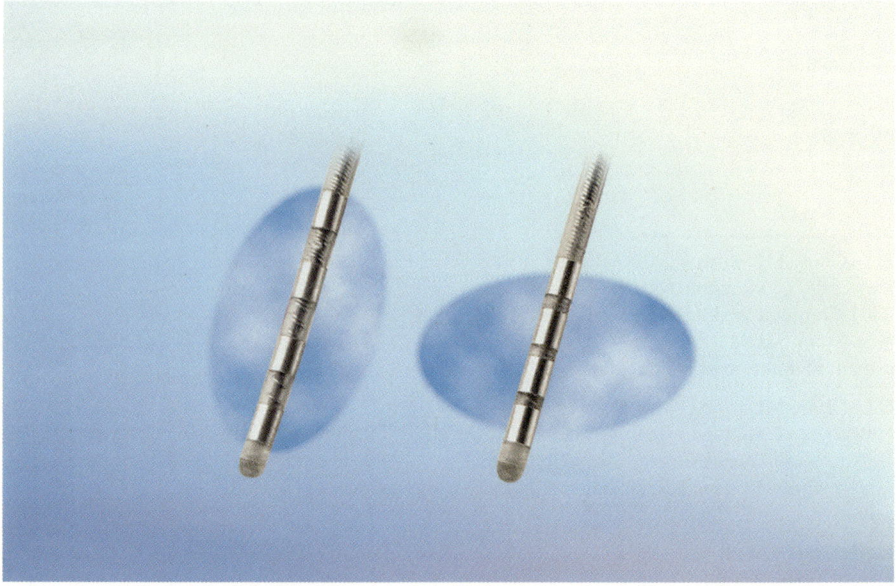

Fig. 5.1 The quadripolar electrodes (leads) used for deep brain stimulation. Each contact on the electrode is 1.5 mm long and 1.27 mm in diameter. On the left is model 3387 (produced by Medtronic), in which the contacts are spaced 1.5 mm apart. On the left is model 3389, in which the contacts are spaced 0.5 mm apart (Reprinted with the permission of Medtronic, Inc. © 2014)

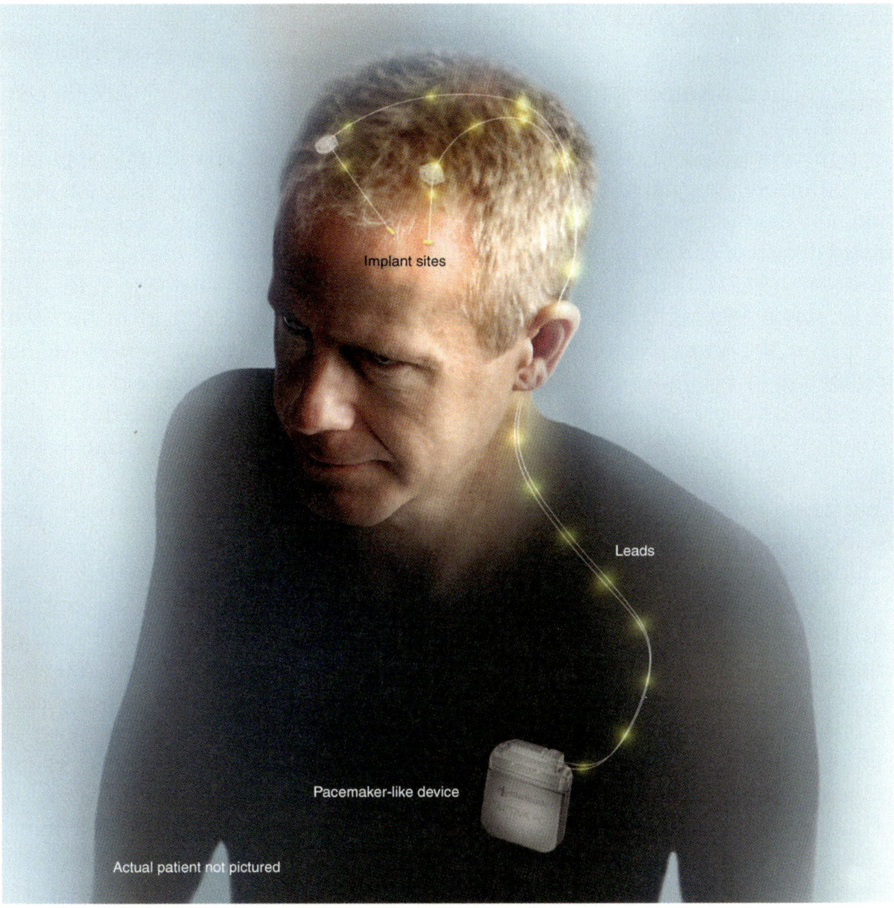

Fig. 5.2 Schematic displaying the implantation of electrodes within the brain. The electrodes are connected by extension wires which travel behind the ear and down to the pulse generator, which is implanted overlying the chest muscles (Reprinted with the permission of Medtronic, Inc. © 2014)

motor complications such as dyskinesias (abnormal involuntary movements) and "wearing off" (recurrence of PD symptoms towards the end of a dose), which can be difficult to manage. DBS markedly improves the wearing off symptoms and dyskinesias in PD. By doing so, a patient's quality of life is also dramatically improved.

DBS is now considered one of the two greatest advances in therapy for the treatment of PD, with the other one being levodopa. In this chapter, we will focus on this life changing therapy for PD. We review how DBS came to be and present the current science behind how DBS works. Clinical indications and clinical outcomes of DBS for PD are presented. Finally, the risks and side effects of DBS, as well as advances in DBS technology are discussed.

History of DBS for Parkinson Disease

Early surgical treatments for movement disorders date to the late nineteenth century. Victor Horsley was a pioneer in this regard and performed cortical motor strip resection to address athetosis and tremor in 1890 [3]. Though this approach helped involuntary movements, it proved undesirable because lesioning the pyramidal system left patients with long-term weakness. The concept of the extrapyramidal system and its possible role in movement disorders was introduced in the 1920s and 1930s, but extrapyramidal structures were not targeted surgically until 1940, when Meyers reported on anterior caudate resections as part of his 1940 series on the treatment of postencephalitic tremor [4]. He demonstrated that tremor could be improved without paresis. However, morbidity and mortality from these open craniotomy procedures remained significant, mainly because of accuracy. The introduction of stereotactically guided frame-based surgery with the first modern stereotactic atlas of the human brain in the late 1940s changed the field of movement disorders surgery [5, 6] because surgery could now be performed with less than 1% mortality [7].

There was a significant increase in stereotactic functional neurosurgery in the 1950s, with Irving Cooper and Rolf Hassler introducing neurosurgical targeting for PD [8]. Part of this rationale emerged after Cooper accidentally tore the anterior choroidal artery during pedunculotomy and observed a dramatic improvement in tremor and rigidity without limb weakness [9]. Cooper concluded that his accident resulted in infarction of the globus pallidus and thalamus, but ligating the anterior choroidal artery did not yield uniform results as the distribution of this artery varied from patient to patient. Spiegel and Wycis are credited with the first direct lesioning of the globus pallidus, though for chorea instead of PD [10, 11]. While clinical effects were somewhat disappointing, the anterodorsal part of the globus pallidus was targeted. Leksell eventually tried the posteroventral pallidum and found that it relieved tremor and rigidity in PD [12]. Around the same time, Hassler and a number of surgeons began to ablate the ventrolateral thalamus at the ventralis oralis anterior/ventralis oralis posterior nuclei (VOA-VOP) to relieve tremor and rigidity for PD [13, 14]. Thalamic lesioning eventually replaced pallidotomy as the surgical treatment for tremor at this time.

Electrical recordings and stimulation began to be used to map out the proximity of other structures in the brain before creating a lesion in the late 1950s and true microelectrode recording was introduced in the early 1960s [15–17]. Because of this, tremorgenic cells, located mostly in the ventralis intermedius (VIM) nucleus, were identified and VIM eventually replaced Voa and Vop as the target for tremor [18]. By the end of the 1960s, microelectrode recording was routinely used for stereotactic movement disorders surgery, but surgery for PD quickly fell out of favor when levodopa was introduced in 1968.

Surgical therapies for PD returned in the 1980s and 1990s because levodopa therapy was associated with debilitating on-off motor fluctuations and dyskinesias as the disease progressed [19]. Laitinen et al., in particular, promoted Leksell's posteroventral pallidotomy as an effective treatment for dyskinesias, rigidity, and bradykinesia in PD [20, 21].

J. Lawrence Pool was the first neurosurgeon to utilize deep brain stimulation in a patient with PD in 1948, stimulating the caudate nucleus. However, the modern era of deep brain stimulation is considered by many to have begun with Alim Louis Benabid, a French neurosurgeon. Benabid and colleagues observed that prolonged high frequency stimulation of the thalamus during lesion localization resulted in a reduction of Parkinsonian tremor [22, 23]. The implantation of deep brain stimulators in the thalamus provided an alternative to lesioning that was reversible, adjustable, and allowed for bilateral treatment [24–26]. However, because only tremor improved with thalamic stimulation, the search for a target that would improve bradykinesia and rigidity ensued.

Laitinen's report of pallidotomy as an effective surgical treatment for PD in 1992 led to increased interest in this target [20, 21]. Before long, many surgeons were trying DBS in the pallidum as an alternative to pallidotomy and reporting good motor outcomes with less risk [27, 28]. At the same time, Benabid's group in Grenoble began targeting the subthalamic nucleus (STN) based on the finding that lesions in this structure in N-methyl-4-phenyl-1,2,3,6-tetrahydropyridine (MPTP) primates dramatically improved tremor, bradykinesia and rigidity without causing ballism [29, 30]. High frequency STN stimulation has since been found to be effective for the cardinal motor symptoms of PD and improve quality of life [31, 32].

How Does DBS Work?

Despite significant advances over the last 10–15 years, explaining how DBS exerts its effect remains an elusive but important goal of translational neuroscience. DBS, while highly successful, does not treat all PD symptoms [33] and may have significant motor and nonmotor side-effects [32]. Furthermore, DBS for investigational indications (e.g., pedunculopontine nucleus stimulation for gait and balance) has shown promise in individuals but inconsistent results at a population level [34]. Finally, observations in DBS patients offer unique insights into extrapyramidal physiology in health and disease, with potential therapeutic implications beyond neuromodulation.

The question of how DBS works may be approached from at least two perspectives. The first is how DBS influences neural elements near the stimulating electrode. When the benefits of DBS were first recognized, their similarity to lesional effects suggested suppression of local neurons. Several experiments support this hypothesis, finding decreased local neuronal firing during or immediately after high frequency pulse trains in rats [35], nonhuman primates [36], and humans [37–40]. Proposed mechanisms include depolarization block [41], somatic hyperpolarization [42], excitation of GABAergic afferents [38], or accumulation (or depletion) of local neuromodulators [37]. Determining which of these mechanisms are responsible for local neuronal inhibition has been difficult, largely because of stimulation artifacts. As it turns out, though, effects on cell bodies may not be the primary determinant of DBS outcomes.

This is because firing rate changes downstream from the stimulated nuclei occur with local neuronal activation. Stimulation of the glutamatergic STN increases globus pallidus, pars externa (GPe) and interna (GPi) firing [43], while stimulating GABAergic nuclei reduces downstream firing. GPi stimulation transiently pauses firing in the basal ganglia recipient thalamus [44, 45], and GPe stimulation suppresses STN and GPi activity [46]. PET [47, 48], fMRI [49], and microdialysis [50] studies are all consistent with increased efferent activity during high frequency DBS. Computational models suggest that somatic hyperpolarization may occur simultaneously with axonal depolarization [42], potentially reconciling local neuronal suppression with efferent activation.

Afferent and passing axons [51] may also be activated by DBS, contributing to somatic inhibition (or excitation) by forcing local neurotransmitter release. More importantly, structures upstream from the target nucleus may be antidromically activated. Recordings consistent with antidromic stimulation have been obtained from motor cortex in animal models [52], as well as patients undergoing thalamic or subthalamic DBS [53–55]. Modeling studies suggest that antidromic stimulation from STN leads is important to modulating network activity [56]. Furthermore, optogenetic experiments in 6-hydroxydopamine (6-OHDA) lesioned mice found that antidromic stimulation of cortical afferents to STN was necessary and sufficient to reduce parkinsonian behavior [57]. It is less clear how pallidal stimulation might antidromically activate motor cortex, though a sparse cortico-pallidal pathway has been identified [58]. Stimulation of passing capsular fibers could also antidromically activate motor cortex [59], but this does not appear to be a significant effect. One study also showed short latency inhibition of motor cortex with pallidal DBS in an MPTP treated monkey [60], though the mechanism and significance of this finding are unclear.

Given that DBS likely activates local afferent, efferent, and passing axons, the next goal is to understand how DBS modulates cortical-basal ganglia-thalamic circuits and motor output. This is a significantly more difficult problem because basal ganglia physiology and pathophysiology are only partially understood. The "rate" model [61, 62], which suggests that basal ganglia neuronal firing rates uniquely determine motor output, has dominated basal ganglia physiology for over 20 years. This model makes many accurate predictions, but is clearly incomplete. In fact, much of the evidence inconsistent with it comes from the surgical treatment of Movement Disorders [63]. For example, the rate model predicts that decreased basal ganglia output should induce uncontrollable movements, but pallidotomy treats chorea and dystonia.

While a comprehensive model of basal ganglia function remains elusive, there are clear differences between normal basal ganglia physiology and the pathophysiology of PD. Patients with PD and dopamine-depleted animals exhibit enhanced neuronal burst firing, oscillations, and synchrony [63]. To variable degrees, DBS restores each of these factors towards their normal state.

Bursts may be defined as brief episodes of high frequency firing against slower background activity, and are found throughout the cortical-basal ganglia-thalamic network in dopamine-depleted subjects [63]. Therapeutic, but not subtherapeutic, GPe [46] and STN [64] DBS reduce GPi bursting. Conversely, low frequency STN DBS, which may exacerbate Parkinsonism, increases GPi bursting [65]. In humans, effective GPi DBS also reduced GPi burst-firing [66], though conflicting results were obtained in MPTP-treated monkeys [67]. Clinically effective STN [65, 68] or GPe [46] DBS is also associated with decreased basal ganglia-recipient thalamic bursting compared to the "off" state. Motor cortical bursting is observed in dopamine-depleted subjects, but has different characteristics compared to basal ganglia bursts [69] and is not diminished by pallidal DBS [59].

Enhanced oscillatory power in single unit and local field potential (LFP) recordings throughout the cortical-basal ganglia-thalamic network are consistently identified in parkinsonian subjects [63]. Oscillations in lower frequencies (~5–20 Hz) are suppressed by subthalamic DBS [68, 70, 71], though the clinical correlates of these oscillations are controversial. Inactivation of the STN in tremulous monkeys eliminates tremor and 8–20 Hz, but not 4–8 Hz, pallidal oscillations [72]. In contrast, single unit oscillations in the cerebellar-recipient thalamus near 5 Hz are highly coherent with rest tremor in humans [73], and correspond temporally to tremor episodes in monkeys [74]. Whether VIM DBS suppresses these low frequency oscillations has not been directly tested, however. Enhanced beta band (~15–30 Hz) power is correlated with bradykinesia and rigidity, and suppressed by both subthalamic [75, 76] and pallidal [59] stimulation coincident with clinical improvement.

"Synchrony" describes two or more events that occur nearly simultaneously, and may refer to single unit spikes, LFP phase across recording sites, or consistent relationships between single unit spikes and LFP phase. Under normal physiologic conditions in awake animals, basal ganglia and motor cortical neurons rarely fire synchronously [77]. After dopamine depletion, however, single unit oscillations in the GPi, GPe, and STN become highly synchronized with each other [71, 78], and basal ganglia-cortical oscillations are more tightly coupled [79]. It has been suggested that excessive synchrony, potentially mediated by neuronal entrainment to enhanced LFP oscillations, limits flexibility in behavioral control [79–81]. For example, if circuits controlling agonist/antagonist muscle pairs cannot operate independently, rigidity would result. Pallidal [59, 67] and subthalamic [79] DBS reduce LFP coherence and single unit synchrony, potentially decoupling pathologically entrained networks. In summary, therapeutic DBS reduces burst firing in the basal ganglia and thalamus (but perhaps not cortex), and suppresses exaggerated oscillations and synchrony throughout the cortical-basal ganglia-thalamic network.

How these physiologic changes translate into clinical improvement is not known, but DBS probably modulates motor function by altering corticospinal activity. In the rate model, motor output is determined by thalamic drive to motor cortex, which is determined by basal ganglia output firing rates. This traditional view of basal ganglia physiology ignores other inputs to "motor" thalamus, especially corticothalamic fibers. Indeed, given the clinical effectiveness of pallidotomy, it appears that recurrent thalamocortical loops can function without pallidal input [though palli-

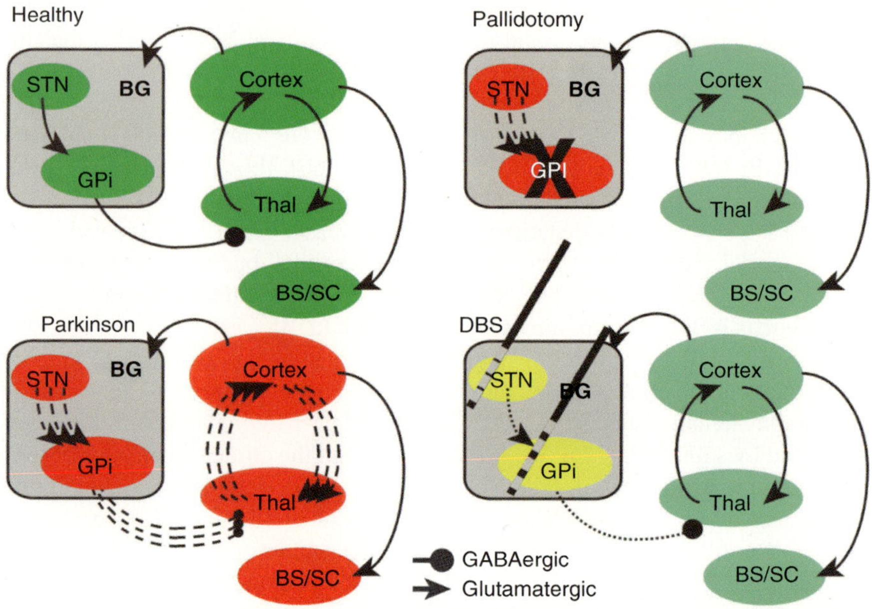

Fig. 5.3 Simplified schematic of possible DBS effects on thalamocortical circuits. In healthy subjects, pallidal input to the thalamus modulates ongoing thalamocortical loops. In PD, synchronized oscillations from the BG disrupt normal thalamocortical function. Eliminating pathologic BG output (pallidotomy) or entraining it to high frequency pallidal or subthalamic stimulation restores thalmocortical circuits toward normal function. This simplified model conveys broad principles of how DBS might work, though it ignores site-specific differences in clinical and physiologic effects. *BS/SC* brain stem/spinal cord, *GPi* globus pallidua, pars interna, *STN* subthalamic nucleus

dotomy patients have specific deficits, particularly in implicit learning – [82]]. It is more likely that pallidothalamic activity regulates the fine timing of thalamic spiking than suppressing it entirely [83, 84]. The bursting, oscillating, synchronous pallidal output of PD disrupts normal thalamocortical function, which can be partially restored by either eliminating pallidal output or entraining it to high frequency stimulation (See Fig. 5.3) [85]. The importance of pallidothalamic spike timing is highlighted by the efficacy of low frequency closed loop DBS, in which pallidal stimulation is triggered by cortical action potentials [86]. Whether direct connections between the basal ganglia and brainstem or antidromic cortical activation also contribute to the clinical effects of DBS is unknown.

The data described above might explain DBS mechanisms for bradykinesia and rigidity, but the physiology of parkinsonian tremor is poorly understood [87]. DBS of the STN, GPi, and VIM thalamus all improve tremor, even when refractory to dopamine replacement. However, VIM thalamus receives its subcortical afferents from the cerebellum. It remains unclear why a (usually) dopa-responsive symptom such as parkinsonian tremor responds to stimulation of cerebellar pathways. Phrased another way, it is not clear why tremor is dopa-responsive when cerebellothalamic pathways are clearly involved in its pathophysiology [88]. Furthermore, neither STN nor GPi are directly connected to VIM thalamus. STN/pallidal stimulation may improve tremor via recently described bidirectional subthalamocerebellar pathways [89]. Alternatively, basal ganglia DBS may activate passing cerebellothalamic axons [33]. Finally, the basal ganglia and cerebellar-recipient thalamus may interact via recurrent connections with motor cortex [63].

Finally, it is not known why certain PD symptoms resolve over different time periods. For example, tremor tends to respond within seconds to DBS, but often returns within weeks of initial programming. Rigidity improves over seconds to minutes, but may continue to improve over weeks. Bradykinesia improves over days to weeks. Presumably delayed effects (or side-effects) result either from alterations in synaptic plasticity or intrinsic neuronal excitability, but how and where this occurs remains unknown.

DBS for Parkinson Disease: Clinical Indications

Successful DBS outcomes result from the selection of appropriate surgical candidates. Because there are risks associated with the surgery, it should only be offered to patients in whom the risk to benefit ratio is favorable. For PD, DBS is typically considered when patients have motor fluctuations that interfere with their quality of life despite optimal medical management. Motor fluctuations include dyskinesias, wearing off, and the on-off phenomena, and tend to occur several years into the disease [90]. It has been common practice to wait until patients are more advanced in their symptoms before referring them for DBS because of the surgical risk. However, a recent trial (the EARLYSTIM study) demonstrated that STN DBS, when performed as soon as motor fluctuations are present, improves motor outcomes as well as quality of life beyond best medical therapy [91]. While there are currently trials investigating the safety of DBS in an even earlier stage of PD (i.e. within a couple of years of diagnosis) [92, 93], with the hope of initiating a larger phase 3 trial to see if DBS can slow down clinical progression, there is no clear evidence to refer patients for this reason at this time. Other appropriate candidates for DBS include those with medication-refractory Parkinsonian tremor [22, 94, 95] or those with dopaminergic medication-induced side effects such as nausea, orthostatic, or impulse-control disorders [96, 97]. Most DBS centers have set protocols for evaluating potential candidates; not all PD patients will be suitable candidates [98, 99].

Surgical candidates should be thoroughly evaluated using a comprehensive, multidisciplinary process [100]. One of these evaluations is a visit with a movement disorders specialist to make sure that the diagnosis is correct and that patients have been tried on appropriate medications. An accurate diagnosis of PD is essential because patients with atypical Parkinsonian syndromes such as progressive supranuclear palsy, multiple system atrophy, dementia with Lewy bodies, corticobasal degeneration, or vascular Parkinsonism respond poorly to DBS [101–104]. Yet, these patients are often referred. Okun et al. reviewed the records of 41 patients at their center who had been characterized as DBS failures and found that 12% had diagnoses other than PD, and would not be expected to respond to DBS [103]. Because of the risk of surgery, it is reasonable to try patients on maximally tolerated doses of levodopa, dopamine agonists, dopamine extenders (catechol-O-methyltransferase (COMT) inhibitors and monoamine oxidase type B (MAO-B) inhibitors) before considering surgery. Amantadine for dyskinesias and trihexyphenidyl or other anticholinergics for tremor should also be considered. Many patients can delay surgery with medication adjustments.

Dopaminergic responsiveness is perhaps the best indicator of a good motor outcome from DBS surgery [99, 105, 106]. The motor symptoms that respond to dopaminergic medication also respond well to DBS. On the other hand, dopaminergic resistant symptoms such as speech, postural instability and freezing of gait are generally unresponsive to DBS. Tremor is the one exception to this rule. Parkinson patients whose primary goals are to improve these symptoms are thus poor candidates. Several long-term studies have shown that speech and postural instability continue to progress after DBS despite changes in stimulation parameters [106–111]. Evaluation of dopaminergic response should be performed in all PD patients being considered for DBS. Patients should first be examined with the Unified Parkinson Disease Rating Scale (UPDRS) or the Movement Disorders Society revision of the Unified Parkinson Disease Rating Scale (MDS-UPDRS) in the medication-off state (practically defined as the condition after not receiving PD medications for 12 h) [112]. After giving a levodopa challenge dose (either suprathreshold or the patient's typical levodopa dose) and the patient reports that the medication is working, the exam is repeated. The best surgical candidates are those whose performance improves significantly (total 25–50% reduction in their motor score) [113].

Exclusionary criteria for DBS in PD include significant cognitive impairment and patients with active psychiatric disease [114, 115]. Patients with dementia and significant cognitive impairment may be unable to provide appropriate feedback during intraoperative testing or postoperative programming. Many aspects of cognition may worsen after DBS and in some PD patients with preexisting cognitive impairment, cognition may worsen irreversibly [116–118]. Because of this, preoperative DBS screening for dementia with neuropsychological testing is a mandatory part of the evaluation. The exact neuropsychological tests that are used to determine dementia may vary from center to center.

Suicidality and depression after DBS for PD has also been reported [119–123]. While the reason for this is unclear, it is typically associated with stimulation of the STN. Additionally, patients with preoperative depression or previous suicide attempts may be more likely to develop postoperative depression [119, 123]. Given this, patients should be screened for psychiatric issues. It is reasonable to delay surgery for patients with active psychiatric illness until their symptoms are stabilized. Furthermore, close monitoring of patients post-operatively who may be at higher risk for suicide should be considered [121, 124].

There have been conflicting studies on whether age affects DBS outcomes. Some centers use 70 or 75 years of age as a cutoff for surgery because many studies have used these ages as cutoffs for inclusion. Additionally, some studies have demonstrated that patients under 70 tend to experience greater motor improvement than patients over 70 [106, 125]. It is also thought that advancing age may be associated with more postoperative complications. However, a recent study found that PD patients older than 75 years of age did not have greater complications at 90 days post-operatively compared to younger patients [126]. This suggests that there should not be an age cutoff for surgery.

DBS for Parkinson Disease: Clinical Outcomes

There are two main DBS targets for PD: the STN and GPi. Both STN and GPi stimulation improve the cardinal symptoms of PD as well as motor fluctuations [32, 127, 128]. Other DBS targets for PD include the VIM thalamus and the pedunculopontine nucleus (PPN). The VIM target reduces parkinsonian tremor [129], but does not significantly improve bradykinesia, rigidity, or motor fluctuations. PPN stimulation is investigational for gait problems and freezing in PD [130–132].

Stimulation of the Subthalamic Nucleus (STN) and Globus Pallidus Interna (GPi)

STN and GPi Stimulation Compared to Best Medical Therapy

Several randomized clinical trials over the last decade have firmly established that both STN and GPi stimulation are effective for patients with moderate to severe PD when compared to best medical therapy [31, 91, 127, 133]. Although stimulation does not improve patients beyond the benefit obtained from dopaminergic medications (best "on" time), DBS can increase the amount of "on" time, reduce wearing off, and reduce dyskinesia.

The first randomized trial showing that stimulation was superior to best medical therapy in PD was published by Deuschl et al. in 2006 [31]. In this landmark trial, 156 advanced PD patients were randomized to either bilateral STN DBS or best medical therapy. The primary outcome of quality of life, as measured by the Parkinson Disease Questionnaire (PDQ-39) was significantly improved at 6 months in the DBS group compared to the medication group. Motor function, as measured by the UPDRS part 3, was also improved in the DBS group at 6 months. However, one limitation of this study was that the evaluations were not blinded. The Veterans Affairs Cooperative Studies Program thus conducted a multicenter, randomized, blinded trial of bilateral deep brain stimulation versus best medical therapy in advanced PD [127]. PD patients who received either STN or GPi stimulation (n = 121) gained 4.6 h per day of additional "on" time without troubling dyskinesias when compared to patients managed with medication alone (n = 134) at 6 months [127]. Additionally, 71% of DBS patients had meaningful clinical improvement in motor function compared to only 32% of those randomized to best medical therapy, and the DBS group had significant improvements in quality-of-life scores. Okun et al. published the results of a constant-current DBS device implanted in the bilateral STN in 136 advanced PD patients [133]. Twenty-five percent of the patients had their stimulation turned on at 3 months instead of immediately. While this was not a blinded study, the immediate stimulation group had 2.51 h of more "on" time at 3 months than the delayed stimulation group. Finally, the EARLYSTIM study demonstrated that STN DBS improved quality of life at 2 years compared to best medical therapy in 251 PD patients (mean age, 52 years and mean disease duration, 7.5 years) within 2 years of experiencing motor fluctuations [91]. Secondary motor outcomes were also improved in the stimulation group at 2 years.

STN Versus GPi Stimulation

A couple of early nonrandomized studies comparing STN to GPi stimulation suggested that the STN might be a better target. The Deep Brain Stimulation for Parkinson's Disease Study Group enrolled 96 patients with STN DBS and 38 patients with GPi DBS [134]. At 3 months, the STN group had a median improvement in UPDRS motor scores of 49% compared to 37% in the GPi group. Another study conducted by Krause et al. suggested that the STN was a superior target for all PD symptoms, while the GPi was the superior target for ameliorating dyskinesias [135]. Many of the early open label studies also suggested that STN stimulation allowed patients to reduce dopaminergic medications and required lower stimulation settings [134, 136], while GPi stimulation appeared to be associated with slightly less cognitive and behavioral side effects [27, 109, 137].

The first randomized prospective trial comparing STN to GPi DBS was performed by Burchiel et al. [138]. They found no difference in off medication UPDRS motor scores between the two groups after 12 months. While dopaminergic doses were able to be decreased in the STN group but not the GPi group, the trial was too small (4 GPi vs. 5 STN patients) to draw firm conclusions. The Veterans Affairs Cooperative Studies Program then conducted a large head-to-head randomized, multicenter trial of STN vs. GPi stimulation in PD [32]. In this trial, 299 subjects were randomized and followed up to 24 months. Both stimulation sites were equally effective on motor symptoms based on the UPDRS motor score, but the STN group had greater decline in processing speed on a cognitive task at 24 months compared to the GPi group. Additionally, the Beck Depression Inventory score worsened by approximately 1 point in the STN group and improved by about 1 point in the GPi group. It is unclear whether or not these differences are clinically meaningful. Similar to earlier nonrandomized and open label studies, the STN stimulation group was able to be titrated to lower doses of dopaminergic medications postoperatively.

The STN group also had lower stimulation amplitudes and pulse widths, which may allow for longer intervals between pulse generator replacement.

Of the 299 subjects in the VA study, 198 consented to be followed for up to 36 months [128]. The amount of improvement in the UPDRS motor score continued, with no difference between the two groups, though changes in quality of life deteriorated after 6 months in both groups. Though on-stimulation/off-medication motor performance was similar between both targets, dopaminergic medications had a less robust benefit in the STN group compared to the GPi group. The mild difference in depression scores seen at 24 months were no longer seen at 36 months. Compared to those undergoing GPi stimulation, STN stimulation patients also had mild worsening in performance on verbal learning testing as well as more rapid decline in Mattis Dementia Rating scale scores at 36 months [128].

Finally, the Netherlands Subthalamic and Pallidal Stimulation (NSTAPS) study was a randomized controlled trial involving 65 patients randomized to GPi and 63 randomized to STN DBS [139]. The primary outcome in this study was functional health, as measured by the weighted Academic Medical Center Linear Disability Scale, and a composite score for cognitive, mood, and behavioral effects. At a year after surgery, there were no differences in these primary outcomes, but the on-stimulation/off-medication motor scores and amount of medication reduction favored the STN group.

Taking all of the above studies into account, it is clear that either target is appropriate for treating the motor symptoms of PD. However, target selection might differ depending on the relative importance of specific non-motor outcomes. As an example, some centers might choose to target GPi rather than STN in a PD patient with mild cognitive impairment or mild depression, while PD patients with side effects from dopaminergic medications might benefit more from STN stimulation because of the ability to reduce medication doses.

Long-Term Outcomes of GPi and STN Stimulation

Though there might be some deterioration in bradykinesia and axial symptoms over time, STN DBS continues to be effective on the three cardinal PD symptoms of tremor, rigidity, and bradykinesia for up to 10 years [107, 140, 141]. Nonetheless, PD continues to progress and patients may develop levodopa unresponsive symptoms such as dementia. Other dopaminergic-resistant features, such as speech, gait, and postural instability, also continue to decline despite long-term stimulation [107, 109, 111, 142].

The longest follow-up study for pallidal stimulation monitored 16 GPi patients at 5–6 years after DBS surgery [143]. The stimulation effect on the motor UPDRS was assessed in the off-medication state in a double blind cross-over fashion (i.e. with stimulation off for 2 h and after 2 h after switching stimulation on [sequence A] or the reverse [sequence B]). GPi DBS was associated with a 20% improvement in the UPDRS motor score in blinded evaluations, and an approximately 35% improvement in unblinded evaluations.

Quality-of-life measures have been shown to improve with DBS of both targets for PD. These improvements can be sustained long-term [144–146], though many initial benefits in quality of life may be lost over time [146]. These improvements may occur because of motor benefit [147], but may also occur because of improvements in mood [120]. Not all PD patients undergoing DBS have satisfactory results. Some may not notice significant improvement in motor function. Some of these deep brain stimulation "failures," may be improved by re-implantation because of suboptimal lead locations [103]. Others may improve with stimulation adjustments by an expert programmer at a DBS center [103, 148]. Unfortunately, 34% of deep brain stimulation "failures" referred to a DBS center could not be improved [103], with the most common reason for failure being implantation in a patient unlikely to benefit from DBS (i.e. misdiagnosis or with symptoms unlikely to improve from stimulation).

Thalamic Stimulation

As mentioned earlier, the modern era of DBS began when Benabid et al. discovered that PD tremor was reduced with high frequency stimulation prior to making a lesion [22, 23]. Less than a decade later, the VIM nucleus of the thalamus became the first US Food and Drug Administration (FDA) approved site for DBS, with an indication for Parkinsonian or other tremor.

The largest series of PD patients undergoing VIM stimulation for Parkinsonian tremor was reported by Limousin and colleagues [149]. In this study, 73 patients with Parkinsonian tremor were enrolled, and tremor scores improved by at least 50% in 85% of the patients at 1 year. Thirty-eight of these patients were re-evaluated at a mean of 6.6 years postoperatively [150]. The tremor contralateral to the DBS electrode in these patients continued to be as well controlled at 6 years as they were a year after surgery. Interestingly, total UPDRS motor scores in this patient population did not change between 1 and 6 years, suggesting that tremor predominant patients have little progression of disease.

In other long-term studies, thalamic DBS has been shown to be safe and effective for parkinsonian tremor, but not bradykinesia or rigidity [95, 151]. Thalamic DBS for PD is mostly done unilaterally, since bilateral stimulation can be associated with significant dysarthria, paresthesias and ataxia [26, 115]. Because STN and GPi stimulation can treat all symptoms of PD and can be done bilaterally with fewer side effects, many DBS centers opt to treat tremor predominant PD patients with STN or GPi stimulation instead.

Pedunculopontine Nucleus (PPN) Stimulation

Because levodopa unresponsive symptoms such as gait and postural instability continue to progress despite pallidal or STN stimulation, there has been interest in exploring other targets for gait dysfunction in PD. The pedunculopontine nucleus (PPN) is thought to mediate gait freezing and postural instability in PD [152]. While no large scale randomized controlled trials have been looked at PPN stimulation, several case series have demonstrated the safety of low-frequency stimulation of the PPN in PD patients. Unfortunately, results for this target are mixed for gait dysfunction [130, 131, 153].

PPN stimulation may also help more than just gait. An open label study of six patients with both PPN and STN electrodes showed fairly similar improvement in UPDRS motor scores with PPN stimulation and STN stimulation alone [154]. When both targets were stimulated simultaneously, there was even more improvement in motor symptoms. Such a synergistic effect was also seen in another open label series with PPN and caudal zona incerta stimulation [155]. PPN stimulation may also affect cognitive and sleep dysfunction in PD [156, 157]. However, because of the small numbers reported in the literature, this target remains experimental. Further studies are needed to better characterize the efficacy of this target on the various symptoms of PD.

Surgical Risks and Side Effects of Stimulation

DBS complications may be related to the surgical procedure, the hardware, or stimulation (see Table 5.1). Due to the lack of standardized guidelines for reporting adverse events, though, the published medical literature may underestimate the prevalence of DBS-related complications [158].

Surgical Risks

A recently published series of over 500 consecutive patients showed an overall procedure complication rate of 11.2 ± 2.03% [159]. Specific complications include those associated with any neurosurgical procedure, such as subdural hematoma, venous infarction, CSF leak, pulmonary embolism, pneumonia, bleeding, wound infection, postoperative seizures, and perioperative confusion. In addition, DBS procedures are associated with a ~3% chance of intracerebral hemorrhage [159, 160]. Only 0.6–1.6% of implantations are associated with neurologic deficit, however [160–162]. Patients with hypertension are at higher risk for intracerebral hemorrhage. The risk also increases with the number of electrode passes needed [134, 163, 164]. While it had previously been thought that risk of hemorrhage increased with age, this was not borne out in at least one study [126].

Hardware-Related Complications

Hardware-related complications have been estimated to occur in 5–9% of patients [159, 165]. Such complications may include infection, device malfunction such as electrode/wire break or implantable pulse generator malfunction, skin erosion, and

Table 5.1 Complications of deep brain stimulation for Parkinson disease

Related to procedure
Intracerebral hemorrhage
Subdural hematoma
Venous infarction
Postoperative seizure
CSF leak
Wound infection
Pulmonary embolisum
Pneumonia
Perioperative confusion
Related to hardware
Infection
Skin erosion
Electrode/wire break
Pulse generator malfunction
Lead migration
Related to stimulation
All targets
Dysarthria
Paresthesias
Motor contractions
Specific to thalamic stimulation
Postural instability
Ataxia
Limb weakness
Specific to GPi stimulation
Blurry vision
Light flashes
Worsening akinesia
Specific to STN stimulation
Diplopia/ocular deviation
Lightheadedness
Sweating
Dyskinesias
Hemiballismus
Dysphagia
Apraxia of eyelid opening
Weight gain
Cognitive impairment
Psychiatric symptoms (depression, suicide, anxiety, apathy, hypomania, impulse control disorders)

lead migration [162, 165]. Diathermy, a form of treatment involving the production of heat in a part of the body by high-frequency electric currents, is contraindicated in someone with a DBS system. In one patient, induction of a radiofrequency current and heating of the electrodes by diathermy caused damage to the brain [166]. In another patient, a brain lesion was produced by the heating of a DBS electrode associated with MRI of the lumbar spine [167]. Thus, MRI of any part of the body other than brain is contraindicated after having DBS. MRI of the brain is believed to be safe in DBS patients as long as the manufacturer's recommendations are followed [168, 169].

Stimulation-Related Effects

Stimulation-related side effects vary with the surgical target, and can often be minimized with reprogramming. Stimulation-related side effects of VIM stimulation include dysarthria, paresthesias, dystonia, postural instability, ataxia, and limb weakness [129, 170, 171]. Stimulation-related side effects related to pallidal stimulation may include blurry vision or light flashes, dysarthria, paresthesias, or motor contractions [134, 172, 173].

Common side effects of STN stimulation include dysarthria, paresthesias, motor contractions, diplopia, lightheadedness, sweating, dyskinesias, or hemiballismus [174–177]. Other side effects of STN stimulation that have been reported include apraxia of eyelid opening, weight gain, cognitive impairment, impaired recognition of emotions, and psychiatric symptoms such as impulse control disorders, depression, anxiety, apathy, and hypomania [109, 111, 178–180]. Apraxia of eyelid opening is infrequent, and the mechanism is poorly understood. The weight gain usually happens in the first 3 months after surgery [181], but may continue in many patients [182, 183]. The underlying mechanism remains unclear but may be related to reduction of energy output, improved alimentation, or a direct influence on lateral hypothalamic function. In a perioperative study evaluating brain metabolism with PET imaging up to 4 months after DBS placement, weight gain was associated with changes in brain metabolism in limbic and associative areas, indicating a possible mechanism [180].

Cognitive and psychiatric effects post-DBS have been well studied in recent years [184–186]. In general, there does not appear to be any major decline in global cognitive functioning after GPi or STN DBS in appropriately selected patients. However, in most studies of STN DBS, verbal fluency and executive dysfunction consistently decline after surgery [128, 187, 188]. Psychiatric effects have also been reported more with STN DBS as opposed to GPi DBS, though it is not always clear if it is due to stimulation or the procedure. Elevated suicide, depression, hypomania and impulse control disorders have all been reported to occur or worsen with STN DBS [121–123, 189, 190]. However, in the head-to-head studies comparing GPi to STN stimulation, GPi has not been unequivocally demonstrated to be a better target with respect to neuropsychological side effects [128, 139].

Future Directions and Advances in DBS Technology

As a technologically intensive therapy, it is logical that many of the advances in DBS would come through technological innovations. Over the past decade, developments in both surgical technique and device design have increased accessibility to the surgery and improved efficiency. Future developments will hopefully improve efficacy and decrease side effects.

Intraoperative Image Guidance for Electrode Insertion

Traditionally, DBS surgery for PD has relied on pre-operative imaging, utilizing a skull-mounted stereotactic frame, and confirmation of electrode placement with microelectrode recording and test stimulation in an awake patient off Parkinson medications. It is therefore difficult to perform the surgery in patients who cannot tolerate their Parkinson symptoms when withdrawn from medications or in those with severe anxiety regarding frame placement or awake surgery. Recent technological breakthroughs now allow the use of real-time intraoperative imaging with MRI or CT to permit accurate DBS electrode placement in patients under general anesthesia [191–193]. Intraoperative visualization of the target utilizing MRI permits adjustments to account for any brain shift that may occur with intracranial air or guide tube placement. Outcomes have been promising. In an early prospective series of patients implanted in the STN utilizing interventional MRI, clinical outcomes, including improvement in UPDRS III score, were similar to published outcomes for traditional DBS electrode placement [194]. The accuracy of DBS electrode placement for CT and MRI guided techniques is reported as 0.8–1.2 mm for MRI and 1.59 mm for CT [191, 194, 195]. Li et al., have proposed the addition of an MR-compatible robotic arm to further enhance the accuracy of electrode placement [196]. While these techniques improve our ability to precisely place an electrode deep within the brain, experience and understanding of the best anatomical target are still required to achieve the best outcomes.

Developments in Implanted Hardware

Current Steering and Field Shaping

Often the therapeutic window of deep brain stimulation is limited by side effects caused by undesirable electrical stimulation of structures surrounding the target of interest. Implantable electrodes currently on the market consist of four cylindrical contacts arranged longitudinally at the distal tip of the lead. By using monopolar or bipolar stimulation through different contacts, the volume of the region stimulated may be controlled. With current lead designs, the volume stimulated is typically arranged symmetrically around the lead, forming a spherical or ellipsoid region of stimulation. Electrodes currently being evaluated have 12–32 contacts at the distal end of the lead, which allows for "directional steering" of the stimulation current [197]. This may help to enhance stimulation at the target while avoiding stimulation of surrounding structures [198].

Closed Loop Stimulation

Current implanted pulse generators for DBS output a constant stream of stimulation, without regard to patients' current symptoms or brain physiology. This may be likened to previous generation cardiac pacemakers, which provided a pacing signal regardless of whether it was needed. Current cardiac pacemakers are capable of analyzing heart rhythms to determine when stimulation is required. Research is progressing to determine what brain signals may be used to provide an appropriate feedback signal [199, 200]. Recordings of local field potentials surrounding the DBS electrode [201, 202] and at the motor cortex [79] have noted abnormal synchronization, particularly in the beta range, in patients with PD. STN DBS has been found to abolish this abnormal synchronization [203]. In a short-term clinical trial of closed loop stimulation using STN beta local field potentials, the amount of time spent with stimulation in the on state was reduced by approximately 50%, with an improvement in motor symptoms similar to continuous DBS [204]. By reducing the time of active stimulation, it may be possible to maintain or improve efficacy while preserving battery life.

Conclusions

DBS has been a revolutionary advance for patients suffering from PD. The discovery that DBS could improve PD symptoms (beginning with tremor) was serendipitous, but we are finally coming to understand how DBS works to exert its effect. DBS improves the cardinal features of tremor, bradykinesia and rigidity, and reduces motor complications from levodopa therapy. While there are certainly risks associated with the procedure, the benefits can be dramatic for appropriately selected patients. Surgical techniques have improved over the years and as more centers are established, patients will have increased accessibility to this life changing procedure. The technology behind DBS hardware continues to improve and we envision that DBS will continue to be a mainstay of PD therapy for years to come.

References

1. Nussbaum RL, Ellis CE. Alzheimer's disease and Parkinson's disease. N Engl J Med. 2003;348(14):1356–64.
2. Dorsey ER, Constantinescu R, Thompson JP, Biglan KM, Holloway RG, Kieburtz K, et al. Projected number of people with Parkinson disease in the most populous nations, 2005 through 2030. Neurology. 2007;68(5):384–6.
3. Horsley V. Remarks on the surgery of the central nervous system. Br Med J. 1890;2(1562):1286–92.

4. Meyers R. Surgical procedures for postencephalitic tremor with notes on the physiology of premotor fibers. Arch Neurol Psychiatry. 1940;44:453–9.
5. Gildenberg PL. Spiegel and Wycis – the early years. Stereotact Funct Neurosurg. 2001;77(1–4):11–6.
6. Speigel EA, Wycis HT, Marks M, Lee AJ. Stereotaxic apparatus for operations on the human brain. Science. 1947;106:349–50.
7. Gildenberg PL. Evolution of basal ganglia surgery for movement disorders. Stereotact Funct Neurosurg. 2006;84(4):131–5.
8. Das K, Benzil DL, Rovit RL, Murali R, Couldwell WT, Irving S. Cooper (1922–1985): a pioneer in functional neurosurgery. J Neurosurg. 1998;89(5):865–73.
9. Cooper IS. Surgical alleviation of Parkinsonism; effects of occlusion of the anterior choroidal artery. J Am Geriatr Soc. 1954;2(11):691–718.
10. Spiegel EA, Wycis HT. Pallidothalamotomy in chorea. Arch Neurol Psychiatry. 1950;64(2):295–6.
11. Wycis HT, Spiegel EA. The effect of thalamotomy and pallidotomy upon involuntary movements in chorea and athetosis. Surg Forum. 1950:329–32.
12. Svennilson E, Torvik A, Lowe R, Leksell L. Treatment of parkinsonism by stereotatic thermolesions in the pallidal region. A clinical evaluation of 81 cases. Acta Psychiatr Scand. 1960;35:358–77.
13. Hassler R, Riechert T, Mundinger F, Umbach W, Ganglberger JA. Physiological observations in stereotaxic operations in extrapyramidal motor disturbances. Brain. 1960;83: 337–50.
14. Redfern RM. History of stereotactic surgery for Parkinson's disease. Br J Neurosurg. 1989;3(3):271–304.
15. Andy OJ, Jurko MF, Sias Jr FR. Subthalamotomy in treatment of Parkinsonian tremor. J Neurosurg. 1963;20:860–70.
16. Schwalb JM, Hamani C. The history and future of deep brain stimulation. Neurotherapeutics. 2008;5(1):3–13.
17. Yamashiro K, Tasker RR. Microstimulation for stereotactic neurosurgery. Stereotact Funct Neurosurg. 1990;54–55:168–71.
18. Tasker RR, Organ LW, Hawrylyshyn P. Sensory organization of the human thalamus. Appl Neurophysiol. 1976;39(3–4):139–53.
19. Narabayashi H, Yokochi F, Nakajima Y. Levodopa-induced dyskinesia and thalamotomy. J Neurol Neurosurg Psychiatry. 1984;47(8):831–9.
20. Laitinen LV, Bergenheim AT, Hariz MI. Leksell's posteroventral pallidotomy in the treatment of Parkinson's disease. J Neurosurg. 1992;76(1):53–61.
21. Laitinen LV, Bergenheim AT, Hariz MI. Ventroposterolateral pallidotomy can abolish all parkinsonian symptoms. Stereotact Funct Neurosurg. 1992;58(1–4):14–21.
22. Benabid AL, Pollak P, Gervason C, Hoffmann D, Gao DM, Hommel M, et al. Long-term `suppression of tremor by chronic stimulation of the ventral intermediate thalamic nucleus. Lancet. 1991;337(8738):403–6.
23. Benabid AL, Pollak P, Louveau A, Henry S, de Rougemont J. Combined (thalamotomy and stimulation) stereotactic surgery of the VIM thalamic nucleus for bilateral Parkinson disease. Appl Neurophysiol. 1987;50(1–6):344–6.
24. Bittar RG, Hyam J, Nandi D, Wang S, Liu X, Joint C, et al. Thalamotomy versus thalamic stimulation for multiple sclerosis tremor. J Clin Neurosci. 2005;12(6):638–42.
25. Pahwa R, Lyons KE, Wilkinson SB, Troster AI, Overman J, Kieltyka J, et al. Comparison of thalamotomy to deep brain stimulation of the thalamus in essential tremor. Mov Disord. 2001;16(1):140–3.
26. Schuurman PR, Bosch DA, Bossuyt PM, Bonsel GJ, van Someren EJ, de Bie RM, et al. A comparison of continuous thalamic stimulation and thalamotomy for suppression of severe tremor. N Engl J Med. 2000;342(7):461–8.
27. Ghika J, Villemure JG, Fankhauser H, Favre J, Assal G, Ghika-Schmid F. Efficiency and safety of bilateral contemporaneous pallidal stimulation (deep brain stimulation) in levodopa-

responsive patients with Parkinson's disease with severe motor fluctuations: a 2-year follow-up review. J Neurosurg. 1998;89(5):713–8.
28. Siegfried J, Lippitz B. Bilateral chronic electrostimulation of ventroposterolateral pallidum: a new therapeutic approach for alleviating all parkinsonian symptoms. Neurosurgery. 1994;35(6):1126–9; discussion 9–30.
29. Aziz TZ, Peggs D, Sambrook MA, Crossman AR. Lesion of the subthalamic nucleus for the alleviation of 1-methyl-4-phenyl-1,2,3,6-tetrahydropyridine (MPTP)-induced parkinsonism in the primate. Mov Disord. 1991;6(4):288–92.
30. Benazzouz A, Gross C, Feger J, Boraud T, Bioulac B. Reversal of rigidity and improvement in motor performance by subthalamic high-frequency stimulation in MPTP-treated monkeys. Eur J Neurosci. 1993;5(4):382–9.
31. Deuschl G, Schade-Brittinger C, Krack P, Volkmann J, Schafer H, Botzel K, et al. A randomized trial of deep-brain stimulation for Parkinson's disease. N Engl J Med. 2006;355(9):896–908.
32. Follett KA, Weaver FM, Stern M, Hur K, Harris CL, Luo P, et al. Pallidal versus subthalamic deep-brain stimulation for Parkinson's disease. N Engl J Med. 2010;362(22):2077–91.
33. Miocinovic S, Somayajula S, Chitnis S, Vitek JL. History, applications, and mechanisms of deep brain stimulation. JAMA Neurol. 2013;70(2):163–71.
34. Morita H, Hass CJ, Moro E, Sudhyadhom A, Kumar R, Okun MS. Pedunculopontine nucleus stimulation: where are we now and what needs to be done to move the field forward? Front Neurol. 2014;5:243.
35. Benazzouz A, Gao DM, Ni ZG, Piallat B, Bouali-Benazzouz R, Benabid AL. Effect of high-frequency stimulation of the subthalamic nucleus on the neuronal activities of the substantia nigra pars reticulata and ventrolateral nucleus of the thalamus in the rat. Neuroscience. 2000;99(2):289–95.
36. Boraud T, Bezard E, Bioulac B, Gross C. High frequency stimulation of the internal Globus Pallidus (GPi) simultaneously improves parkinsonian symptoms and reduces the firing frequency of GPi neurons in the MPTP-treated monkey. Neurosci Lett. 1996;215(1):17–20.
37. Birdno MJ, Tang W, Dostrovsky JO, Hutchison WD, Grill WM. Response of human thalamic neurons to high-frequency stimulation. PLoS One. 2014;9(5):e96026.
38. Dostrovsky JO, Levy R, Wu JP, Hutchison WD, Tasker RR, Lozano AM. Microstimulation-induced inhibition of neuronal firing in human globus pallidus. J Neurophysiol. 2000;84(1):570–4.
39. Filali M, Hutchison WD, Palter VN, Lozano AM, Dostrovsky JO. Stimulation-induced inhibition of neuronal firing in human subthalamic nucleus. Exp Brain Res. 2004;156(3):274–81.
40. Welter ML, Houeto JL, Bonnet AM, Bejjani PB, Mesnage V, Dormont D, et al. Effects of high-frequency stimulation on subthalamic neuronal activity in parkinsonian patients. Arch Neurol. 2004;61(1):89–96.
41. Beurrier C, Bioulac B, Audin J, Hammond C. High-frequency stimulation produces a transient blockade of voltage-gated currents in subthalamic neurons. J Neurophysiol. 2001;85(4):1351–6.
42. McIntyre CC, Grill WM, Sherman DL, Thakor NV. Cellular effects of deep brain stimulation: model-based analysis of activation and inhibition. J Neurophysiol. 2004;91(4):1457–69.
43. Hashimoto T, Elder CM, Okun MS, Patrick SK, Vitek JL. Stimulation of the subthalamic nucleus changes the firing pattern of pallidal neurons. J Neurosci. 2003;23(5):1916–23.
44. Anderson ME, Postupna N, Ruffo M. Effects of high-frequency stimulation in the internal globus pallidus on the activity of thalamic neurons in the awake monkey. J Neurophysiol. 2003;89(2):1150–60.
45. Montgomery Jr EB. Effects of GPi stimulation on human thalamic neuronal activity. Clin Neurophysiol. 2006;117(12):2691–702.
46. Vitek JL, Zhang J, Hashimoto T, Russo GS, Baker KB. External pallidal stimulation improves parkinsonian motor signs and modulates neuronal activity throughout the basal ganglia thalamic network. Exp Neurol. 2012;233(1):581–6.

47. Hershey T, Revilla FJ, Wernle AR, McGee-Minnich L, Antenor JV, Videen TO, et al. Cortical and subcortical blood flow effects of subthalamic nucleus stimulation in PD. Neurology. 2003;61(6):816–21.
48. Perlmutter JS, Mink JW, Bastian AJ, Zackowski K, Hershey T, Miyawaki E, et al. Blood flow responses to deep brain stimulation of thalamus. Neurology. 2002;58(9):1388–94.
49. Jech R, Urgosik D, Tintera J, Nebuzelsky A, Krasensky J, Liscak R, et al. Functional magnetic resonance imaging during deep brain stimulation: a pilot study in four patients with Parkinson's disease. Mov Disord. 2001;16(6):1126–32.
50. Boulet S, Lacombe E, Carcenac C, Feuerstein C, Sgambato-Faure V, Poupard A, et al. Subthalamic stimulation-induced forelimb dyskinesias are linked to an increase in glutamate levels in the substantia nigra pars reticulata. J Neurosci. 2006;26(42):10768–76.
51. Johnson MD, McIntyre CC. Quantifying the neural elements activated and inhibited by globus pallidus deep brain stimulation. J Neurophysiol. 2008;100(5):2549–63.
52. Li S, Arbuthnott GW, Jutras MJ, Goldberg JA, Jaeger D. Resonant antidromic cortical circuit activation as a consequence of high-frequency subthalamic deep-brain stimulation. J Neurophysiol. 2007;98(6):3525–37.
53. Walker HC, Huang H, Gonzalez CL, Bryant JE, Killen J, Cutter GR, et al. Short latency activation of cortex during clinically effective subthalamic deep brain stimulation for Parkinson's disease. Mov Disord. 2012;27(7):864–73.
54. Walker HC, Huang H, Gonzalez CL, Bryant JE, Killen J, Knowlton RC, et al. Short latency activation of cortex by clinically effective thalamic brain stimulation for tremor. Mov Disord. 2012;27(11):1404–12.
55. Kuriakose R, Saha U, Castillo G, Udupa K, Ni Z, Gunraj C, et al. The nature and time course of cortical activation following subthalamic stimulation in Parkinson's disease. Cereb Cortex. 2010;20(8):1926–36.
56. Santaniello S, McCarthy MM, Montgomery Jr EB, Gale JT, Kopell N, Sarma SV. Therapeutic mechanisms of high-frequency stimulation in Parkinson's disease and neural restoration via loop-based reinforcement. Proc Natl Acad Sci U S A. 2015;112(6):E586–95.
57. Gradinaru V, Mogri M, Thompson KR, Henderson JM, Deisseroth K. Optical deconstruction of parkinsonian neural circuitry. Science. 2009;324(5925):354–9.
58. Smith Y, Wichmann T. The cortico-pallidal projection: an additional route for cortical regulation of the basal ganglia circuitry. Mov Disord. 2015;30(3):293–5.
59. McCairn KW, Turner RS. Pallidal Stimulation Suppresses Pathological Dysrhythmia in the Parkinsonian Motor Cortex. J Neurophysiol. 2015;113(7):2537–48. doi:10.1152/jn.00701.2014.
60. Johnson MD, Vitek JL, McIntyre CC. Pallidal stimulation that improves parkinsonian motor symptoms also modulates neuronal firing patterns in primary motor cortex in the MPTP-treated monkey. Exp Neurol. 2009;219(1):359–62.
61. Albin RL, Young AB, Penney JB. The functional anatomy of basal ganglia disorders. Trends Neurosci. 1989;12(10):366–75.
62. DeLong MR. Primate models of movement disorders of basal ganglia origin. Trends Neurosci. 1990;13(7):281–5.
63. Ellens DJ, Leventhal DK. Review: electrophysiology of basal ganglia and cortex in models of Parkinson disease. J Parkinsons Dis. 2013;3(3):241–54.
64. Hahn PJ, Russo GS, Hashimoto T, Miocinovic S, Xu W, McIntyre CC, et al. Pallidal burst activity during therapeutic deep brain stimulation. Exp Neurol. 2008;211(1):243–51.
65. Dorval AD, Russo GS, Hashimoto T, Xu W, Grill WM, Vitek JL. Deep brain stimulation reduces neuronal entropy in the MPTP-primate model of Parkinson's disease. J Neurophysiol. 2008;100(5):2807–18.
66. Cleary DR, Raslan AM, Rubin JE, Bahgat D, Viswanathan A, Heinricher MM, et al. Deep brain stimulation entrains local neuronal firing in human globus pallidus internus. J Neurophysiol. 2013;109(4):978–87.

67. McCairn KW, Turner RS. Deep brain stimulation of the globus pallidus internus in the parkinsonian primate: local entrainment and suppression of low-frequency oscillations. J Neurophysiol. 2009;101(4):1941–60.
68. Xu W, Russo GS, Hashimoto T, Zhang J, Vitek JL. Subthalamic nucleus stimulation modulates thalamic neuronal activity. J Neurosci. 2008;28(46):11916–24.
69. Pasquereau B, Turner RS. Primary motor cortex of the parkinsonian monkey: differential effects on the spontaneous activity of pyramidal tract-type neurons. Cereb Cortex. 2011;21(6):1362–78.
70. McConnell GC, So RQ, Hilliard JD, Lopomo P, Grill WM. Effective deep brain stimulation suppresses low-frequency network oscillations in the basal ganglia by regularizing neural firing patterns. J Neurosci. 2012;32(45):15657–68.
71. Meissner W, Leblois A, Hansel D, Bioulac B, Gross CE, Benazzouz A, et al. Subthalamic high frequency stimulation resets subthalamic firing and reduces abnormal oscillations. Brain. 2005;128(Pt 10):2372–82.
72. Wichmann T, Bergman H, DeLong MR. The primate subthalamic nucleus. III. Changes in motor behavior and neuronal activity in the internal pallidum induced by subthalamic inactivation in the MPTP model of parkinsonism. J Neurophysiol. 1994;72(2):521–30.
73. Lenz FA, Tasker RR, Kwan HC, Schnider S, Kwong R, Murayama Y, et al. Single unit analysis of the human ventral thalamic nuclear group: correlation of thalamic "tremor cells" with the 3-6 Hz component of parkinsonian tremor. J Neurosci. 1988;8(3):754–64.
74. Guehl D, Pessiglione M, Francois C, Yelnik J, Hirsch EC, Feger J, et al. Tremor-related activity of neurons in the 'motor' thalamus: changes in firing rate and pattern in the MPTP vervet model of parkinsonism. Eur J Neurosci. 2003;17(11):2388–400.
75. Moran A, Stein E, Tischler H, Bar-Gad I. Decoupling neuronal oscillations during subthalamic nucleus stimulation in the parkinsonian primate. Neurobiol Dis. 2012;45(1):583–90.
76. Ray NJ, Jenkinson N, Wang S, Holland P, Brittain JS, Joint C, et al. Local field potential beta activity in the subthalamic nucleus of patients with Parkinson's disease is associated with improvements in bradykinesia after dopamine and deep brain stimulation. Exp Neurol. 2008;213(1):108–13.
77. Bar-Gad I, Heimer G, Ritov Y, Bergman H. Functional correlations between neighboring neurons in the primate globus pallidus are weak or nonexistent. J Neurosci. 2003;23(10):4012–6.
78. Rivlin-Etzion M, Elias S, Heimer G, Bergman H. Computational physiology of the basal ganglia in Parkinson's disease. Prog Brain Res. 2010;183:259–73.
79. de Hemptinne C, Ryapolova-Webb ES, Air EL, Garcia PA, Miller KJ, Ojemann JG, et al. Exaggerated phase-amplitude coupling in the primary motor cortex in Parkinson disease. Proc Natl Acad Sci U S A. 2013;110(12):4780–5.
80. Brittain JS, Brown P. Oscillations and the basal ganglia: motor control and beyond. Neuroimage. 2014;85(Pt 2):637–47.
81. Leventhal DK, Gage GJ, Schmidt R, Pettibone JR, Case AC, Berke JD. Basal ganglia beta oscillations accompany cue utilization. Neuron. 2012;73(3):523–36.
82. Obeso JA, Jahanshahi M, Alvarez L, Macias R, Pedroso I, Wilkinson L, et al. What can man do without basal ganglia motor output? The effect of combined unilateral subthalamotomy and pallidotomy in a patient with Parkinson's disease. Exp Neurol. 2009;220(2):283–92.
83. Goldberg JH, Farries MA, Fee MS. Basal ganglia output to the thalamus: still a paradox. Trends Neurosci. 2013;36(12):695–705.
84. Seeger-Armbruster S, Bosch-Bouju C, Little ST, Smither RA, Hughes SM, Hyland BI, et al. Patterned, but not tonic, optogenetic stimulation in motor thalamus improves reaching in acute drug-induced Parkinsonian rats. J Neurosci. 2015;35(3):1211–6.
85. Rubin JE, McIntyre CC, Turner RS, Wichmann T. Basal ganglia activity patterns in parkinsonism and computational modeling of their downstream effects. Eur J Neurosci. 2012;36(2):2213–28.

86. Rosin B, Slovik M, Mitelman R, Rivlin-Etzion M, Haber SN, Israel Z, et al. Closed-loop deep brain stimulation is superior in ameliorating parkinsonism. Neuron. 2011;72(2):370–84.
87. Hallett M. Tremor: pathophysiology. Parkinsonism Relat Disord. 2014;20(Suppl 1):S118–22.
88. Helmich RC, Hallett M, Deuschl G, Toni I, Bloem BR. Cerebral causes and consequences of parkinsonian resting tremor: a tale of two circuits? Brain. 2012;135(Pt 11):3206–26.
89. Bostan AC, Dum RP, Strick PL. Cerebellar networks with the cerebral cortex and basal ganglia. Trends Cogn Sci. 2013;17(5):241–54.
90. Olanow CW. Can we achieve neuroprotection with currently available anti-parkinsonian interventions? Neurology. 2009;72(7 Suppl):S59–64.
91. Schuepbach WM, Rau J, Knudsen K, Volkmann J, Krack P, Timmermann L, et al. Neurostimulation for Parkinson's disease with early motor complications. N Engl J Med. 2013;368(7):610–22.
92. Charles PD, Dolhun RM, Gill CE, Davis TL, Bliton MJ, Tramontana MG, et al. Deep brain stimulation in early Parkinson's disease: enrollment experience from a pilot trial. Parkinsonism Relat Disord. 2012;18(3):268–73.
93. Charles D, Konrad PE, Neimat JS, Molinari AL, Tramontana MG, Finder SG, et al. Subthalamic nucleus deep brain stimulation in early stage Parkinson's disease. Parkinsonism Relat Disord. 2014;20(7):731–7.
94. Deuschl G, Bain P. Deep brain stimulation for tremor: patient selection and evaluation. Mov Disord. 2002;17(Suppl 3):S102–11.
95. Kumar R, Lozano AM, Sime E, Lang AE. Long-term follow-up of thalamic deep brain stimulation for essential and parkinsonian tremor. Neurology. 2003;61(11):1601–4.
96. Bandini F, Primavera A, Pizzorno M, Cocito L. Using STN DBS and medication reduction as a strategy to treat pathological gambling in Parkinson's disease. Parkinsonism Relat Disord. 2007;13(6):369–71.
97. Molina JA, Sainz-Artiga MJ, Fraile A, Jimenez-Jimenez FJ, Villanueva C, Orti-Pareja M, et al. Pathologic gambling in Parkinson's disease: a behavioral manifestation of pharmacologic treatment? Mov Disord. 2000;15(5):869–72.
98. Morgante L, Morgante F, Moro E, Epifanio A, Girlanda P, Ragonese P, et al. How many parkinsonian patients are suitable candidates for deep brain stimulation of subthalamic nucleus? Results of a questionnaire. Parkinsonism Relat Disord. 2007;13(8):528–31.
99. Pahwa R, Factor SA, Lyons KE, Ondo WG, Gronseth G, Bronte-Stewart H, et al. Practice parameter: treatment of Parkinson disease with motor fluctuations and dyskinesia (an evidence-based review): report of the Quality Standards Subcommittee of the American Academy of Neurology. Neurology. 2006;66(7):983–95.
100. Abboud H, Mehanna R, Machado A, Ahmed A, Gostkowski M, Cooper S, et al. Comprehensive, multidisciplinary deep brain stimulation screening for Parkinson patients: no room for "short cuts". Mov Disord Clin Pract (Hoboken). 2014;1(4):336–41.
101. Shih LC, Tarsy D. Deep brain stimulation for the treatment of atypical parkinsonism. Mov Disord. 2007;22(15):2149–55.
102. Chou KL, Forman MS, Trojanowski JQ, Hurtig HI, Baltuch GH. Subthalamic nucleus deep brain stimulation in a patient with levodopa-responsive multiple system atrophy. Case report. J Neurosurg. 2004;100(3):553–6.
103. Okun MS, Tagliati M, Pourfar M, Fernandez HH, Rodriguez RL, Alterman RL, et al. Management of referred deep brain stimulation failures: a retrospective analysis from 2 movement disorders centers. Arch Neurol. 2005;62(8):1250–5.
104. Visser-Vandewalle V, Temel Y, Colle H, van der Linden C. Bilateral high-frequency stimulation of the subthalamic nucleus in patients with multiple system atrophy–parkinsonism. Report of four cases. J Neurosurg. 2003;98(4):882–7.
105. Kleiner-Fisman G, Herzog J, Fisman DN, Tamma F, Lyons KE, Pahwa R, et al. Subthalamic nucleus deep brain stimulation: summary and meta-analysis of outcomes. Mov Disord. 2006;21(Suppl 14):S290–304.

106. Welter ML, Houeto JL, Tezenas du Montcel S, Mesnage V, Bonnet AM, Pillon B, et al. Clinical predictive factors of subthalamic stimulation in Parkinson's disease. Brain. 2002;125(Pt 3):575–83.
107. Castrioto A, Lozano AM, Poon YY, Lang AE, Fallis M, Moro E. Ten-year outcome of subthalamic stimulation in Parkinson disease: a blinded evaluation. Arch Neurol. 2011;68(12):1550–6.
108. Kleiner-Fisman G, Fisman DN, Sime E, Saint-Cyr JA, Lozano AM, Lang AE. Long-term follow up of bilateral deep brain stimulation of the subthalamic nucleus in patients with advanced Parkinson disease. J Neurosurg. 2003;99(3):489–95.
109. Krack P, Batir A, Van Blercom N, Chabardes S, Fraix V, Ardouin C, et al. Five-year follow-up of bilateral stimulation of the subthalamic nucleus in advanced Parkinson's disease. N Engl J Med. 2003;349(20):1925–34.
110. Lubik S, Fogel W, Tronnier V, Krause M, Konig J, Jost WH. Gait analysis in patients with advanced Parkinson disease: different or additive effects on gait induced by levodopa and chronic STN stimulation. J Neural Transm. 2006;113(2):163–73.
111. Schupbach WM, Chastan N, Welter ML, Houeto JL, Mesnage V, Bonnet AM, et al. Stimulation of the subthalamic nucleus in Parkinson's disease: a 5 year follow up. J Neurol Neurosurg Psychiatry. 2005;76(12):1640–4.
112. Chou KL, Taylor JL, Patil PG. The MDS-UPDRS tracks motor and non-motor improvement due to subthalamic nucleus deep brain stimulation in Parkinson disease. Parkinsonism Relat Disord. 2013;19(11):966–9.
113. Yu H, Neimat JS. The treatment of movement disorders by deep brain stimulation. Neurotherapeutics. 2008;5(1):26–36.
114. Bronstein JM, Tagliati M, Alterman RL, Lozano AM, Volkmann J, Stefani A, et al. Deep brain stimulation for Parkinson disease: an expert consensus and review of key issues. Arch Neurol. 2011;68(2):165.
115. Lang AE, Houeto JL, Krack P, Kubu C, Lyons KE, Moro E, et al. Deep brain stimulation: preoperative issues. Mov Disord. 2006;21(Suppl 14):S171–96.
116. Hariz MI, Johansson F, Shamsgovara P, Johansson E, Hariz GM, Fagerlund M. Bilateral subthalamic nucleus stimulation in a parkinsonian patient with preoperative deficits in speech and cognition: persistent improvement in mobility but increased dependency: a case study. Mov Disord. 2000;15(1):136–9.
117. Morrison CE, Borod JC, Perrine K, Beric A, Brin MF, Rezai A, et al. Neuropsychological functioning following bilateral subthalamic nucleus stimulation in Parkinson's disease. Arch Clin Neuropsychol. 2004;19(2):165–81.
118. Saint-Cyr JA, Trepanier LL, Kumar R, Lozano AM, Lang AE. Neuropsychological consequences of chronic bilateral stimulation of the subthalamic nucleus in Parkinson's disease. Brain. 2000;123(Pt 10):2091–108.
119. Houeto JL, Mesnage V, Mallet L, Pillon B, Gargiulo M, du Moncel ST, et al. Behavioural disorders, Parkinson's disease and subthalamic stimulation. J Neurol Neurosurg Psychiatry. 2002;72(6):701–7.
120. Troster AI, Fields JA, Wilkinson S, Pahwa R, Koller WC, Lyons KE. Effect of motor improvement on quality of life following subthalamic stimulation is mediated by changes in depressive symptomatology. Stereotact Funct Neurosurg. 2003;80(1–4):43–7.
121. Appleby BS, Duggan PS, Regenberg A, Rabins PV. Psychiatric and neuropsychiatric adverse events associated with deep brain stimulation: a meta-analysis of ten years' experience. Mov Disord. 2007;22(12):1722–8.
122. Soulas T, Gurruchaga JM, Palfi S, Cesaro P, Nguyen JP, Fenelon G. Attempted and completed suicides after subthalamic nucleus stimulation for Parkinson's disease. J Neurol Neurosurg Psychiatry. 2008;79(8):952–4.
123. Voon V, Krack P, Lang AE, Lozano AM, Dujardin K, Schupbach M, et al. A multicentre study on suicide outcomes following subthalamic stimulation for Parkinson's disease. Brain. 2008;131(Pt 10):2720–8.

124. Saint-Cyr JA, Albanese A. STN DBS in PD: selection criteria for surgery should include cognitive and psychiatric factors. Neurology. 2006;66(12):1799–800.
125. Charles PD, Van Blercom N, Krack P, Lee SL, Xie J, Besson G, et al. Predictors of effective bilateral subthalamic nucleus stimulation for PD. Neurology. 2002;59(6):932–4.
126. DeLong MR, Huang KT, Gallis J, Lokhnygina Y, Parente B, Hickey P, et al. Effect of advancing age on outcomes of deep brain stimulation for Parkinson disease. JAMA Neurol. 2014;71(10):1290–5.
127. Weaver FM, Follett K, Stern M, Hur K, Harris C, Marks Jr WJ, et al. Bilateral deep brain stimulation vs best medical therapy for patients with advanced Parkinson disease: a randomized controlled trial. JAMA. 2009;301(1):63–73.
128. Weaver FM, Follett KA, Stern M, Luo P, Harris CL, Hur K, et al. Randomized trial of deep brain stimulation for Parkinson disease: thirty-six-month outcomes. Neurology. 2012;79(1):55–65.
129. Pahwa R, Lyons KE, Wilkinson SB, Simpson Jr RK, Ondo WG, Tarsy D, et al. Long-term evaluation of deep brain stimulation of the thalamus. J Neurosurg. 2006;104(4):506–12.
130. Ferraye MU, Debu B, Fraix V, Goetz L, Ardouin C, Yelnik J, et al. Effects of pedunculopontine nucleus area stimulation on gait disorders in Parkinson's disease. Brain. 2010;133(Pt 1):205–14.
131. Ostrem JL, Christine CW, Glass GA, Schrock LE, Starr PA. Pedunculopontine nucleus deep brain stimulation in a patient with primary progressive freezing gait disorder. Stereotact Funct Neurosurg. 2010;88(1):51–5.
132. Thevathasan W, Cole MH, Graepel CL, Hyam JA, Jenkinson N, Brittain JS, et al. A spatiotemporal analysis of gait freezing and the impact of pedunculopontine nucleus stimulation. Brain. 2012;135(Pt 5):1446–54.
133. Okun MS, Gallo BV, Mandybur G, Jagid J, Foote KD, Revilla FJ, et al. Subthalamic deep brain stimulation with a constant-current device in Parkinson's disease: an open-label randomised controlled trial. Lancet Neurol. 2012;11(2):140–9.
134. Deep Brain Stimulation for Parkinson's Disease Study Group. Deep-brain stimulation of the subthalamic nucleus or the pars interna of the globus pallidus in Parkinson's disease. N Engl J Med. 2001;345(13):956–63.
135. Krause M, Fogel W, Heck A, Hacke W, Bonsanto M, Trenkwalder C, et al. Deep brain stimulation for the treatment of Parkinson's disease: subthalamic nucleus versus globus pallidus internus. J Neurol Neurosurg Psychiatry. 2001;70(4):464–70.
136. Volkmann J, Allert N, Voges J, Weiss PH, Freund HJ, Sturm V. Safety and efficacy of pallidal or subthalamic nucleus stimulation in advanced PD. Neurology. 2001;56(4):548–51.
137. Volkmann J, Allert N, Voges J, Sturm V, Schnitzler A, Freund HJ. Long-term results of bilateral pallidal stimulation in Parkinson's disease. Ann Neurol. 2004;55(6):871–5.
138. Burchiel KJ, Anderson VC, Favre J, Hammerstad JP. Comparison of pallidal and subthalamic nucleus deep brain stimulation for advanced Parkinson's disease: results of a randomized, blinded pilot study. Neurosurgery. 1999;45(6):1375–82; discussion 82–4.
139. Odekerken VJ, van Laar T, Staal MJ, Mosch A, Hoffmann CF, Nijssen PC, et al. Subthalamic nucleus versus globus pallidus bilateral deep brain stimulation for advanced Parkinson's disease (NSTAPS study): a randomised controlled trial. Lancet Neurol. 2013;12(1):37–44.
140. Bang Henriksen M, Johnsen EL, Sunde N, Vase A, Gjelstrup MC, Ostergaard K. Surviving 10 years with deep brain stimulation for Parkinson's disease – a follow-up of 79 patients. Eur J Neurol. 2016;23(1):53–61.
141. Janssen ML, Duits AA, Tourai AM, Ackermans L, Leentjes AF, van Kranen-Mastenbroek V, et al. Subthalamic nucleus high-frequency stimulation for advanced Parkinson's disease: motor and neuropsychological outcome after 10 years. Stereotact Funct Neurosurg. 2014;92(6):381–7.
142. Rodriguez-Oroz MC, Obeso JA, Lang AE, Houeto JL, Pollak P, Rehncrona S, et al. Bilateral deep brain stimulation in Parkinson's disease: a multicentre study with 4 years follow-up. Brain. 2005;128(Pt 10):2240–9.

143. Moro E, Lozano AM, Pollak P, Agid Y, Rehncrona S, Volkmann J, et al. Long-term results of a multicenter study on subthalamic and pallidal stimulation in Parkinson's disease. Mov Disord. 2010;25(5):578–86.
144. Lyons KE, Pahwa R. Long-term benefits in quality of life provided by bilateral subthalamic stimulation in patients with Parkinson disease. J Neurosurg. 2005;103(2):252–5.
145. Siderowf A, Jaggi JL, Xie SX, Loveland-Jones C, Leng L, Hurtig H, et al. Long-term effects of bilateral subthalamic nucleus stimulation on health-related quality of life in advanced Parkinson's disease. Mov Disord. 2006;21(6):746–53.
146. Volkmann J, Albanese A, Kulisevsky J, Tornqvist AL, Houeto JL, Pidoux B, et al. Long-term effects of pallidal or subthalamic deep brain stimulation on quality of life in Parkinson's disease. Mov Disord. 2009;24(8):1154–61.
147. Lagrange E, Krack P, Moro E, Ardouin C, Van Blercom N, Chabardes S, et al. Bilateral subthalamic nucleus stimulation improves health-related quality of life in PD. Neurology. 2002;59(12):1976–8.
148. Moro E, Poon YY, Lozano AM, Saint-Cyr JA, Lang AE. Subthalamic nucleus stimulation: improvements in outcome with reprogramming. Arch Neurol. 2006;63(9):1266–72.
149. Limousin P, Speelman JD, Gielen F, Janssens M. Multicentre European study of thalamic stimulation in parkinsonian and essential tremor. J Neurol Neurosurg Psychiatry. 1999;66(3):289–96.
150. Hariz MI, Krack P, Alesch F, Augustinsson LE, Bosch A, Ekberg R, et al. Multicentre European study of thalamic stimulation for parkinsonian tremor: a 6 year follow-up. J Neurol Neurosurg Psychiatry. 2008;79(6):694–9.
151. Lyons KE, Koller WC, Wilkinson SB, Pahwa R. Long term safety and efficacy of unilateral deep brain stimulation of the thalamus for parkinsonian tremor. J Neurol Neurosurg Psychiatry. 2001;71(5):682–4.
152. Pahapill PA, Lozano AM. The pedunculopontine nucleus and Parkinson's disease. Brain. 2000;123(Pt 9):1767–83.
153. Plaha P, Gill SS. Bilateral deep brain stimulation of the pedunculopontine nucleus for Parkinson's disease. Neuroreport. 2005;16(17):1883–7.
154. Stefani A, Lozano AM, Peppe A, Stanzione P, Galati S, Tropepi D, et al. Bilateral deep brain stimulation of the pedunculopontine and subthalamic nuclei in severe Parkinson's disease. Brain. 2007;130(Pt 6):1596–607.
155. Khan S, Javed S, Mooney L, White P, Plaha P, Whone A, et al. Clinical outcomes from bilateral versus unilateral stimulation of the pedunculopontine nucleus with and without concomitant caudal zona incerta region stimulation in Parkinson's disease. Br J Neurosurg. 2012;26(5):722–5.
156. Alessandro S, Ceravolo R, Brusa L, Pierantozzi M, Costa A, Galati S, et al. Non-motor functions in parkinsonian patients implanted in the pedunculopontine nucleus: focus on sleep and cognitive domains. J Neurol Sci. 2010;289(1–2):44–8.
157. Lim AS, Moro E, Lozano AM, Hamani C, Dostrovsky JO, Hutchison WD, et al. Selective enhancement of rapid eye movement sleep by deep brain stimulation of the human pons. Ann Neurol. 2009;66(1):110–4.
158. Videnovic A, Metman LV. Deep brain stimulation for Parkinson's disease: prevalence of adverse events and need for standardized reporting. Mov Disord. 2008;23(3):343–9.
159. Patel DM, Walker HC, Brooks R, Omar N, Ditty B, Guthrie BL. Adverse events associated with deep brain stimulation for movement disorders: analysis of 510 consecutive cases. Neurosurgery. 2015;11(Suppl 2):190–9.
160. Binder DK, Rau GM, Starr PA. Risk factors for hemorrhage during microelectrode-guided deep brain stimulator implantation for movement disorders. Neurosurgery. 2005;56(4):722–32; discussion –32.
161. Bhatia S, Oh M, Whiting T, Quigley M, Whiting D. Surgical complications of deep brain stimulation. A longitudinal single surgeon, single institution study. Stereotact Funct Neurosurg. 2008;86(6):367–72.

162. Kenney C, Simpson R, Hunter C, Ondo W, Almaguer M, Davidson A, et al. Short-term and long-term safety of deep brain stimulation in the treatment of movement disorders. J Neurosurg. 2007;106(4):621–5.
163. Ben-Haim S, Asaad WF, Gale JT, Eskandar EN. Risk factors for hemorrhage during microelectrode-guided deep brain stimulation and the introduction of an improved microelectrode design. Neurosurgery. 2009;64(4):754–62; discussion 62–3.
164. Zrinzo L, Foltynie T, Limousin P, Hariz MI. Reducing hemorrhagic complications in functional neurosurgery: a large case series and systematic literature review. J Neurosurg. 2012;116(1):84–94.
165. Baizabal Carvallo JF, Mostile G, Almaguer M, Davidson A, Simpson R, Jankovic J. Deep brain stimulation hardware complications in patients with movement disorders: risk factors and clinical correlations. Stereotact Funct Neurosurg. 2012;90(5):300–6.
166. Nutt JG, Anderson VC, Peacock JH, Hammerstad JP, Burchiel KJ. DBS and diathermy interaction induces severe CNS damage. Neurology. 2001;56(10):1384–6.
167. Henderson JM, Tkach J, Phillips M, Baker K, Shellock FG, Rezai AR. Permanent neurological deficit related to magnetic resonance imaging in a patient with implanted deep brain stimulation electrodes for Parkinson's disease: case report. Neurosurgery. 2005;57(5):E1063; discussion E.
168. Tagliati M, Jankovic J, Pagan F, Susatia F, Isaias IU, Okun MS. Safety of MRI in patients with implanted deep brain stimulation devices. Neuroimage. 2009;47(Suppl 2):T53–7.
169. Zrinzo L, Yoshida F, Hariz MI, Thornton J, Foltynie T, Yousry TA, et al. Clinical safety of brain magnetic resonance imaging with implanted deep brain stimulation hardware: large case series and review of the literature. World Neurosurg. 2011;76(1–2):164–72; discussion 69–73.
170. Anderson WS, Lenz FA. Surgery insight: deep brain stimulation for movement disorders. Nat Clin Pract Neurol. 2006;2(6):310–20.
171. Obwegeser AA, Uitti RJ, Witte RJ, Lucas JA, Turk MF, Wharen RE, Jr. Quantitative and qualitative outcome measures after thalamic deep brain stimulation to treat disabling tremors. Neurosurgery. 2001;48(2):274–81; discussion 81–4.
172. Isaias IU, Alterman RL, Tagliati M. Deep brain stimulation for primary generalized dystonia: long-term outcomes. Arch Neurol. 2009;66(4):465–70.
173. Loher TJ, Capelle HH, Kaelin-Lang A, Weber S, Weigel R, Burgunder JM, et al. Deep brain stimulation for dystonia: outcome at long-term follow-up. J Neurol. 2008;255(6):881–4.
174. Hamani C, Richter E, Schwalb JM, Lozano AM. Bilateral subthalamic nucleus stimulation for Parkinson's disease: a systematic review of the clinical literature. Neurosurgery. 2008;62(Suppl 2):863–74.
175. Hariz MI. Complications of deep brain stimulation surgery. Mov Disord. 2002;17(Suppl 3):S162–6.
176. Pollak P, Krack P, Fraix V, Mendes A, Moro E, Chabardes S, et al. Intraoperative micro- and macrostimulation of the subthalamic nucleus in Parkinson's disease. Mov Disord. 2002;17(Suppl 3):S155–61.
177. Umemura A, Jaggi JL, Hurtig HI, Siderowf AD, Colcher A, Stern MB, et al. Deep brain stimulation for movement disorders: morbidity and mortality in 109 patients. J Neurosurg. 2003;98(4):779–84.
178. Deuschl G, Herzog J, Kleiner-Fisman G, Kubu C, Lozano AM, Lyons KE, et al. Deep brain stimulation: postoperative issues. Mov Disord [Review]. 2006;21:S219–S37.
179. Peron J, Grandjean D, Le Jeune F, Sauleau P, Haegelen C, Drapier D, et al. Recognition of emotional prosody is altered after subthalamic nucleus deep brain stimulation in Parkinson's disease. Neuropsychologia. 2010;48(4):1053–62.
180. Sauleau P, Le Jeune F, Drapier S, Houvenaghel JF, Dondaine T, Haegelen C, et al. Weight gain following subthalamic nucleus deep brain stimulation: a PET study. Mov Disord. 2014;29(14):1781–7.
181. Tuite PJ, Maxwell RE, Ikramuddin S, Kotz CM, Billington CJ, Laseski MA, et al. Weight and body mass index in Parkinson's disease patients after deep brain stimulation surgery. Parkinsonism Relat Disord. 2005;11(4):247–52.

182. Guehl D, Cuny E, Benazzouz A, Rougier A, Tison F, Machado S, et al. Side-effects of subthalamic stimulation in Parkinson's disease: clinical evolution and predictive factors. Eur J Neurol. 2006;13(9):963–71.
183. Sauleau P, Leray E, Rouaud T, Drapier S, Drapier D, Blanchard S, et al. Comparison of weight gain and energy intake after subthalamic versus pallidal stimulation in Parkinson's disease. Mov Disord. 2009;24(14):2149–55.
184. Doshi PK, Chhaya N, Bhatt MH. Depression leading to attempted suicide after bilateral subthalamic nucleus stimulation for Parkinson's disease. Mov Disord. 2002;17(5):1084–5.
185. Rothlind JC, Cockshott RW, Starr PA, Marks Jr WJ. Neuropsychological performance following staged bilateral pallidal or subthalamic nucleus deep brain stimulation for Parkinson's disease. J Int Neuropsychol Soc. 2007;13(1):68–79.
186. Temel Y, Kessels A, Tan S, Topdag A, Boon P, Visser-Vandewalle V. Behavioural changes after bilateral subthalamic stimulation in advanced Parkinson disease: a systematic review. Parkinsonism Relat Disord. 2006;12(5):265–72.
187. Okun MS, Fernandez HH, Wu SS, Kirsch-Darrow L, Bowers D, Bova F, et al. Cognition and mood in Parkinson's disease in subthalamic nucleus versus globus pallidus interna deep brain stimulation: the COMPARE trial. Ann Neurol. 2009;65(5):586–95.
188. Zangaglia R, Pacchetti C, Pasotti C, Mancini F, Servello D, Sinforiani E, et al. Deep brain stimulation and cognitive functions in Parkinson's disease: a three-year controlled study. Mov Disord. 2009;24(11):1621–8.
189. Funkiewiez A, Ardouin C, Caputo E, Krack P, Fraix V, Klinger H, et al. Long term effects of bilateral subthalamic nucleus stimulation on cognitive function, mood, and behaviour in Parkinson's disease. J Neurol Neurosurg Psychiatry. 2004;75(6):834–9.
190. Porat O, Cohen OS, Schwartz R, Hassin-Baer S. Association of preoperative symptom profile with psychiatric symptoms following subthalamic nucleus stimulation in patients with Parkinson's disease. J Neuropsychiatry Clin Neurosci. 2009 Fall;21(4):398–405.
191. Burchiel KJ, McCartney S, Lee A, Raslan AM. Accuracy of deep brain stimulation electrode placement using intraoperative computed tomography without microelectrode recording. J Neurosurg. 2013;119(2):301–6.
192. Martin AJ, Larson PS, Ostrem JL, Keith Sootsman W, Talke P, Weber OM, et al. Placement of deep brain stimulator electrodes using real-time high-field interventional magnetic resonance imaging. Magn Reson Med. 2005;54(5):1107–14.
193. Starr PA, Martin AJ, Larson PS. Implantation of deep brain stimulator electrodes using interventional MRI. Neurosurg Clin N Am. 2009;20(2):193–203.
194. Ostrem JL, Galifianakis NB, Markun LC, Grace JK, Martin AJ, Starr PA, et al. Clinical outcomes of PD patients having bilateral STN DBS using high-field interventional MR-imaging for lead placement. Clin Neurol Neurosurg. 2013;115(6):708–12.
195. Martin AJ, Larson PS, Ostrem JL, Starr PA. Interventional magnetic resonance guidance of deep brain stimulator implantation for Parkinson disease. Top Magn Reson Imaging. 2009;19(4):213–21.
196. Li G, Su H, Cole G, Shang W, Harrington K, Camilo A, et al. Robotic system for MRI-guided stereotactic neurosurgery. IEEE Trans Biomed Eng. 2015;62(4):1077–88.
197. Contarino MF, Bour LJ, Verhagen R, Lourens MA, de Bie RM, van den Munckhof P, et al. Directional steering: a novel approach to deep brain stimulation. Neurology. 2014;83(13):1163–9.
198. Pollo C, Kaelin-Lang A, Oertel MF, Stieglitz L, Taub E, Fuhr P, et al. Directional deep brain stimulation: an intraoperative double-blind pilot study. Brain. 2014;137(Pt 7):2015–26.
199. Hammond C, Bergman H, Brown P. Pathological synchronization in Parkinson's disease: networks, models and treatments. Trends Neurosci. 2007;30(7):357–64.
200. Hebb AO, Zhang JJ, Mahoor MH, Tsiokos C, Matlack C, Chizeck HJ, et al. Creating the feedback loop: closed-loop neurostimulation. Neurosurg Clin N Am. 2014;25(1):187–204.
201. Hohlefeld FU, Huchzermeyer C, Huebl J, Schneider GH, Nolte G, Brucke C, et al. Functional and effective connectivity in subthalamic local field potential recordings of patients with Parkinson's disease. Neuroscience. 2013;250:320–32.

202. Yang AI, Vanegas N, Lungu C, Zaghloul KA. Beta-coupled high-frequency activity and beta-locked neuronal spiking in the subthalamic nucleus of Parkinson's disease. J Neurosci. 2014;34(38):12816–27.
203. Eusebio A, Thevathasan W, Doyle Gaynor L, Pogosyan A, Bye E, Foltynie T, et al. Deep brain stimulation can suppress pathological synchronisation in parkinsonian patients. J Neurol Neurosurg Psychiatry. 2011;82(5):569–73.
204. Little S, Pogosyan A, Neal S, Zavala B, Zrinzo L, Hariz M, et al. Adaptive deep brain stimulation in advanced Parkinson disease. Ann Neurol. 2013;74(3):449–57.

Chapter 6
Electrical Stimulation for the Treatment of Dysphagia

Sue Pownall, Pam Enderby, and Lise Sproson

Abstract Dysphagia is the term used to describe swallowing disorders usually resulting from a neurological or physical impairment of the oral, pharyngeal or oesophageal mechanisms. Difficulty with swallowing may have life threatening consequences and can lead to an impaired quality of life. Electrical stimulation has recently become of interest to clinicians working with people presenting with dysphagia due to its rehabilitation potential especially for pharyngeal stage swallowing disorders. The electro-therapies for dysphagia can be divided into two main groups; those that are peripherally delivered and those where the stimulation is delivered cortically. This chapter outlines a number of electro-therapies as treatment approaches for dysphagia. The rationale for the use of each technique in the treatment of dysphagia is explained and an overview of the current published literature reported.

Keywords Dysphagia • Electrical stimulation • Electro-therapies • Neuro-muscular electrical stimulation • Repetitive transcranial magnetic stimulation

Introduction

Dysphagia is the term used to describe a swallowing disorder usually resulting from a neurological or physical impairment of the oral, pharyngeal or oesophageal mechanisms. The significance of dysphagia has only relatively recently been appreciated. It has a marked impact on survival, general health and quality of life. There are a

S. Pownall, PhD, BSc (Hons), FRCSLT (✉)
Sheffield Teaching Hospitals NHS Foundation Trust,
Speech and Language Therapy Department, Sheffield, UK
e-mail: Sue.pownall@sth.nhs.uk

P. Enderby, PhD, DSc (Hon), MSc, FRCSLT
University of Sheffield, School of Health and Related Research, Sheffield, UK
e-mail: p.m.enderby@sheffield.ac.uk

L. Sproson, MSc, B.Med.Sci (Hons), MRCSLT
Sheffield Teaching Hospitals NHS Foundation Trust, NIHR Devices for Dignity HTC,
Sheffield, UK
e-mail: lise.sproson@nhs.net

A. Majid (ed.), *Electroceuticals*, DOI 10.1007/978-3-319-28612-9_6

range of approaches to the assessment of dysphagia which is important given that aspiration (food or liquid entering the lungs) as a result of impaired swallowing can be easily overlooked, and if untreated may result in the person developing pneumonia. The most significant method of improving dysphagia is by detecting its presence, nature and severity through appropriate assessment. Without this, appropriate interventions cannot be implemented and, conversely inappropriate interventions may not be avoided.

Dysphagia can be a transient, persistent or a progressively worsening symptom according to the underlying pathology. The normal swallow has four interconnected physiological phases:

1. oral preparatory phase
2. oral phase
3. pharyngeal phase
4. oesophageal phase

The first three of these together are termed the oropharyngeal phase [1]. The 'normal' swallow needs the respiratory, oral, pharyngeal, laryngeal and oesophageal anatomical structures to function in synchrony, which is dependent upon the cognitive, motor and sensory nervous system being intact. Disorders of swallowing are associated with increased likelihood of aspiration, chest infections, and under nutrition. Pneumonia is common sequelae of dysphagia and is associated with higher costs of care [2].

Incidence and Prevalence of Dysphagia

Disordered swallowing has been recognised as a significant problem following stroke. Whilst stroke is the third most common cause of death and the most important cause of long-term disability most stroke-related deaths are due to medical complications of the stroke, rather than directly due to the neurological damage. Only 10% of stroke-related deaths are caused by neurological deficits, while 30% of post-stroke deaths are due to pneumonia [3]. In 67% of patients pneumonia manifests within 48 h of admission [4]. Clinical studies show evidence of dysphagia in over 70% of stroke patients [5]. In 75% of patients with early swallowing problems dysphagia will continue to be moderate to severe, and in 15% it will remain profound [6]. Preventing pneumonia with early and effective treatment of dysphagia could have a significant impact on survival, patient experience, functional recovery and costs.

Dysphagia is a common symptom associated with progressive neurological disease with 200/100,000 UK population having difficulties with swallowing associated with Parkinson's disease [7]. Furthermore, more than 90% of those with motor neurone disease (ALS) will develop this symptom at some point in the course of the disorder. Sixty-eight percent of those with dementia in nursing homes have been reported as having difficulty swallowing and this is considered a low estimate [8].

Suckling and swallowing are common problems associated with cerebral palsy (57 and 38%) in the first 12 months of life [9].

Dysphagia is, also, now recognised as a symptom of concern in many other conditions such as COPD [10], head and neck cancer [11], thermal burn injury [12] and acquired brain injury [13]. A study of those having cervical discectomy and fusion indicated an incidence of dysphagia in 50.3% of patients [14].

Impact of Dysphagia

Dysphagia can present in many ways, and the patient may demonstrate one or several of the following symptoms:

- Food spillage from lips
- Taking a long time to finish a meal
- Poor chewing ability
- Dry mouth
- Drooling
- Nasal regurgitation
- Food sticking in the throat
- Poor oral hygiene
- Coughing and choking
- Regurgitation
- Weight loss
- Repeated chest infections

Difficulty with swallowing may have life threatening consequences and can lead to an impaired quality of life. This may be due to embarrassment and lack of enjoyment of food, which can have profound social consequences for both the person and members of the family.

Role of the Speech and Language Therapist in the Management of Dysphagia

Speech and language therapists/speech pathologists have a unique role in the assessment, diagnosis and management of oropharyngeal dysphagia. The aims and objectives of speech and language therapy interventions for dysphagia depend on the type and nature of the dysphagia, the underlying cause, and the needs and preferences of the individual. Considering the safety of the swallow, managing aspiration and preventing complications are of paramount concern. In children the aims and objectives will change as appropriate to the age as the child's anatomy and neurological abilities alter with growth and development [15].

The overall aims of the speech and language therapist working with an individual with dysphagia include:

- accurate assessment (there may be multiple assessments over time) leading to accurate diagnosis of dysphagia which may assist with the differential medical diagnosis.
- ensuring safety (reducing or preventing aspiration) with regards to swallowing function.
- balancing these factors with quality of life, taking into account the individual's preferences and beliefs.
- working with other members of the team, particularly dieticians, to optimise nutrition and hydration.
- stimulating improved swallowing with oral motor/sensory exercises, swallow techniques and positioning.

Speech and language therapists (SLTs) will often provide education and training for those responsible for providing nutrition, hydration and mealtime support (family, professionals, and relevant others) and maintain links with the multi-disciplinary team to ensure good communication. SLTs are pivotal in the team supporting long-term management of those with dysphagia associated with a long-term chronic or progressive condition. There is evidence that some individuals discharged with a percutaneous endoscopic gastrostomy (PEG) tube can have these removed once swallowing improves. The speech and language therapist has a role in monitoring change of swallowing over time. Appropriate insertion or removal of PEGs is associated with improved quality of life and reduced health and social care costs.

Management of dysphagia frequently requires environmental modifications, safe swallowing advice, appropriate dietary modification, and the application of swallowing strategies, which improve the efficiency of swallow function and reduce the risk of aspiration [16–18].

Many of these interventions are designed to minimise symptoms of dysphagia rather than aimed at restoring physiological deficits, and thus are only providing compensatory management. Successful rehabilitation of the pharyngeal phase impairments remains a unique challenge to clinicians. Research into electrical stimulation techniques is gaining interest due to its rehabilitation potential especially for pharyngeal stage swallowing disorders.

Electrical Stimulation in Dysphagia

Electrical stimulation became of interest to clinicians working with people presenting with dysphagia following its successful use as a treatment intervention by physiotherapists for disorders such as foot drop and facial paralysis, where muscles are stimulated to enhance their function and performance [19]. There are, however, a number of different electrico-therapeutic interventions which have been proposed as treatment options for dysphagia and it is necessary to differentiate between them.

We will address the following:

- transcutaneous neuromuscular electrical stimulation (NMES or TNMES), via stimulation to sensory nerve fibres, which primarily supports circulation to the swallowing muscles; or where a muscle contraction is stimulated primarily to strengthen the muscles of swallowing via stimulation to motor nerve fibres
- palatal electrical stimulation, where the palate is stimulated with a specific training device
- pharyngeal electrical stimulation (PES), where an intraluminal catheter is placed in the pharynx as a source of peripheral sensorimotor input
- Functional magnetic stimulation (FMS) a non-invasive method of stimulating the muscles and nerves of swallowing via a coil rather than electrodes
- repetitive transcranial magnetic stimulation (rTMS), a non-invasive method of stimulating the brain, which is thought to be effective in controlling the excitability of the motor cortex
- transdirect current stimulation (tDCS), where a weak electrical current is passed over the brain by the use of surface electrodes
- paired associative stimulation, where pharyngeal electrical stimulation (PES) is paired with direct transcranial electrical stimulation

Each treatment approach will be outlined. The rationale for the use in the treatment of dysphagia will be explained and an overview of the current evidence for each intervention will be reported. The electro-therapies for dysphagia can be divided into two main groups; peripherally delivered and cortically delivered stimulation.

Peripherally Delivered Stimulation Approaches

Transcutaneous Neuromuscular Electrical Stimulation

Transcutaneous neuromuscular electrical stimulation is a relatively new therapeutic intervention for the treatment of swallowing disorders and was first approved by the Food and Drug Administration in USA in 2001 as a treatment for dysphagia. Although it is used as a treatment modality in the USA, it is currently not used in routine clinical practice in the UK and other European countries although the efficacy of NMES for the treatment of dysphagia is being investigated in a small number of research studies.

Transcutaneous neuro-muscular electrical stimulation can be defined as "the external control of innervated but paretic or paralytic muscles by electrical stimulation of the corresponding intact peripheral nerves" [20]. It is referred to in the literature by a potentially confusing variety of acronyms (NMES, TNMES, EMS, TES, TC and the trademarks VitalStim and AMPCARE™). For the consistency for this chapter, the acronym NMES will be used.

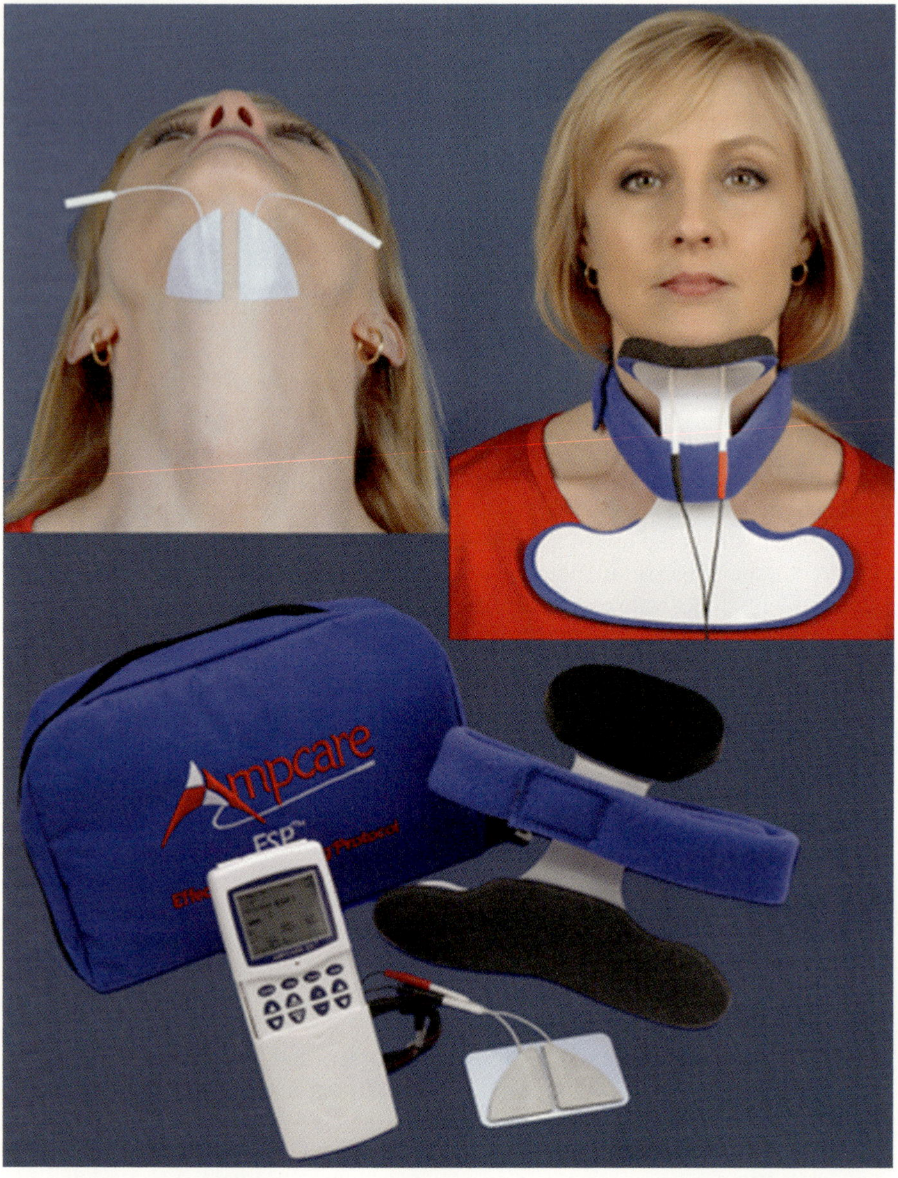

Fig. 6.1 Equipment and placement site of the Ampcare™ Effective Swallowing Protocol device (With permission from Professor Patrick McAdoo)

NMES is a non-invasive technique, involving application of an electrical current to the targeted muscle groups via the skin using electrodes placed on the skin surface. The source of the electrical current is usually from a battery powered hand held stimulator unit (see Fig. 6.1).

The hypothesis of transcutaneous electrical stimulation for the treatment of dysphagia is two-fold. Firstly, that by targeting the musculature of the oropharynx with electrical current, the muscles required for swallowing will be strengthened. It is postulated that by increasing the intensity of the electrical current, the electrical field penetrates deeper and depolarizes nerve endings in muscles to produce a muscle contraction. This process aims to strengthen the innervated muscles [21] and may protect striated muscles from atrophy [22, 23]. Secondly, stimulation of the sensory pathways may promote reorganization of the motor cortex and enhance motor relearning.

During volitional muscle contraction that occurs in traditional exercise, type I motor unit fibres are typically recruited first whereas in NMES, the fast twitch muscle fibres (type II motor unit fibres) are activated first and it is postulated that this pattern of recruitment will lead to enhanced muscle strengthening [22, 23]. This is considered to be a positive aspect of NMES in the treatment of dysphagia since a number of the muscles of swallowing are thought to have a higher proportion of type II motor unit fibres; for example the digastric muscle and middle pharyngeal constrictor muscles. However, although muscle strength may be gained during NMES, the carryover to functional activities is not thought to be as great as that of active exercises due to this manner of motor recruitment being opposite to usual recruitment [24]. This is thought to be especially true when the exercise is tailored to match the motor unit activation pattern of the desired movement.

When NMES is combined with traditional swallow exercises, the simultaneous recruitment of both types I and II muscle fibres during the combined therapy is thought to generate larger swallowing muscle force and enhance the therapeutic effect above that of NMES or exercise alone in dysphagia treatment. The greatest gains may thus be obtained when NMES is paired with resistance training and/or functional activities [25]. When using NMES as an adjunct treatment technique, an individual often produces more numerous and more frequent swallows during the treatment session than with exercise alone and this repetitive action of swallowing may help to explain the improved overall therapeutic effect which has been found in some studies [26–29]. Additionally, the electrical stimulation combined with swallowing practise and exercise can increase swallowing excitability in the motor cortex of the brain and facilitate motor learning.

The placement of electrodes during electrical stimulation for treating dysphagia is an area of some controversy particularly as the muscles involved in swallowing are small and many are overlapping. Suprahyoid muscles including the anterior belly of the digastric, the mylohyoid, and the geniohyoid muscles are responsible for the anterior and superior movement of the hyoid. Whilst the infrahyoid muscles such as the sternohyoid, omohyoid, and sternothyroid muscles depress the hyoid.

When swallowing, the movement of the larynx in both an upward and forward direction is critical for closure of the laryngeal vestibule and the reduction in the risk of aspiration occurring during the swallow process. Reduced elevation and superior motion of the larynx, which are common occurrences in people presenting with dysphagia, is usually as a result of reduced hyoid movement.

When the electrodes are placed on the group of infrahyoid muscles, the electrical current is thought to reach the sternohyoid and omohyoid muscles first, because the sternohyoid muscle is larger and closer to the surface than the thyrohyoid muscle. However, as the sternohyoid and omohyoid muscles pull the hyoid bone downwards, this site of electrode placement has been found to result in a downward movement of the hyoid [30, 31]. It is suggested that this could be a detrimental movement to patients who present with dysphagia? as it may put them at greater risk of aspiration as a result of the airway remaining open during the swallowing process [30]. This is especially likely if the individual is consuming diet and/or fluid at the same time as the stimulation is being received.

However, a further theory explored in the literature [30] is that such a movement during swallowing, may produce a resistance against upward displacement of the hyolaryngeal structures and so may strengthen the suprahyoid muscles and thyrohyoid muscle which lift the larynx. With this debate in mind some may thus consider that the electrode placement on the suprahyoid muscles may be a safer placement to achieve hyolaryngeal elevation in dysphagic patients with weak muscles and reduced hyolaryngeal elevation.

One of the most commonly used NMES techniques in the USA for treating patients with dysphagia incorporates electrode placements which stimulate both the suprahyoid and infrahyoid muscles [22]. This technique was developed by a team based in Chattanooga, USA and is marketed under the trade name of VitalStim Therapy. The intervention uses a pair of electrodes usually positioned bilaterally on the digastric muscles and the other on the thyrohyoid muscle. The electrical current is delivered via a hand held stimulator unit for a period of up to 60 min whilst the patient produces voluntary swallows. At regular intervals throughout each treatment session, patients are asked whether they can tolerate greater current intensity. Use of increased intensities facilitates progressively stronger muscle contractions, with the aim of achieving maximum treatment outcomes.

Studies reported in the literature have used the protocol over an intervention period of up to 5 days a week, for up to approximately 4 weeks of intervention. Some authors use this electrode placement with a current intensity at a sensory level only whilst others set the intensity at both a sensory and motor level. Different nerves are thought to be stimulated by increasing the intensity of the electrical stimulation. At the lower levels, the electrical current will stimulate just the afferent nerves (sensory nerves). The patient is reported to feel the electrical stimulation perhaps as a 'tingling sensation' but no muscles are contracting. As the intensity increases, some of the efferent nerves (motor nerves) will be stimulated resulting in a muscle contraction. During the treatment sessions, patients are generally encouraged to swallow boluses of oral intake via voluntary swallowing activity.

In contrast, a further protocol cleared by the FDA in USA for the treatment of dysphagia uses electrodes positioned only on the submental musculature, in order to target the anterior digastric, mylohyoid and geniohyoid muscles (the suprahyoid muscles) as these protract and elevate the hyoid bone and raise the larynx. This protocol is marketed under the trade name of the Ampcare Effective Swallowing Protocol.™

This protocol uses different electrode placement and different treatment parameters to the previously described protocol (Fig. 6.1). However, the electrical current is also provided via a hand held stimulator unit. The stimulus is set according to the maximum patient tolerance level and aims to produce a motor unit response level muscle contraction. This protocol differs from the previously described technique, as the patient is encouraged to carryout simultaneous laryngeal exercises during the stimulation period rather than taking oral intake. The exercises are produced against resistance, by incorporating a specially designed neck brace, which acts as a resistive device for the patient to work against. Pulse duration/width is an adjustable parameter during this technique, allowing the clinician to select the most comfortable parameter for the patient. Treatments are generally 5 days a week for a period of around 4–6 weeks.

The parameters are adjusted during the intervention period to encourage the individual to work harder during the sessions. In Week 1, treatment involves a total of 60 stimulations (each lasting 5 s) during which the patients carry out exercises and then swallow. In Week 2, the rest period between pulses of stimulation is reduced, so that patients receive a total of 72 stimulations during the session. In Weeks 3 and 4, patients receive a total of 90 stimulations.This procedure is postulated to encourage progressive muscle strengthening. The exercises completed during each pulse of stimulation are specifically selected to target hyoid and laryngeal elevation.

The aim of combining the resistive exercises simultaneously with the stimulation aims to strengthen and improve functional swallowing movement patterns through muscle contraction against resistance. It also aims to improve cortical reorganization and neurovascular coupling, and provide an overload principle to muscles, to increase range of motion and strength.

Since an initial study by Freed et al. [22], there have been a considerable number of studies investigating the therapeutic effect of NMES on swallow function. The majority of these have focussed on dysphagia post stroke. Baijens and colleagues [32] have looked at Parkinson's disease and found no significant effects when compared to traditional therapy – however they only used a single session of stimulation. Ryu et al. [33] looked at dysphagia following head and neck cancer and found no significant differences between NMES and traditional therapy.

Within the stroke dysphagia population, there have been conflicting findings within the literature. This may in part be due to the heterogeneity of the treatment protocol across studies – some have used NMES alone versus traditional therapy techniques, whereas others have used it as an adjunct. Differing electrode types have been used, with different electrode application sites and different treatment parameters. Many studies have also been criticised for use of small sample sizes, lack of randomised controls and lack of blinding or inter-rater reliability controls [22, 28, 34].

These limitations make meta-analysis a challenge and so there remains a need for large scale, randomised controlled trials using explicit reporting of electrode type, placement and treatment parameters before decisions regarding clinical adoption of this technique can be made. Several systematic reviews [35, 21] and meta-analysis studies [36–38] have been completed, although they each acknowledge the limitations inherent in combining studies with significant heterogeneity. A Cochrane review in 2012 [39] summarises the position, stating that the evidence on NMES (as with the other electrical stimulation approaches) “remains unclear”.

Given the cautionary notes above regarding the difficulty in extrapolating definitive answers from the current evidence base regarding NMES and treatment efficacy post stroke dysphagia, Table 6.1 summarises the main points from the available literature to date.

Palatal Electrical Stimulation

Electrical stimulation via a palatal prosthesis as a treatment for post stroke dysphagia has been explored in a small number of patients who present with delayed triggering of the swallow. This technique involves fitting each patient with an individually made palatal appliance (constructed from a dental impression). Electrodes extend posteriorly from an acrylic plate and are designed to contact the soft palate. The electrodes are not placed at a specific point on the soft palate; rather the aim is to deliver general stimulation to the palate.

Palatal electrical stimulation is founded upon the hypothesis that the stimulation will excite sensory feedback and so result in stimulation of an involuntary swallow reflex. Electrical stimulation is generally provided at 1-s intervals and the patients are asked to swallow a bolus during stimulation [40].

This technique has been explored in a very small number of studies [40, 41] which developed from earlier work on mechanical/thermal stimulation of the faucial arches in order to trigger swallowing. Following a failure to demonstrate treatment efficacy of mechanical/thermal stimulation, these studies investigated whether electrical stimulation to the palate might prove more effective. The earlier study by Park [40] concluded that palatal electrical stimulation had improved swallow function in 2 out of 4 patients in a case series; however the Power study [41] used a real versus sham design on 16 patients with post stroke dysphagia and found no evidence of functional change. The technique has received little attention since this period and is unlikely to be adopted into routine clinical practice, as other electro-therapeutic approaches have offered more promising results.

Pharyngeal Electrical Stimulation

The use of pharyngeal electrical stimulation (PES), as a treatment for dysphagia has been explored primarily by Hamdy and colleagues [42–44], mainly via trials on healthy volunteers and then on patients with dysphagia post stroke.

In this approach, the electrical input is provided via an intraluminal pharyngeal catheter, placed into the pharynx via either the nasal or oral cavity. The catheter is connected to an electrical stimulator base unit, which generates a stimulus according to set parameters.

Table 6.1 Summary points of literature regarding Neuro-muscular electrical stimulation (NMES) in the treatment of dysphagia

Summary of current consensus in the literature on NMES		
Statement	Supporting evidence	Qualifying notes
NMES as an adjunct to targeted traditional therapy techniques is more effective in treating post stroke dysphagia then traditional therapy alone	Lim et al. (2009) [26] Park et al. (2012) [27] Kushner et al. (2013) [28] Lee et al. (2014) [29]	Clarity is required on optimal dose intensity, optimal electrode sites, treatment protocols and timing of therapy post stroke
There is insufficient evidence that NMES alone is effective	In favour of NMES: Freed et al. (2001) [22] Permsirivanich et al. (2009) [69] Gallas et al. (2010) [34] Against NMES: Bulow et al. (2008) [70]	It should be noted that the 2001 and 2010 studies have been strongly criticised for having weak study design, whereas the Bulow study was a multi-centre, randomised controlled trial
Summary of gaps in the current evidence		
Evidence required	Supporting evidence	Qualifying notes
Systematic reviews and meta- analyses have not been able to reach definitive agreement regarding the treatment efficacy of NMES	Systematic reviews in favour of NMES: Carnaby-Mann et al. (2007) [36] Huckabee et al. (2007) [20] Langdon et al. (2010) [71] Tan et al. (2013) [37] Chen et al. (2015) [38] Systematic reviews against NMES: Reviews concluding the evidence is insufficient to answer this: Ayala et al. (2008) [35] Clark et al. (2009) [21] Geeganage et al. (2012) [39]	Authors who have felt that they can reach a conclusion acknowledge that their meta analyses are limited by the heterogeneity of treatment approaches used (eg as an adjunct to traditional therapy or used alone), relatively small number of studies for inclusion, plus study design weaknesses
Further research is required to determine optimum treatment parameters (eg stimulation intensity) and electrode placement	Geeganage et al. (2012) [39] Poorjavad et al. (2014) [68] National Institute for Health and Care Excellence (NICE) (2014) [72]	Clarity is required regarding whether sensory or motor stimulation levels are more effective, also to determine which muscle groups should be targeted for which dysphagic symptoms, and to define electrode placement accordingly
Further research is required to determine the patient groups for which NMES might be effective (eg Stroke, degenerative neurology, cancer)	NICE (2014) [72]	Much of the published studies have focussed on stroke

The stimulation in this technique is described as a sensorimotor input which primarily activates the afferent nerves. However, when given at higher intensities the stimulation can “evoke small twitches of the pharyngeal musculature” ([45] p8). This approach is designed to exploit neuroplasticity by enhancing the excitability and organisation of the motor cortex in the brain. Stimulation is described in studies as being for around 10 min a day for a period of 1–3 days [46].

Much of the earlier research into PES and dysphagia has focussed on stroke – and specifically on the acute phase of stroke [46]. However, Vasant [47] looked at PES in more chronic post stroke dysphagia; concluding that data collection at 3 months post stroke showed that PES expedited recovery of swallow function in comparison to traditional therapy. A Cochrane review by Geeganage et al. [39] reported that PES “reduced pharyngeal transit time” of the bolus during swallowing and this approach therefore justifies further larger randomised controlled trials, particularly studies which evaluate the economic efficacy of this approach, and its longer term health outcomes.

Functional Magnetic Stimulation

A much more recently investigated type of neurorehabilitation of swallowing is functional magnetic stimulation (FMS). This type of neuromodulation involves a current pulse passing through a coil to generate a magnetic field (Fig. 6.2), causing stimulation to nerves and muscles, in FMS the current is applied peripherally, over targeted muscle groups.

FMS stimulates nerves and muscles by changing the electrical potential of the nerve cell wall and if this change is large enough, an action potential in the nerve will be generated. If the nerve is a motor nerve a muscle fibre is activated.

The principles behind FMS can be thought of as largely similar to those for neuromuscular electrical stimulation, but FMS is postulated by some to achieve a greater range of depth to stimulate deep tissue without pain [48].

With FMS it is speculated that it may be possible to induce improved contractibility of pharyngeal muscle groups and neuro-modulation of swallowing-related muscle groups by stimulation of the pharyngeal muscles and their dominant nerves through FMS [49]. One of the afferent pathways of the swallowing reflex is the sensory branch of the vagus nerve from the pharyngeal mucosa. It is speculated that if the vagus nerve is stimulated, it is possible that afferent input from the oropharynx could act on the swallowing reflex centre in the medulla oblongata and on the cerebral cortex. As research protocols using FMS have not involved oral intake, it is thought that this intervention can be carried out safely even for patients with severe dysphagia [49].

It should be noted that currently, this technique has only been investigated by a very small group of researchers, through research studies using small numbers of subjects. These studies have often included uncontrolled trial designs and therefore more research – including larger, randomised controlled trials – will be required before this technique could be considered for translation into clinical practice.

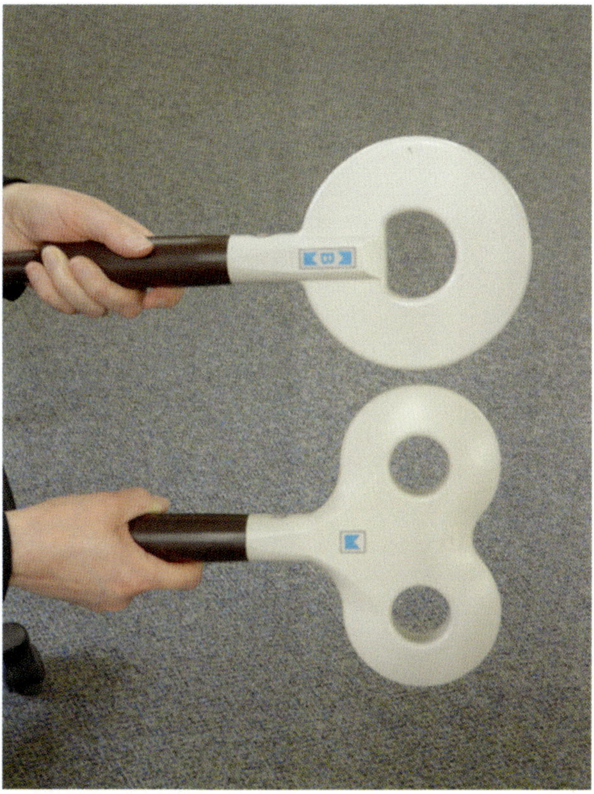

Fig. 6.2 Circular and figure of eight coils for delivery of cortical stimulation (With permission from Professor A.T. Barker)

Cortically Delivered Stimulation Approaches

Repetitive transcranial magnetic stimulation (rTMS) and transcranial direct current stimulation (tDCS) deliver stimulation to the cerebral cortex and have also been investigated as potential tools for facilitating recovery of swallowing function. These two different interventions are considered to be non-invasive and appear to be safe when used according to established safety guidelines [50].

Repetitive Transcranial Magnetic Stimulation

Repetitive transcranial magnetic stimulation (rTMS) is a non-invasive method of stimulating the brain and it is thought to be effective in controlling the excitability of the motor cortex and in reducing the inhibitory imbalance between the hemispheres after stroke [26].

Stimulation is usually via a figure-of-eight coil positioned over one of the two hemispheres of the brain (Figs. 6.2 and 6.3). High frequency magnetic stimulation of an affected hemisphere is postulated to increase the excitability of the cortex,

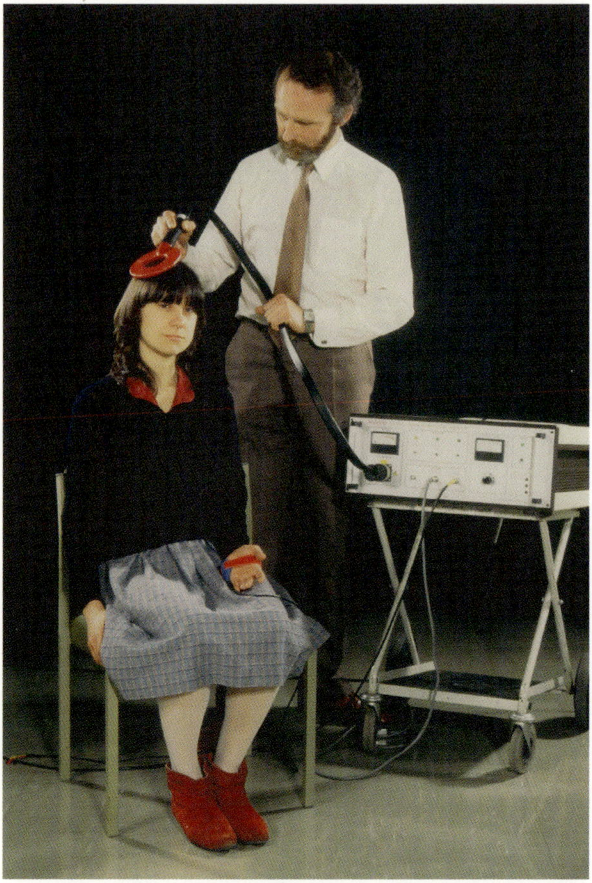

Fig. 6.3 The first repetitive transcranial magnetic stimulation (rTMS) system developed in Sheffield, UK (With permission from Professor A. Barker)

whereas low-frequency stimulation of the unaffected hemisphere lowers cortical excitability, which might decrease the imbalance between the hemispheres [26, 51, 52]. The stimulation of neuronal networks is thought to outlast the actual stimulation period by 30–60 min [53, 54]. However, the exact recovery mechanism of rTMS is currently unclear. Positive effects of rTMS in stroke patients with dysphagia have been reported in some studies [55–59]. However, each study uses a different magnetic stimulation frequency with no definitely established protocol.

Some of the current evidence regarding rTMS relates to studies on normal subjects, or on virtual lesions [60] a number of small studies have investigated the potential of rTMS to rehabilitate swallow function either by use of rTMS alone [55–58] or in combination with intensive traditional swallow rehabilitation exercises [59]. Each of these studies found positive effects of rTMS on swallow function (although using varying outcome measures). Caution should be applied to these findings however as very small sample sizes have been used to date and several of the studies used uncontrolled designs. Evidence based guidelines for the use of rTMS [61] have included stroke within the clinical applications they evaluated, however their conclusions relate to the effects on general motor deficit, aphasia and hemineglect rather than dysphagia.

Transcranial Direct Current Stimulation

Transcranial direct current stimulation (tDCS) is an additional non-invasive technique that has been investigated in a small number of studies [62–66]. During tDCS a weak electrical current is passed over the brain via two surface electrodes placed on the scalp to produce changes in neuronal excitability [62]. The effects of tDCS are dependent on the direction of the current flow. Doeltgen ([63] p209) suggests that "anodal stimulation of the motor cortex generally produces facilitation of motor cortical excitability, whereas cathodal stimulation reduces it".

It is postulated that the application of tDCS to the cortical motor and sensory pharyngeal areas can improve swallowing function when combined with traditional swallowing activities [45, 60, 62]. Shigematsu et al. [50] showed beneficial effects of tDCS in conjunction with traditional dysphagia therapy exercises post stroke.

Although tDCS is cheaper and easier to carryout than rTMS, and there have been several studies which have shown favourable results, the sample sizes have been small and there remain unanswered questions regarding the optimum dose for stimulating the motor cortex and also the optimal site for electrode placement over the cerebral cortex.

Many of the studies so far on clinical populations have focussed on stroke. However, Restivo [64] investigated the effects of tDCS versus pharyngeal electrical stimulation (PES) on multiple sclerosis related dysphagia. Patients who received real versus sham tDCS made significantly greater improvement on measures of swallow function and also penetration-aspiration scales under videofluoroscopy, however there was no significant difference between tDCS and PES groups, although the authors reported that tDCS was better tolerated than PES.

Consideration of the timing of the measurement of any beneficial effects must also be made; Yang [65] found no significant difference between tDCS plus traditional therapy versus sham stimulation plus traditional therapy immediately after treatment, however at 3 months, the tDCS group showed improvement on dysphagia outcome measures (when factors of age, time post onset etc. were controlled for). Further research is therefore required to determine whether this intervention should be adopted into clinical practice.

Paired Associative Stimulation (PAS)

Michou and colleagues [66] looked at pairing pharyngeal electrical stimulation with direct transcranial electrical stimulation. They first tested the technique on virtual lesions in healthy volunteers, which they created by repetitive transcranial magnetic stimulation over the pharyngeal cortex. They reported reversing the lesions with

10 min of paired stimulation (compared to sham stimulation) and then went on to evaluate the effects of PAS in a proof-of principle study on six patients with dysphagia post stroke. They found that PAS to the contralesional pharyngeal motor cortex "increased excitability of the unaffected hemisphere," (p 37) accompanied by a reduction in severity of aspiration and/or laryngeal penetration and reduced bolus flow times through the pharynx. This is currently early phase research on a small sample size and the authors acknowledge further research will be required into the potential treatment efficacy of this approach. It is also interesting to speculate whether other stimulation approaches might be paired and to what effect in future studies.

Future Direction

With the application of electrical stimulation techniques to the treatment of dysphagia the aim is to improve or recover swallowing function. The outcome for the patient is likely improved nutritional status and quality of life and the prevention of deleterious health outcomes; moreover the outcome for the health economy is likely reduced costs, due to reduction in occurrence of dysphagia related complications such as aspiration pneumonia and reduction in hospital admissions which are costly to the health economy. Many of the electrical stimulation techniques described in this chapter are showing positive trends as treatment approaches for oropharyngeal dysphagia however before they can be translated into routine clinical practice further research is indicated to answer the emerging questions around dose response effects, standardised protocols for intervention and evidence around which patient populations respond maximally to each method, particularly over the longer term. Many of the studies discussed have included functional changes to the swallow as an outcome measure for example the Functional Oral Intake Scale (FOIS) [67] which describes on a seven point scale the foods and drinks that a person is able to take orally or via a PEG. However fewer studies have included specific physiological measures which could objectively quantify changes in the swallowing biomechanics eg measures of laryngeal elevation or airway closure timings following the e-stimulation intervention.

The positive effects being described in the literature regarding the efficacy of the different electrical stimulation techniques for treating oropharyngeal dysphagia may yield exciting benefits for patients in the coming years. Carefully controlled and fully powered trials are needed to ensure clinical practise is evidence based and targeted at providing maximal clinical benefits to patients.

The selection of a specific modality for an individual patient will need to be based on the underlying physiological features of the swallowing deficit. Knowing the specific features for remediation from detailed assessment procedures will allow specific therapeutic protocols to be developed and specific outcome measures to be utilised. The identification and clear understanding of stimulation effects on the underlying pathophysiology of swallowing disorders and on the central nervous system organisation will allow individualised treatment protocols to be designed [68].

Before we can apply these promising treatments more widely to the general dysphagia population we need to improve our understanding of the efficacy of each individual technique. The challenge for both clinicians and researchers is to complete large scale robust research trials which incorporate control groups, randomisation processes and clear outcome measures on homogeneous samples of patients. Only then can the full potential of electrical stimulation for the treatment of dysphagia be fully determined.

References

1. Logemann J. Evaluation and treatment of swallowing disorders. San Diego: College-Hill Press Inc; 1983.
2. Katzan IL, Dawson NV, Thomas ME, Votruba ME, Cebul RD. The cost of pneumonia after acute stroke. Neurology. 2007;68:1938–43.
3. Heuschmann PU, Kolominsky-Rabas PL, Roether J, Misselwitz B, Lowitzsch K, Heidrich J, et al. Predictors of in-hospital mortality in patients with acute ischemic stroke treated with thrombolytic therapy. JAMA. 2004;292(15):1831–8.
4. Hassan A, Khealani BA, Shafgat S, Aslam M, Salahuddin N, Syed NA, et al. Stroke-associated pneumonia: microbiological data and outcome. Singapore Med J. 2006;47(3):204–7.
5. Martino R, Foley N, Bhogal S, Diamant N, Speechley M, Teasell R. Dysphagia after stroke: incidence, diagnosis, and pulmonary complications. Stroke. 2005;36(12):2756–63.
6. Mann G, Hankey GJ, Cameron D. Swallowing function after stroke. Prognosis and prognostic factors at six months. Stroke. 1999;30(4):744–8.
7. Hartelius L, Svensson P. Speech and swallowing symptoms associated with Parkinson's disease and multiple sclerosis: a survey. Folia Phoniatr. 1994;46(1):9–17.
8. Steele C, Greenwood C, Ens I, Robertson C, Seidman-Carlson C. Mealtime difficulties in a home for the aged: not just dysphagia. Dysphagia. 1997;12:43–50.
9. Reilly S, Skuse D, Poblete X. Prevalence of feeding problems and oral motor dysfunction in children with cerebral palsy: a community survey. J Pediatr. 1996;129(6):877–82.
10. McKinstry M, Tranter M, Sweeney J. Outcomes of dysphagia intervention in a pulmonary rehabilitation program. Dysphagia. 2010;25(2):104–11.
11. McCabe D, Ashford J, Wheeler-Hegland K, Frymark T, Mullen R, Musson N, et al. Evidence-based systematic review: Oropharyngeal dysphagia behavioral treatments. Part IV- Impact of dysphagia treatment on individuals' postcancer treatments. 2 J Rehabil Res Dev. 2009;46(2): 205–14.
12. Ward E, Uriate M, Conroy A. Duration of dysphagic symptoms and swallowing outcomes after thermal burn injury. J Burn Care Rehabil. 2001;22(6):441–53.
13. Ward E, Green K, Morton A. Patterns and predictors of swallowing resolution following adult traumatic brain injury. J Head Trauma Rehabil. 2007;22(3):184–91.
14. Frempong-Boadu A, Houton JK, Osborn B, Opulencia J, Kells L, Guida DG, Roux P. Swallowing and speech dysfunction in patients undergoing anterior cervical discectomy and fusion: a prospective, objective preoperative and post-operative assessment. J Spinal Disord Tech. 2002;15(5):362–8.
15. Logemann J. Evaluation and treatment of swallowing disorders. (rev. ed). Austin: PRO-ED and St. Tammany Parish Schools Dysphagia Team; 1998.
16. Crary M, Groher M. Introduction to adult swallowing disorders. Philadelphia: Butterworth-Heinemann; 2003.
17. Costa Bandeira A, Azevedo E, Vartanian JG, Nishimoto I, Kowalski L, Carrara-de AE. Quality of life related to swallowing after tongue cancer treatment. Anna Karinne Dysphagia. 2008;23(2):183.

18. Rosenvinge S, Starke I. Improving care for patients with dysphagia. Age Ageing. 2005;34(6):587–93.
19. Robbins SM, Houghton PE, Woodbury MG, Brown JL. The therapeutic effect of functional and transcutaneous electric stimulation on improving gait speed in stroke patients: a meta-analysis. Arch Phys Med Rehabil. 2006;87:853–9.
20. Huckabee ML, Doeltgen S. Emerging modalities in dysphagia rehabilitation: neuromuscular electrical stimulation. N Z Med J. 2007;120:U2744.
21. Clark H, Lazarus C, Arvedson J, Schooling T, Frymark T. Evidence-based sustematic review: effects of neuromuscular electrical stimulation on swallowing and neural activation. Am J Speech Lang Pathol. 2009;18:361–75.
22. Freed ML, Freed L, Chatburn RL, Christian M. Electrical stimulation for swallowing disorders caused by stroke. Respir Care. 2001;46(5):466–74.
23. Blumenfeld L, Hahn Y, LePage A, Leonard R, Belafsky PC. Transcutaneous electrical stimulation versus traditional dysphagia therapy: a nonconcurrent cohort study. Otolaryngol Head Neck Surg. 2006;135(5):754–7.
24. Clark HM. Neuromuscular treatments for speech and swallowing: a tutorial. Am J Speech Lang Pathol. 2003;12(4):400–15.
25. Mysiw WJ, Jackson RD. Electrical stimulation. In: Braddom RL, editor. Physical medicine and rehabilitation. Philadelphia: Saunders; 1996. p. 464–87.
26. Lim KB, Lee HJ, Lim SS, Choi YI. Neuromuscular electrical and thermal-tactile stimulation for dysphagia caused by stroke: a randomized controlled trial. J Rehabil Med. 2009;41:174–8.
27. Park JW, Kim Y, Oh JC, Lee HJ. Effortful swallowing training combined with electrical stimulation in post stroke dysphagia: a randomized controlled study. Dysphagia. 2012;27:521–7.
28. Kushner DS, Peters K, Eroglu S, Perless-Carroll M, Johnson-Greene D. Neuromuscular electrical stimulation in acute stoke feeding tube-dependent dysphagia during inpatient rehabilitation. Am J Phys Med Rehabil. 2013;92(6):486–95.
29. Lee KW, Kim SB, Lee JH, Lee SJ, Ri JW, Park JG. The effect of early neuromuscular electrical stimulation therapy in acute/subacute ischaemic stroke patients with dysphagia. Ann Rehabil Med. 2014;38(2):153–9.
30. Ludlow C, Humbert I, Saxon K, Poletto C, Sonies B, Crujido L. Effects of surface electrical stimulation in chronic pharyngeal dysphagia. Dysphagia. 2007;22:1–10.
31. Humbert IA, Poletto CJ, Saxon KG, Kearney PR, Crujido L, Wright-Harp W, et al. The effect of surface electrical stimulation on hyolaryngeal movement in normal individuals at rest and during swallowing. J Appl Physiol. 2006;101:1657–63.
32. Baijens LW, Speyer R, Passos VL, Pilz W, Van der Kruis J, Haarmans S, Desjardins-Rombouts C. Surface electrical stimulation in dysphagic Parkinson patients: a randomized clinical trial. Laryngoscope. 2013;123(11):38–44.
33. Ryu JS, Kang JK, Park JY, Nam SY, Choi SH, Roh JL, et al. The effect of electrical stimulation therapy on dysphagia following treatment for head and neck cancer. Oral Oncol. 2009;45:665–8.
34. Gallas S, Marie JP, Leroi AM. Sensory transcutaneous electrical stimulation improves post-stroke dysphagic patients. Dysphagia. 2010;25:291–7.
35. Ayala KJ, Cruz KJ. Transcutaneous electrical stimulation in dysphagia treatment: is there sufficient evidence? Tex J Audiol Speech Lang Pathol. 2008;31:37–54.
36. Carnaby-Mann G, Crary M. Examining the evidence on neuromuscular electrical stimulation for swallowing, a meta-analysis. Arch Otolaryngol Head Neck Surg. 2007;133:564–71.
37. Tan C, Liu Y, Li W, Liu J, Chen L. Transcutaneous neuromuscular electrical stimulation can improve swallowing function in patients with dysphagia caused by non-stroke diseases: a meta-analysis. J Oral Rehabil. 2013;40:472–80.
38. Chen YW, Chang KH, Chen HC, Liang WM, Wang YH, Lin YN. The effects of surface neuromuscular electrical stimulation on post-stroke dysphagia: a systematic review and meta-analysis. Clin Rehabil. 2015. doi:10.1177/0269215515571681

39. Geeganage C, Beavan J, Ellender S, Bath PM. Interventions for dysphagia and nutritional support in acute and subacute stroke. Cochrane Database Syst Rev. 2012;10:CD000323.
40. Park CL, O'Neill PA, Martin DF. A pilot exploratory study of oral electrical stimulation on swallow function after stroke: an innovative technique. Dysphagia. 1997;12(3):161–6.
41. Power M, Fraser CH, Hobson A, Singh S, Tyrell P, Nicholson D, Turnbull I, Thompson DG, Hamdy S. Evaluating oral stimulation as a treatment for dysphagia after stroke. Dysphagia. 2006;21:49–55.
42. Hamdy S, Rothwell JC, Aziz Q, Singh KD, Thompson DG. Long term re-organization of human motor cortex driven by short term sensory stimulation. Nat Neurosci. 1998;1(1):64–8.
43. Hamdy S, Aziz Q, Rothwell JC. Recovery of swallowing after dysphagic stroke realtes to functional reorganization in the intact motor cortex. Gastroenterology. 1998;115(5):1104–12.
44. Hamdy S, Rothwell JC, Aziz Q, Thompson DG. Organization and reorganization of human swallowing motor cortex: implications for recovery after stroke. Clin Sci. 2000;99(2):151–7.
45. Mistry S, Michou E, Vasant D, Ghannouchi I, Verin E, Hamdy S. New techniques – future. J Gastroenterol Hepatol. 2014;3(5):1080–7.
46. Jayasekeran V, Singh S, Tyrrell P, Michou E, Jefferson S, Mistry S, et al. Adjunctive functional pharyngeal electrical stimulation reverses swallowing disability following brain lesions. Gastroenterology. 2010;138(5):1737–46.
47. Vasant DH, Michou E, Tyrrell P, Mistry S, Jayasekeran V, Hamdy S. Pharyngeal electrical stimulation (PES) expedites swallowing recovery in dysphagia post-acute stroke: a phase II double-blinded randomised controlled trial. Gastroenterology. 2014;146(5):S-77.
48. Momosaki R, Abo M, Watanabe S, Kakuda W, Yamada N, Mochio K. Functional magnetic stimulation using a parabolic coil for dysphagia after stroke. Neuromodulation. 2014;17(7):637–41.
49. Momosaki R, Abo M, Watanabe S, Kakuda W, Yamada N. Functional magnetic stimulation over suprahyoid muscle can induce plastic change in swallowing motor cortex. Arch Phys Med Rehabil. 2014;95 10(e91–e92):0003–9993.
50. Shigematsu T, Fujishima I, Ohno K. Transcranial direct current stimulation improves swallowing function in stroke patients. Neurorehabil Neural Repair. 2013;27(4):363–9.
51. Hummel F, Celnik P, Giraux P, Floel A, Wu WH, Gerloff C, et al. Effects of non-invasive cortical stimulation on skilled motor function in chronic stroke. Brain. 2005;128(pt3):490–9.
52. Hummel FC, Cohen LG. Non-invasive brain stimulation: a new strategy to improve neurorehabilitation after stroke? Lancet Neurol. 2006;5:708–12.
53. Stefan K, Kunesch E, Cohen LG, Benecke R, Classen J. Induction of plasticity in the human motor cortex by paired associative stimulation. Brain. 2000;123:572–84.
54. Huang YZ, Edwards MJ, Rounis E, Bhatia KP, Rothwell JC. Theta burst stimulation of the human motor cortex. Neuron. 2005;45:201–6.
55. Verin E, Leroi AM. Poststroke dysphagia rehabilitation by repetitive transcranial magnetic stimulation: a non-controlled pilot study. Dysphagia. 2009;24(2):204–10.
56. Khedr EM, Abo-Elfetoh N. Therapeutic role of rTMS on recovery of dysphagia in patients with lateral medullary syndrome and brainstem infarction. J Neurol Neurosurg Psychiatry. 2010;81(5):495–9.
57. Kim L, Chun MH, Kim BR, Lee SJ. Effect of repetitive transcranial magnetic stimulation on patients with brain injury and dysphagia. Ann Rehabil Med. 2011;35:765–71.
58. Cheng IK, Chan KM, Wong CS, Cheung RT. Preliminary evidence of the effects of high-frequency repetitive transcranial magnetic stimulation (rTMS) on swallowing functions in post-stroke individuals with chronic dysphagia. Int J Lang Commun Disord. 2015;50(3):389–96. doi:10.1111/1460-6984.12144.
59. Momosaki R, Abo M, Kakuda W. Bilateral repetitive transcranial magnetic stimulation combined with intensive swallowing rehabilitation for chronic stroke dysphagia: a case series study. Case Rep Neurol. 2014;6(1):60–7.
60. Jefferson S, Mistry S, Michou E, Singh S, Rothwell JC, Hamdy S. Reversal of a virtual lesion in human pharyngeal motor cortex by high frequency contralesional brain stimulation. Gastroenterology. 2009;137:841–9.

61. Lefaucheur JP, Obadia NA, Antal A, Ayache SS, Baeken C, Benninger D, et al. Evidence based guidelines on the therapeutic use of repetitive transcranial magnetic stimulation. Clin Neurophysiol. 2014;125(11):2150–206.
62. Kumar S, Wagner CW, Frayne C, Zhu L, Selim M, Feng W, et al. Noninvasive brain stimulation may improve stroke-related dysphagia: a pilot study. Stroke. 2011;42:1035–40.
63. Doeltgen S, Huckabee ML. Swallowing rehabilitation: from the research laboratory to routine clinical application. Arch Phys Med Rehabil. 2012;93:207–13.
64. Restivo DA, Casabona A, Marchese-Ragona R. Transcranial direct current stimulation (TDCS) for dysphagia associated to multiple sclerosis. Clin Neurophysiol. 2014;125:1–205.
65. Yang EJ, Baek SR, Shin J, Lim JY, Jang HJ, Kim YK, Paik NJ. Effects of transcranial direct current stimulation (tDCS) on post-stroke dysphagia. Restor Neurol Neurosci. 2012;30(4):303–11.
66. Michou E, Mistry S, Jefferson S, Singh S, Rothwell J, Hamdy S. Targeting unlesioned pharyngeal motor cortex improves swallowing in healthy individuals and after dysphagic stroke. Gastroenterology. 2012;142:29–38.
67. Crary MA, Carnaby-Mann GD, Groher M. Initial psychometric assessment of a functional oral intake scale for dysphagia in stroke patients. Arch Phys Med Rehabil. 2005;86(8):1516–20.
68. Poorjavad M, Moghadam ST, Ansari NN, Daemi M. Surface electrical stimulation for treating swallowing disorders after stroke: a review of the stimulation intensity levels and the electrode placements. Stroke Res Treat. 2014;24:918057. HTTP://DXDOI.ORG/10.1155/2014/918057.
69. Permsirivanich W, Tipchatyotin S, Wongchai M, Leelanmit V, Setthawacharawanich S, Sathirapanya P, et al. Comparing the effects of rehabilitation swallowing therapy vs. neuromuscular electrical stimulation therapy among stroke patients with persistent pharyngeal dysphagia: a randomized controlled study. J Med Assoc Thia. 2009;92(2):259–65.
70. Bulow M, Speyer R, Baijens L, Woisard V, Ekberg O. Neuromuscular electrical stimulation (NMES) in stroke patients with oral and pharyngeal dysfunction. Dysphagia. 2008;23:302–9.
71. Langdon C, Backer D. Dysphagia in stroke: a new solution. Stroke Res Treat. 2010:570403. doi:10.4061/2010/570403.
72. National Institute for Health and Care Excellence. Transcutaneous neuromuscular electrical stimulation for oropharyngeal dysphagia. NICE interventional procedure guidance (IPG490). 2014. ISBN 978-1-4731-0529-4.

Chapter 7
Vagal Nerve Stimulation for the Treatment of Heart Failure

Emma J. Radcliffe and Andrew W. Trafford

Abstract Despite the availability of several different therapies, heart failure remains a leading cause of death worldwide, with high mortality and morbidity rates. One prognostically important feature of heart failure, that remains unaltered by conventional therapy, is vagal withdrawal. Vagal nerve stimulation (VNS) allows the direct manipulation of vagal tone, via implantable pulse generators. Deemed both safe and tolerable for human use, pre-clinical and clinical data indicate promising improvements of left ventricular function with chronic VNS therapy. Despite several proposed mechanisms, little is understood about how the cardioprotective effect is mediated, leaving several unanswered questions for ongoing research and clinical trials.

Keywords Heart failure • Systolic dysfunction • Vagus • Nerve • Vagal nerve stimulation • Left ventricle • Ejection fraction • Heart rate • Heart rate variability • Inflammation

Introduction

Heart failure represents a significant global health problem, affecting almost 23 million people worldwide [1]. In the United Kingdom alone it is estimated that around 550,000 people are living with heart failure [2]. The prevalence of heart failure increases considerably with age, and in particular there is a much higher disease prevalence in those over 75 [2]. Given our aging population, and that more effective treatments for acute cardiovascular events are now in place, heart failure represents a final common pathway for the growing number of patients surviving initial cardiac insults [3].

E.J. Radcliffe, Bsc(Hons), PhD (✉) • A.W. Trafford, BVSc, Cert VA, PhD, MRCVS
Institute of Cardiovascular Science, School of Medicine, University of Manchester, Manchester, UK
e-mail: emma.radcliffe@manchester.ac.uk; andrew.w.trafford@manchester.ac.uk

A. Majid (ed.), *Electroceuticals*, DOI 10.1007/978-3-319-28612-9_7

Defining Heart Failure

Heart failure is a term used in general to refer to some form of ventricular dysfunction. On the whole it describes a number of overlapping cardiac conditions and is often associated with terms such as acute, transient, chronic, diastolic and systolic. A more pertinent definition of heart failure has been proposed by the European Society of Cardiology (ESC) [4]; they term heart failure as a syndrome with which patients present with both the clinical signs and symptoms consistent with heart failure (see Table 7.1), and evidence of structural or functional abnormalities at rest.

For the purpose of this chapter the term heart failure will be used to describe chronic heart failure with reduced left ventricular ejection fraction as this accounts for around 80% of heart failure hospitalisations [4].

Heart Failure Pathology

Heart failure is characterised not only by left ventricular dysfunction but also by chronic neurohumoral activation [5]. Sympathetic drive is increased in a bid to improve cardiac output, leading to a spill over of cardiac catecholamines and resultant increase in circulating catecholamine levels [6]. Reduced cardiac output and the associated reduction in systemic blood pressure also lead to activation of the renin-angiotensin-aldosterone system, leading to abnormally high angiotensin II levels [7]. Initially this acts as a compensatory mechanism by both enhancing cardiac output and maintaining perfusion pressure. However, chronic catecholamine exposure ultimately leads to deleterious remodelling of the cardiac ß-adrenergic axis; ß-receptors levels are down regulated [8] and desensitised due to downstream uncoupling [9], rendering the heart non-responsive to any increased metabolic demands. This is also paralleled by a reduction of parasympathetic control over the

Table 7.1 Defining heart failure; heart failure patients will present with evidence from all three categories [2]

Category	Example
Clinical symptoms	Breathlessness at rest or during exercise Fatigue Tiredness Ankle swelling
Clinical signs	Tachycardia Tachypnoea Pulmonary rales Pleural effusion Raised jugular venous pressure
Objective evidence of structural or functional abnormality at rest	Cardiomegaly Third heart sound Cardiac murmurs Echocardiogram abnormality Raised natriuretic peptide concentration

heart [10], resulting predominantly from loss of transduction at the level of the cardiac parasympathetic ganglion [11]. In combination, enhance sympathetic drive and vagal withdrawal result in notable autonomic imbalance in heart failure. In end-stage heart failure the loss of sympathetic responsiveness and parasympathetic tone can be so severe that comparisons have been drawn between end-stage failing hearts and the de-innervated hearts of a transplant patient [12]. Further neurohumoral activation subsequently increases the demand on the non-responsive heart, increasing cardiac stress and thereby driving the progressive deterioration of cardiac function [13].This degeneration affects the muscular, conduction and connective tissues of the heart, resulting in extensive remodelling of the left ventricle (Fig. 7.1).

This vicious cycle of progressive decline in ejection fraction is ultimately fatal. Typically, there is only a 50% survival rate 4 years from the time of diagnosis, with 40% of patients being re-hospitalised within the first year [14]. Although this is a poor prognosis, the time course of the disease does allow for chronic health care interventions to be instigated, with the aim of preventing further cardiac deterioration or preferably improving cardiac function in cardiac function.

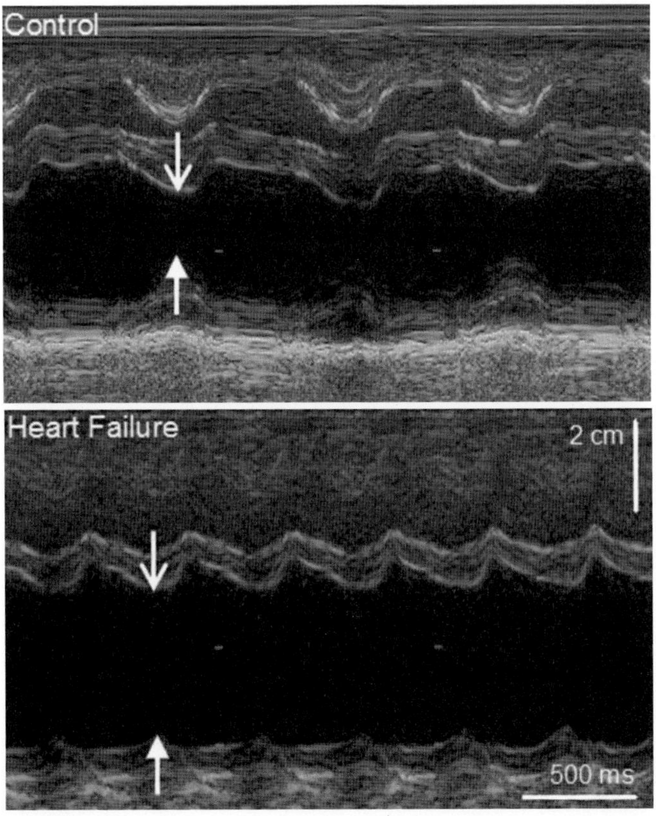

Fig. 7.1 Heart failure is characterised by a drastic left ventricular remodelling; left ventricular dilation, wall thinning and reduced contractility in both the septum (*open arrows*) and free wall (*closed arrows*) can be observed using echocardiography

Treating Heart Failure

Current Guidelines

The currently recommended treatment for heart failure with reduced left ventricular ejection fraction can be split into three major categories: (1) treatments targeting the underlying cause of heart failure, (2) pharmacological and (3) non-pharmacological heart failure therapies. Many cardiac conditions such as coronary artery disease, valvular disease, various cardiomyopathies and atrial fibrillation can all lead to the development of chronic heart failure. Consequently, the first line of heart failure treatment is to target these underlying conditions. Given the wide variety of these disorders it is beyond the scope of this chapter to discuss their specific treatment guidelines. However, it is important to recognise the impact that optimal management of these conditions could have on the development and progression of heart failure, and also in the context of VNS because these treatments can entail modulation of the autonomic nervous system (e.g. ß-blockers, see below). The guidelines for the treatment of developed chronic heart failure are outline in Fig. 7.2.

Pharmacological Treatments

The primary aim of pharmacological heart failure therapies is to target and counteract the excessive neurohumoral activation. Modulation of the renin-angiotensin-aldersterone system is achieved using angiotensin converting enzyme (ACE) inhibitors, angiotensin receptor blockers (ARB's) and mineralocorticoid receptor (MR) antagonists, whilst hyperactivity of the sympathetic nervous system is tackled at the level of the heart using β-blocker therapy. Recent reports suggest that around 75% of patients admitted for coronary heart disease, the major cause of heart failure, are subsequently prescribed β-blockers and ACE inhibitors [15], a figure which appear to be on the increase [2]. Other pharmacological treatments include, diuretics to relieve congestion and ivabradine and digoxin to reduce heart rate and myocardial oxygen consumption. Despite the profound ability of such pharmacological agents to affect the target organ, the prognosis for heart failure patients remains poor; this raises the question – is there a need for a less organ-specific, more systemic level treatments to be brought to clinic?

Non-pharmacological Treatments

Non-pharmacological therapies, such as cardiac resynchronisation therapy (CRT) and implantable cardioverter-defibrillators (ICD's) are also available for qualifying patients. These treatments can be used to improve cardiac pump efficiency and protect against cardiac arrhythmias, which otherwise cause high rate of sudden cardiac death amongst the heart failure population.

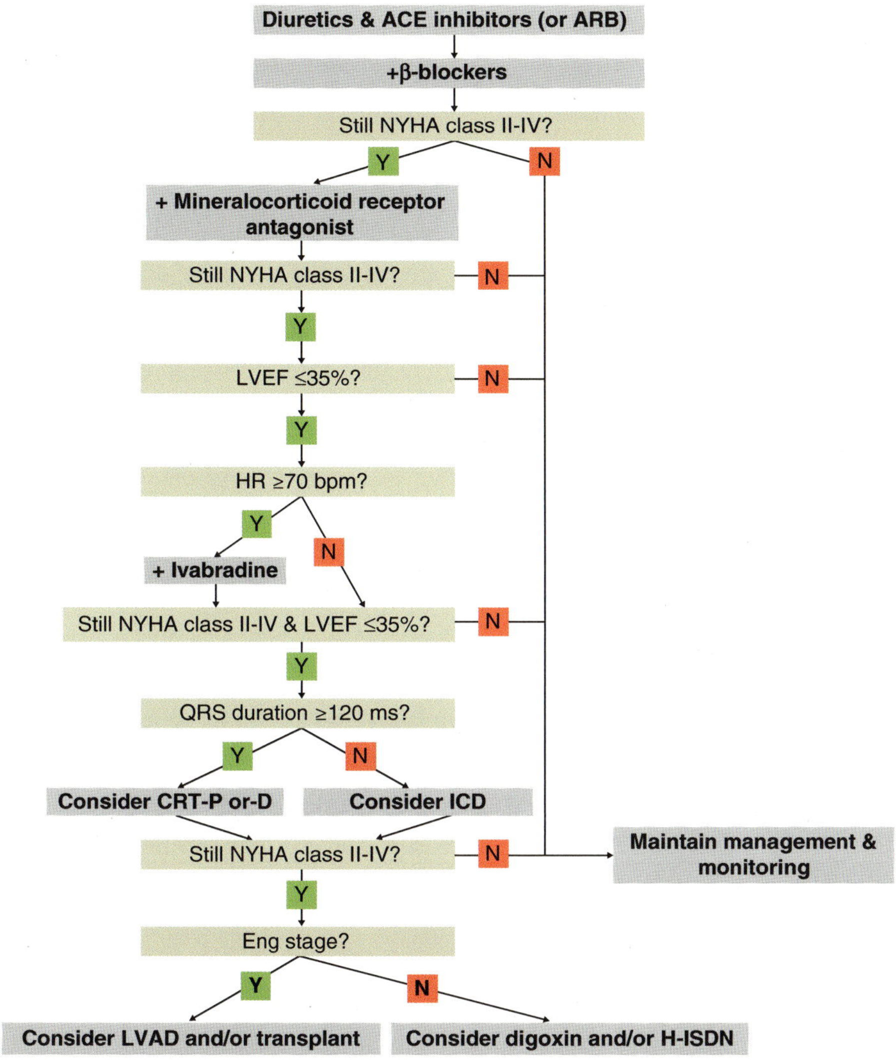

Fig. 7.2 The current European guidelines for the treatment of chronic systolic heart failure (Adapted from [2]). *ACE* angiotensin converting enzyme, *ARB* angiotensin receptor blocker, *NYHA* New York Heart Association, *LVEF* left ventricular ejection fraction, *HR* heart rate, *CRT- P* cardiac resynchronisation therapy pacemaker, *CRT–D* cardiac resynchronisation therapy defibrillator, *ICD* implantable cardioverter-defibrillator, *LVAD* left ventricular assist device, *H-ISDN* hydralazine and isosorbide dinitrate (With permission © Jobn Wiley and Sons. [4])

The availability of these treatments is likely the explanation for improvements in heart failure prognosis reported since there incorporation into clinical practice [16, 17]. However, not all patients qualify for CRT and despite their availability, mortality rates still remain high.

Is there a Role for Vagal Nerve Stimulation?

Over recent years attention has turned to targeting the parasympathetic nervous system. This hypothesis stemmed from the observation of parasympathetic withdrawal in heart failure [18], and that this shares a significant correlation with the progressive loss of left ventricular function [19].Furthermore, this prognostically important characteristic of the disease remains unaltered by current heart failure therapies [20].Vagal nerve stimulation (VNS) provides a means of directly addressing parasympathetic tone, thus representing a new, emerging and promising step in the treatment of heart failure.

It is the purpose of this chapter to firstly introduce the concept of VNS, what it is, and how it is implemented specifically to treat cardiac disease. Subsequently, pre-clinical and clinical data for the use of VNS will be discussed, as will the proposed mechanisms of the treatment. Finally, the future of VNS in clinical practice and heart failure treatment will be considered.

Vagal Nerve Stimulation

The first reported case of VNS can be traced back as far as 1883; when the neurologist James L. Corning described a form of manual external VNS for seizure suppression [21]. VNS is still in use, and is probably best known for its applications in the treatment of epilepsy [22]. However, inevitable scientific advances mean that VNS now has applications in the treatment of several other conditions including depression [23], obesity [24] and heart failure. Technological advances have also lead to the development of much more sophisticated and specific stimulation protocols.

What Is Vagal Nerve Stimulation?

VNS now describes the direct application of small electrical pulses to stimulate the vagus nerve. This is achieved using small, implantable, pacemaker-like devices and specially designed leads that allow direct contact between the electrodes and the nerve. In contrast to its use in epilepsy patients, VNS for the treatment of cardiac disease is predominantly performed on the right side. Right sided stimulation was initially used as the right nerve has a more potent effect on heart rate than the left [25]. In studies comparing right and left-sided stimulation, measures of cardiac function, such as improvements in left ventricular end systolic volume, left ventricular end systolic diameter and aerobic exercise capacity, seem to favour right-sided VNS, although the differences are minor [26]. Stimulation leads are implanted at the level of the cervical vagus, 2–3 cm below the carotid artery bifurcation, with the cathode directed towards the heart (Fig. 7.3).

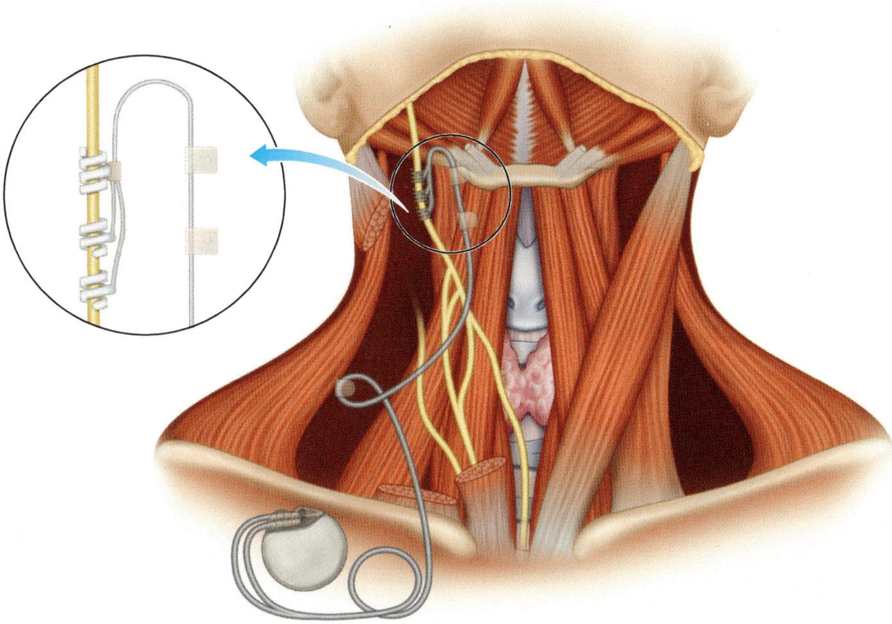

Fig. 7.3 A schematic of the placement of a VNS lead and generator for the treatment of heart failure. VNS leads are implanted around the right cervical vagus. Tie downs are used to relieve any strain on the lead and the pulse generator is sealed in a subcutaneous pocket. *VNS* vagal nerve stimulation

Stimulation Parameters

Modern day devices allow the manipulation of several stimulation parameters; current amplitude, pulse width, stimulation frequency, and the duty cycle can all be altered so that VNS treatment can be personalised for each case. Table 7.2 indicates the variation in stimulation parameters that have been used to date in the treatment of heart failure.

Current amplitude can be manipulated in order to selectively recruit the specific fibre groups of the nerve. Erlanger and Gasser were the first to distinguish three categories of nerve fibre; A fibres with a diameter of 5–20 μm, B fibres with a diameter of <3 μm and C fibres with a diameter of 0.4–2μm [27]. They found the threshold for action potential initiation to be inversely proportional to the square of the fibre diameter. Hence, with increasing current amplitudes fibres are recruited sequentially, in the order of A, B and C [27]. Specifically within the vagus, activation thresholds are 0.02–0.2 mA for A fibres, 0.04–0.6 mA for B fibres and greater than 2.0 mA for C fibres [28]. Both experimental and clinical stimulation amplitudes vary somewhat, with those used in animal studies typically sufficient to decrease heart rate by around 5–17% [29, 30]. VNS used in clinical practice is initiated at low

Table 7.2 A summary of previously reported experimental and clinical stimulation parameters

Study	Species/model	Lead position	Frequency (Hz)	Pulse width (ms)	Amplitude (mA)	HR reduction (bpm)	Duty cycle
Li et al. (2004) [29]	Rat/MI	Right cervical	20	0.2	0.1–0.3	20–30	10 s on 50 s off (~17%)
Sabbah et al. (2010) [33]	Dog/microembolism	Right cervical	20	0.3	1.5–2.0	–	10 s on 50 s off (~17%)
Zhang et al. (2009) [30]	Dog/tachypaced	Right cervical	20	0.5	0.75–2.5	20	14 s on 12 s off (~54%)
Schwartz et al. (2008) [31] and De Ferrari et al. (2011) [38]	Human	Right cervical	–	1.0	1.1–5.5	5–10	2–10 s on 6–30 s off (25%)
Premchand et al. (2014) (ANTHEM-HF) [26]	Human	Left and right cervical	10	0.13	1.4–2.6	4–6	14 s on 66 s off (~18%)
Zannad et al. (2014) (NECTAR-HF) [43]	Human	Right cervical	20	0.3	0.5–1.98	–	10 s on 50 s off (~17%)

HR heart rate, *MI* myocardial infarction

amplitudes before the current output is increased incrementally. This up titration period is usually dictated or limited by patient comfort and/or the presence of undesirable side effects such as cough and hoarseness. Typically slightly smaller heart rate reductions are achieved in clinical practice [31]; something that in isolation may have little relevance to VNS induced improvements in cardiac function (see below for more detail), but may instead be indicative of the level of VNS dosing.

Although to date there is no real evidence for which combination of stimulation parameters are most effective in the treatment of heart failure, some factors have been identified as potentially harmful. For example, stimulation frequencies of 50 Hz and above can cause irreversible neuronal damage [32]. Consequently, only stimulation frequencies of 20–30 Hz have been approved for use by the United States Food and Drug Administration. Similarly, stimulation amplitudes of 4 mA should not be exceeded as above this point stimulation may become harmful. The risk of neuronal damage can also be reduced by using an intermittent or on/off stimulation protocol that is known as a duty cycle. 'Off' periods of as little as 5 s have been shown to reduce neuronal damage by as much as 75% [32], and in general reducing the stimulation percentage of the duty cycle reduces risk of neuronal damage.

Evidence for the Use of Vagal Nerve Stimulation to Treat Heart Failure

Given that VNS is still a somewhat emergent therapy for the treatment of heart failure, much of what is known is derived from pre-clinical or animal studies. The following section will review the experimental evidence supporting the use of VNS in heart failure, which has collectively led to its implementation in human clinical trials.

Animal Studies of Vagal Nerve Stimulation

One of the first, pivotal studies of VNS for the treatment of heart failure was performed by Li et al. (2004). VNS (Table 7.2) was used in a rat, myocardial infarction (MI) model of heart failure. Six weeks of treatment reduced mortality rates from 50% in sham treated controls to 14% at a 20 week follow up [29]. Of particular note in this study is that the cardioprotective effects of VNS were shown to extend beyond the termination of the treatment period. Improvements in survival were accompanied by improvements in left ventricular function; the increased end-diastolic left ventricular pressure observed in heart failure (23.5 ± 4.2 mmHg) was reduced with VNS (17.1 ± 5.9 mmHg), and heart failure induced reductions in dp/dt_{max} (1987 ± 192 mmHg/s) were also reversed with treatment (4152 ± 237 mmHg/s) [29].

VNS induced improvements in left ventricular function have since been reported in several other models of heart failure, including larger animals. For example, VNS has been shown to improve left ventricular ejection fraction by around 10% when compared to untreated controls (40.1 ± 0.9 and 31.7 ± 1.1% respectively) in a canine model of coronary microembolisation induced ischemic heart failure [33]. Zhang et al. (2009) also showed that VNS treatment reduces both end-systolic and end-diastolic pressures and increases left ventricular ejection fraction in a tachypaced canine model of heart failure [30]. More recently, it has also been shown that low-level VNS, insufficient to bring about acute heart rate reductions, can also improve left ventricular function. Low-level VNS significantly reduces end-systolic volume and increases left ventricular ejection fraction in dogs with failing hearts [34]. Together these studies indicate that the cardioprotective effects of VNS may extend beyond its acute effect on heart rate and haemodynamic function (see below for more detail). However, regardless of the underlying mechanism, this experimental data indicates the efficacy of VNS in larger animal models of heart failure; together these findings support VNS can be used to attenuate or in some instances even reverse deleterious left ventricular dysfunction. Larger animals share more closely matched anatomical [35] and electrophysiological [36] characteristics with the human heart, therefore this data collectively provides a vital platform from which theory can be translated into clinical practice. As a consequence, the first human trials for the use of VNS for the treatment of heart failure began in 2008 [31].

Clinical Evidence for the Use of Vagal Nerve Stimulation to Treat Heart Failure

Animal models of heart failure have provided strong experimental evidence of the potential of VNS therapy in chronic heart failure [29, 30, 33]. Given the established practice for the use of VNS in other patient groups, such as those with epilepsy [37] and depression [38], human clinical trials for VNS in the treatment of heart failure were quickly established and importantly for the first time were able to assess the effects of VNS alongside otherwise optimally managed treatment regimes.

The first 'in human' VNS trail for the treatment of heart failure was carried out in a small group of eight patients, with the aim of ascertaining whether VNS was feasible, safe and effective [31]. Patients received chronic stimulation (Table 7.2) and were followed up at 1, 3 and 6 months. Reported side effects of the treatment included cough, pain at the site of stimulation, mandibular pain and voice alterations, although no side effects were deemed severe and all resolved over the course of the trial. Clinical outcomes of the treatment looked promising; left ventricular end-systolic volume was reduced from 208 ± 71 mls at baseline to 190 ± 83 mls following 6 months treatment. This was accompanied by a reduction in New York Heart Association (NYHA) classification, and increases in both quality of life scores and exercise capacity [31]. Given the success of the study it was extended to include a 12-month follow up, in a larger cohort of 32 patients [39]. Beneficial outcomes were maintained over the longer treatment period, and were even extended to include a significant improvement in left ventricular ejection fraction, from 21.1 ± 7.5% at baseline to 34.1 ± 12.5 at 12 month follow up [39]. This work was the first to indicate the potential for translation of experimental findings into the clinical setting. Consequently, following this initial success, larger scale trials were established to determine if such promising findings could be reproduced in the wider heart failure population. Subsequently, 3 multi-centre trials were set up: the Increase Of Vagal TonE in Heart Failure (INOVATE-HF) [40], the Autonomic Neural regulation Therapy to Enhance Myocardial function in Heart Failure (ANTHEM-HF) [41] and the NEuroCardiac TherApy foR Heart Failure study (NECTAR-HF) [42], all of which are ongoing.

The NECTAR-HF trial was similarly designed to assess the effects of VNS on ventricular function, ventricular dimensions, exercise capacity and quality of life [42], this time in a cohort of 96 patients [43]. Inclusion criteria included a left ventricular ejection fraction of ≤35%, left ventricular end-diastolic diameter of ≥55 mm, and NYHA classification of II or III. Patients were randomised 2:1 into either the active treatment or control group, all of which partook in the 30-day titration period. Subsequently, interim results were released when patients reached the 6-month time point. In this instance, no favourable changes in left ventricular dimensions or function were reported. Changes in left ventricular end-diastolic and -systolic diameter, and left ventricular ejection fraction were similar to those of patients in the control group. No significant changes were found in either exercise capacity, measured as peak VO_2, or brain natriuretic peptide (BNP) levels. However, this study did demonstrate that VNS could improve both patient quality of life and NYHA classification, in the larger cohort. Given the lack of measurable functional improvements, this could be attributed to a placebo effect, particularly because improvements were only made in self-reported measures and blinding throughout the trial was deemed compromised by the presence/ lack of stimulation related side effects [43]. The 18-month follow up results are still anticipated.

The primary objective of the INOVATE-HF study is to evaluate the safety and efficacy of VNS in heart failure patients by assessing the 'time to first event', defined as any unplanned hospitalisation for heart failure and all-cause mortality. They aim to enlist up to 650 patients displaying <40% left ventricular ejection fraction, NYHA Class III symptoms and with a QRS duration of <120 ms. Patients will be randomised 3:2 into an active VNS or standard optimal care treatment group. The study enrolled its first patient in April 2011, and the first outcome reports are anticipated during 2015 [40].

The ANTHEM-HF study instead aims to probe some of the key unanswered questions relating to the methodology such as whether left and right sided stimulation have similar effects on left ventricular remodelling, whether the same outcomes can be achieved with lower level stimulation, reducing the risk to benefit ratio, and whether the effects of VNS are additive to conventional β-blocker therapy and independent of the heart rate effect? [41] 60 subjects were enrolled between July 2012 and July 2013, all with left ventricular ejection fraction ≤ 40%, left ventricular end-diastolic volume between 50-80 mm, NYHA classification II-III and receiving optimal pharmacological care. All patients received VNS treatment but were randomised on a 1:1 ratio into active VNS treatment via either the left or right cervical vagus nerve. Patients then underwent a 10-week titration period and were subsequently followed up at 6 months [26]. In keeping with earlier clinical observations [18, 31] left ventricular function was enhanced following treatment; left ventricular ejection fraction was increased by 4.5% when left and right-sided stimulation data was grouped. NYHA classification was improved in 77% of patients, with none showing worsening, which may be otherwise expected due to the progressive nature of the condition. The only significant difference observed between patients receiving right and left sided stimulation was an attenuated improvement in exercise capacity, as measured by 6-min walk test, in the left-sided group. Other efficacy measures, including left ventricular ejection fraction, end-systolic and -diastolic volumes, all appeared to favour right-sided stimulation. However, differences were not great enough to draw definitive conclusions [26].

Overall, clinical trials of VNS have repeatedly shown the treatment to positively impact upon left ventricular function and quality of life in patients receiving otherwise optimal care, the only exception being the NECTAR trail. The failing of this study to improve structural or functional outcome measures of left ventricular function was unexpected, and contradictory. In this study up-titration of stimulation amplitude was not as great as in other trials (see Table 7.2). Consequently, the lack of improvement in outcome measures was attributed in part to a general lack of understanding of optimal stimulation parameters and dosing [43]. This highlights a key limiting factor to advances in cardiac VNS therapy- little is truly understood about the parameters contributing to and mechanisms mediating the cardioprotective effect.

Proposed Mechanisms of VNS

VNS and Vagal Tone

The primary rationale behind the use of VNS in the treatment of chronic heart failure is to directly target autonomic imbalance by upregulating parasympathetic drive. Direct measures of vagal tone are possible, but highly invasive, with the risk often outweighing the reward. Consequently, the use of direct measures is restricted to experimental studies, where alternatives will not suffice. Several less invasive indirect measures of vagal tone do exist, including measures of baroreflex sensitivity [44] and heart rate variability (HRV) [45].

Heart Rate Variability

Time Domain Heart Rate Variability

HRV describes the study of the variation in time interval between cardiac beats. Commonly reported simplistic measures include the standard deviation of consecutive RR intervals (SDNN), the standard deviation from the average RR interval

(SDANN) and the mean number of times consecutive RR intervals exceeds 50 milliseconds (pNN50). These are termed 'time-domain' measures as they are solely concerned with the time between beats. SDNN is reduced in chronic heart failure patients [46] and time domain HRV has been routinely shown to have a significant prognostic importance in those with cardiac disease; reduced SDNN is a significant predictor of cardiac events, even once other risk factors such as age, smoking status and left ventricular hypertrophy are accounted for [47]. More specifically, SDNN was found to be the most powerful predictor of risk of death due to heart failure progression, when compared to several measures of left ventricular remodelling [48]. Many studies of VNS in the treatment of heart failure have therefore assessed HRV as an outcome measure. Increases in SNDD [30], pNN50 [39] and SDANN [43] have all been reported with VNS treatment. Although time-domain HRV has a strong prognostic value, and was previously thought to be a measure predominantly influenced by vagal activity, sympathetic action and heart rate [49] can also have a profound effect on all HRV parameters. Consequently, all HRV data should be interpreted carefully with consideration for these factors. Vagal activity can be assessed in more isolation by using frequency domain parameters of HRV.

Frequency Domain Heart Rate Variability

Frequency domain aspects of HRV can be assessed by transforming RR interval data into frequency power spectra, most commonly by using a fast Fourier transformation (FFT). Frequency data can then be split into frequency categories, representing different autonomic influences on the heart. Sympathetic activity is mediated by noradrenaline, activating G-protein coupled receptors and the subsequent initiation of an intracellular second messenger signalling cascade. However, parasympathetic, acetylecholine mediated activation occurs via muscarinic receptors and its effect is facilitated by proteins predominantly situated in the cell membrane [50]. In combination with the quicker reuptake of acetylecholine than noradrenaline [51], this results in changes in parasympathetic activation influencing heart rate more rapidly than sympathetic activity. Consequently, low frequency (LF, 0.04–0.15 Hz) HRV changes are often attributed to sympathetic activity, whereas high frequency (HF, 0.15–1.0 Hz) changes are attributed to vagal activity [45]. As would be expected with the autonomic imbalance observed in heart failure, during the compensatory state there is an increase in LF HRV and a reduction in HF HRV [12], representative of chronic sympathetic activation and vagal withdrawal. The limited data for the effects of VNS on frequency domain HRV suggests that it is capable of both reducing LF HRV and increasing HF HRV to produce a more favourable LF:HF ratio [30]. However, in light of the knowledge that VNS affects heart rate, appropriate corrections for heart rate changes do need to be incorporated into these studies before true conclusions on changes in vagal tone can be drawn.

Preferential changes in both time- and frequency-domain HRV parameters, along with chronic heart rate changes [26, 29, 31, 34, 39], and enhanced baroreflex sensitivity [30] all suggest that VNS treatment can chronically alter parasympathetic tone, thereby restoring a more favourable autonomic balance. Although clearly beneficial in a prognostic sense, it is the mechanistic implications of this, which remain less well understood.

Enhanced parasympathetic tone could act on the heart in a variety of way; benefits could be attributed to cross-talk between the parasympathetic and sympathetic systems, causing reductions in the adrenergic hyperactivity. However, the therapeutic effect of VNS is still seen in patients receiving optimal β-blocker therapy [26, 39, 43, 52]. Indeed, it is not yet clear whether the effects are mediated through stimulation of efferent fibres having a direct cardiac effect or through vagal afferents and the central cardiac control centres. This section will therefore go on to discuss some of the potential mechanisms that have been proposed, as outlined in Fig. 7.4.

VNS, Heart Rate and Haemodynamics

One very simplistic explanation for the therapeutic effects of VNS in heart failure is that the stimulation may induce a chronic heart rate reduction, similar to those seen with existing therapies such as β-blockers and ivabradine [53]. In this instance rate reduction is allows time for more efficient ventricular filling and consequently larger stroke volumes. Indeed both animal [29] and human [26, 31] studies have shown chronic heart rate reductions with VNS, even when acute heart rate reductions are only modest [39] or non-existent [34]. However, beneficial outcomes have still been reported in the absence of chronic heart rate changes [30, 43]. One study in particular, using a tachypaced model of heart failure, completely eliminated the effects of VNS upon heart rate. Improvements of left ventricular function were still observed under these conditions [30]. Hence, it appears likely that the effects of VNS upon heart rate are not crucial to mediating its therapeutic effect. However, it has been suggested that the presence of a heart rate reduction may magnify the therapeutic effect of VNS [34]. This could explain the lack of reversal of left ventricular dysfunction reported in the NECTAR-HF trial where no chronic heart rate changes were observed [43]. It has also been suggested that heart rate changes may simply represent a preferential shift in autonomic balance towards parasympathetic dominance [31]. Regardless, it is clear that further understanding of the contribution of heart rate in VNS is vital, and consequently this is a major ongoing aim of current clinical trials [41].

VNS and Inflammation

An additional factor with may contribute to the therapeutic effects of VNS in heart failure are its anti-inflammatory capabilities. Heart failure is associated with both chronic cardiac and systemic inflammation. Consequently, the supression of this inflammatory response could contribute to the therapeutic outcomes observed with VNS treatment.

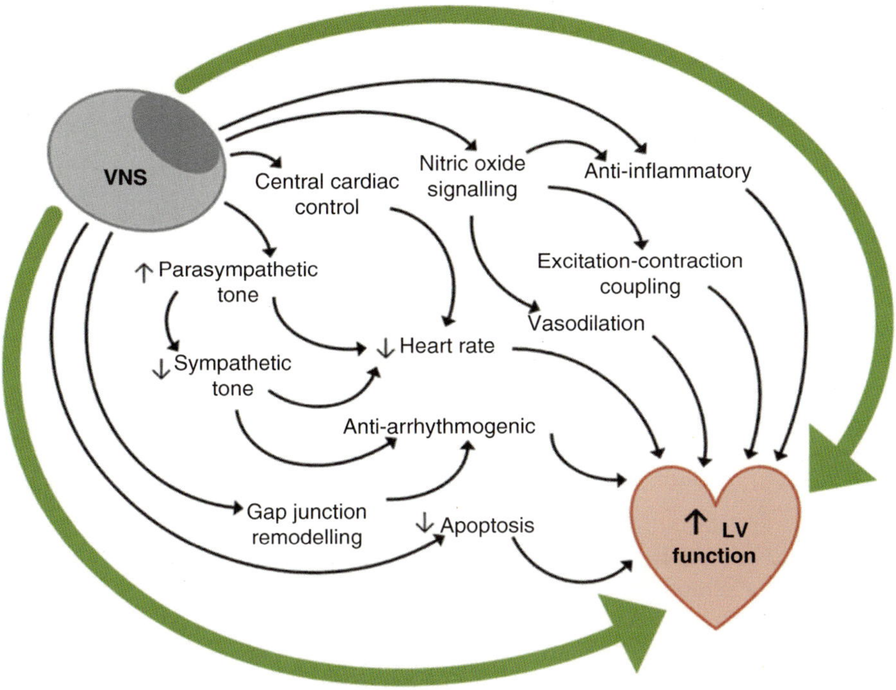

Fig. 7.4 The proposed mechanisms underlying the cardioprotective effects of VNS are extensive and highly interlinked. *VNS* vagal nerve stimulation, *LV* left ventricular

Patients with chronic heart failure display with elevated levels of circulating inflammatory markers such as tumour necrosis factor (TNF) α, interleukin (IL) -1β and IL-6 [54–57]. Increased levels of inflammatory cytokines have been reported in the myocardium itself [58] and are thought to be produced in response to the increased left ventricular end diastolic wall stress in the failing heart [59]. Overspill of the heightened myocardial cytokine levels into the coronary circulation may contribute to the elevated circulating levels [60]. Several other organs and cell types have also been implicated in contributing, including the liver, lungs, leukocytes and endothelial cells [59]. Importantly, levels of circulating cytokines have been shown to share a significant correlation with NYHA classification and left ventricular dysfunction [56, 57, 60], raising the possibility that, rather than merely reflecting a more severely diseased state, they may play an active role in the pathophysiology of progressive cardiac dysfunction [59].

Several studies have examined the effects of VNS on circulating cytokine levels in chronic heart failure. Experimentally, VNS reduces both myocardial and plasma IL-6 and TNFα levels in multiple models of heart failure at a 3 month follow up [61]. The first in-man trial of VNS for the treatment of heart failure demonstrated that chronic stimulation was also capable of reducing plasma IL-6 levels in humans. However, the positive findings observed at 3 months were not maintained at the full

6-month follow up. This was attributed to the deterioration of a subset of patients at the latter time point [31]. Subsequently, others have shown that VNS is can cause sustained longe- term alterations in inflammatory marker expression. Hamann et al. (2013) showed that reductions in both IL-6 and TRNα reported at 3 months of treatment could be maintained and even slightly enhanced at a later 6 month follow up [34].

Strong evidence exists for the pathway of vagal involvement in inflammation suppression in macrophages [62], whereby acetylcholine released from the nerve binds nicotinic receptors, inhibiting TNF release; an effect mediated by the nicotinic receptor α7 subunit [63]. It therefore appears likely that activation of this pathway may be responsible for some of the downregulation in circulating cytokines observed in VNS treated heart failure. However, given that myocardial TNFα and IL-6 levels are also reduced with VNS, it seems plausible that other yet unidentified pathways may also contribute.

In many instances the cardioprotective effects of VNS have been attributed to its anti-inflammatory actions. However it is important to consider that anti-TNF treatments for chronic heart failure have also been subject to large-scale multicentre trails with limited positive and even negative outcomes [64, 65]. Consequently, although reduction in IL-6 and TNFα levels may represent a prognostic improvement in heart failure patients, their role in mediating the cardioprotective effect remains questionable. More recently attentions have turned to the more promising role of VNS in macrophage control following acute ischemic injury [66].

VNS and Electrophysiological Remodelling

As the severity of left ventricular dysfunction increases in chronic heart failure patients so too does the occurrence of ventricular arrhythmias [67]. Normal cardiac rhythm is dependent on the electrical coupling of myocytes to allow synchronous contraction. In heart failure there are a number of mechanisms that can disrupt this and so contribute to the onset of arrhythmias; these include structural cardiac remodelling, such as scar formation and cellular remodelling, ion channel remodelling and alterations in calcium homeostasis. In the following sections we will consider how some of these may be beneficially altered by VNS and thus give rise to a potential antiarrhythmic effect of VNS. It is also worth considering that by reducing inflammation, VNS may also be limiting the formation of pro-arrhythmic substrates within the heart and thus VNS may be acting at multiple levels as a cardioprotective, anti-inflammatory, antiarrhythmic and inotropic factor.

Electrical coupling of cardiomyocytes is achieved by connexins, small channels in the plasma membrane, which allow a physical continuation of cytoplasm between adjoining cells [68]. Heart failure is associated with a degree of gap junction remodelling; distribution is shifted from the intercalated disks to the lateral borders of the cell [69], and there is a reduction in both connexin-43 mRNA and protein levels [70, 71]. Heterogeneous reductions in connexin-43, to a similar extent reported in the failing human heart [71], are sufficient to increase arrhythmia susceptibility in failing canine hearts [72]. Increased arrhythmogenesis is attributed to the degree of action potential dispersion and transmural conduction slowing, which can allow for conduction block and re-entrant circuits to form [72]. Such alterations in electrophysiological function may affect heart failure progression on two fronts: (1) dsynchronous contraction in the absence of arrhythmia may reduce pumping efficiency and further reduce left ventricular ejection fraction and (2) arrhythmias often result in sudden cardiac death [73], severely impacting on mortality rates.

Consequently, some studies of VNS for the treatment of heart failure have also examined the effects of VNS on gap junction remodelling. Three months VNS therapy has been shown to increase connexin-43 mRNA levels, and increase protein expression by roughly 25% in heart failure dogs, when compared to untreated controls. mRNA and protein expression for connexins -40 and -45 were also reduced in heart failure, and improved with VNS treatment [74]. No cases of sudden death were reported in either the control or treated groups, however VNS treatment was associated with an approximately 10% improvement in left ventricular ejection fraction in the same model [33]. There is limited clinical data for the effects of VNS on reducing sudden cardiac death in heart failure. Trials thus far have reported lower overall death rates in VNS treated (1/63) compared to control (2/32) patients. However, these were not attributed to sudden cardiac death and no differences were found between ICD shock rate and anti-tachy pacing in the two groups [43]. Given that VNS therapy has been demonstrated to have a desirable effect on gap junction remodelling in heart failure, it is possible that larger cohort studies, such as the ongoing INOVATE-HF trail [40], may be required to detect any significant changes in sudden cardiac death rates.

VNS and Nitric Oxide Production

An alternative mechanism through which VNS may regulate cardiac function in heart failure is through changes in nitric oxide (NO) signalling.

NO is synthesised in the heart and the vasculature, by the enzyme nitric oxide synthase (NOS), in the following reaction:

$$1-\text{arginine}+\text{NADPH} \leftrightarrow \text{citrulline}+\text{nitric oxide}$$

Three isoforms of NOS have been identified: neuronal NOS (nNOS, NOS-1 or NOS-I), inducible NOS (iNOS, NOS-2 or NOS-II), and endothelial NOS (eNOS, NOS-3 or NOS-III).

Inducible Nitric Oxide Synthase

iNOS is expressed predominantly in inflammatory cell types but also in cardiomyocytes and produces NO in response to inflammatory stimuli [75]. As would be expected with the level of systemic inflammation observed in heart failure, iNOS expression is upregulated in both experimental and human heart failure [61, 76]. Transgenic overexpression of iNOS, specifically within the myocardium, can cause significant left ventricular dilation, the associated congestive heart failure phenotype and sudden cardiac death in mice [77]. Chronic VNS treatment has previously been shown to normalise the heart failure induced upregulation of iNOS in canine hearts [61], although such findings are yet to be corroborated in the human condition.

Constitutive Nitric Oxide Synthase

eNOS expression is reduced and nNOS expression increased in failing hearts [61, 78], both of which are reversed with chronic VNS treatment [61]. Acute VNS has also been shown to cause NO production, in a frequency dependant manner, via nNOS in the ventricular myocardium [79]. There is therefore direct evidence for the role of VNS in modulating cardiac NO activity. In cardiomyocytes themselves eNOS is situated on the sarcolemmal membrane [80, 81], where it interacts with the L-type calcium channel via the β-adrenergic signalling cascade [80, 82]. nNOS is also present in cardiomyocytes; it is situated on the sarcoplasmic reticulum where it is closely associated with both the Ryanodine receptor and sarcoplasmic reticulum calcium ATPase (SERCA) [83]. Given the crucial role of calcium in regulating cellular contraction [84], the association of eNOS and nNOS with calcium handling proteins, is suggestive of a role for NO regulating cardiac contraction. Indeed, NO has been shown to have both positively and negatively inotropic effects on isolated cardiomyocytes [see [85] for review]. The differential effects of NO are likely due to its divergent signalling pathways [86] and highly compartmentalised effects [75]. However, independently of its effects, the link between VNS, NO and calcium handling may provide a mechanistic link contributing to the cardioprotective effects of this treatment.

Is There a Future for VNS?

Vagal nerve stimulation clearly provides a means to alter parasympathetic influence on the diseased heart, as evidenced through increased HRV and baroreflex sensitivity in those receiving treatment. Importantly the means to do so has until now been lacking from all other available heart failure therapies. The significance of targeting this aspect of the disease is highlighted not only it the prognostic value of vagal withdrawal, but for the first time in the body of evidence demonstrating the improvements in left ventricular function that are possible with VNS treatment. In light of this, VNS represents a promising new complementary approach to heart failure treatment.

However, for the development of optimal VNS patient therapy to continue, several key questions remain to be answered; specifically questions surrounding aspects of the level nervous activation required to mediate the cardioprotective effects, and how stimulation parameters can be monitored to target this.

Looking to the future, technological advances in VNS delivery may create more questions than answers in this area. Transcutaneous VNS devices have recently been brought to the market. This bypasses the need for invasive implantation. However patients take responsibility for delivering the treatment themselves. The benefits of VNS in heart failure have been linked with chronic opposed to acute bouts of stimulation; consequently the use of such devices may not be appropriate in this setting. Furthermore factors such as patients training and compliance are more likely to influence the overall effectiveness of any treatment regimens when the stimulation is required more frequently.

Finally, only with a more in depth understanding of the mechanisms underpinning the structural and functional changes seen with treatment will it be possible to identify optimum stimulation programs. Extended follow up results of ongoing large scale trials are necessary before VNS for the treatment of heart failure can be recommended outside of the experimental setting.

References

1. Go AS, Mozaffarian D, Roger VL, Benjamin EJ, Berry JD, Borden WB, et al. Heart disease and stroke statistics-2013 update a report from the American Heart Association. Circulation. 2013;127(1):E6–E245.
2. Townsend N, Williams J, Bhatnagar P, Wickramasinghe K, Rayner M. Cardiovascular disease statistics 2014. London: British Heart Foundation; 2014.
3. Ezekowitz JA, Kaul P, Bakal JA, Armstrong PW, Welsh RC, McAlister FA. Declining in-hospital mortality and increasing heart failure incidence in elderly patients with first myocardial infarction reply. J Am Coll Cardiol. 2009;55(1):81.
4. McMurray JJV, Adamopoulos S, Anker SD, Auricchio A, Bohm M, Dickstein K, et al. ESC guidelines for the diagnosis and treatment of acute and chronic heart failure 2012 the task force for the diagnosis and treatment of acute and chronic heart failure 2012 of the European Society of Cardiology. Developed in collaboration with the Heart Failure Association (HFA) of the ESC. Eur J Heart Fail. 2012;14(8):803–69.
5. Francis GS, Goldsmith SR, Levine TB, Olivari MT, Cohn JN. The neurohumoral axis in congestive heart-failure. Ann Intern Med. 1984;101(3):370–7.
6. Cohn JN, Levine TB, Olivari MT, Garberg V, Lura D, Francis GS, et al. Plasma norepinephrine as a guide to prognosis in patients with chronic congestive heart-failure. N Engl J Med. 1984;311(13):819–23.
7. Dzau VJ, Colucci WS, Hollenberg NK, Williams GH. Relation of the renin-angiotensin-aldosterone system to clinical state in congestive heart-failure. Circulation. 1981;63(3):645–51.

8. Bristow MR, Minobe WA, Raynolds MV, Port JD, Rasmussen R, Ray PE, et al. Reduced beta (1) receptor messenger-RNA abundance in the failing human heart. J Clin Invest. 1993; 92(6):2737–45.
9. Ungerer M, Bohm M, Elce JS, Erdmann E, Lohse MJ. Altered expression of beta-adrenergic-receptor kinase and beta-1-adrenergic receptors in the failing human heart. Circulation. 1993;87(2):454–63.
10. Eckberg DL, Drabinsky M, Braunwald E. Defective cardiac parasympathetic control in patients with heart disease. N Engl J Med. 1971;285(16):877–83. Epub 1971/10/14
11. Bibevski S, Dunlap ME. Ganglionic mechanisms contribute to diminished vagal control in heart failure. Circulation. 1999;99(22):2958–63. Epub 1999/06/09
12. Sztajzel J. Heart rate variability: a noninvasive electrocardiographic method to measure the autonomic nervous system. Swiss Med Wkly. 2004;134(35–36):514–22.
13. Francis GS, Benedict C, Johnstone DE, Kirlin PC, Nicklas J, Liang CS, et al. Comparison of neuroendocrine activation in patients with left-ventricular dysfunction with and without congestive-heart-failure - a substudy of the Studies of Left-Ventricular Dysfunction (Solvd). Circulation. 1990;82(5):1724–9.
14. Dickstein K, Cohen-Solal A, Filippatos G, McMurray JJV, Ponikowski P, Poole-Wilson PA, et al. ESC guidelines for the diagnosis and treatment of acute and chronic heart failure 2008 the task force for the diagnosis and treatment of acute and chronic heart failure 2008 of the European Society of Cardiology. Developed in collaboration with the Heart Failure Association of the ESC (HFA) and endorsed by the European Society of Intensive Care Medicine (ESICM). Eur J Heart Fail. 2008;10(10):933–89.
15. Nichols M, Townsend N, Luengo-Fernandez R, Leal L, Gray A, Sacrborough P, Rayner M. European cardiovascular disease statistics 2012. Brussels: European Heart Network, European Society of Cardiology. Sophia Antipolis; 2012.
16. MacIntyre K, Capewell S, Stewart S, Chalmers JWT, Boyd J, Finlayson A, et al. Evidence of improving prognosis in heart failure - trends in case fatality in 66 547 patients hospitalized between 1986 and 1995. Circulation. 2000;102(10):1126–31.
17. Cleland JGF, Daubert J, Erdmann E, Freemantle N, Gras D, Kappenberger L, et al. The effect of cardiac resynchronization on morbidity and mortality in heart failure. N Engl J Med. 2005;352(15):1539–49.
18. Binkley PF, Nunziata E, Haas GJ, Nelson SD, Cody RJ. Parasympathetic withdrawal is an integral component of autonomic imbalance in congestive-heart-failure - demonstration in human-subjects and verification in a paced canine model of ventricular failure. J Am Coll Cardiol. 1991;18(2):464–72.
19. Nolan J, Flapan AD, Capewell S, Macdonald TM, Neilson JMM, Ewing DJ. Decreased cardiac parasympathetic activity in chronic heart-failure and Its relation to left-ventricular function. Br Heart J. 1992;67(6):482–5.
20. Desai MY, Watanabe MA, Laddu AA, Hauptman PJ. Pharmacologic modulation of parasympathetic activity in heart failure. Heart Fail Rev. 2011;16(2):179–93.
21. Corning JL. Considerations on the pathology and therapeutics of epilepsy. J Nerv Ment Dis. 1883;10(2):243–8.
22. Ben-Menachem E. Vagus-nerve stimulation for the treatment of epilepsy. Lancet Neurol. 2002;1(8):477–82. Epub 2003/07/10
23. Tisi G, Franzini A, Messina G, Savino M, Gambini O. Vagus nerve stimulation therapy in treatment-resistant depression: a series report. Psychiatry Clin Neurosci. 2014;68(8):606–11.
24. Bodenlos JS, Schneider KL, Oleski J, Gordon K, Rothschild AJ, Pagoto SL. Vagus nerve stimulation and food intake: effect of body mass index. J Diabetes Sci Technol. 2014;8(3):590–5. Epub 2014/05/31
25. Randall WC, Ardell JL. Selective parasympathectomy of automatic and conductile tissues of the canine heart. Am J Physiol. 1985;248(1):H61–H8.
26. Premchand RK, Sharma K, Mittal S, Monteiro R, Dixit S, Libbus I, et al. Autonomic regulation therapy via left or right cervical vagus nerve stimulation in patients with chronic heart failure: results of the ANTHEM-HF trial. J Card Fail. 2014;20(11):808–16.

27. Erlanger J, Gasser HS. The action potential in fibers of slow conduction in spinal roots and somatic nerves. Am J Physiol. 1930;92(1):43–82.
28. Woodbury DM, Woodbury JW. Effects of vagal-stimulation on experimentally induced seizures in rats. Epilepsia. 1990;31:S7–S19.
29. Li M, Zheng C, Sato T, Kawada T, Sugimachi M, Sunagawa K. Vagal nerve stimulation markedly improves long-term survival after chronic heart failure in rats. Circulation. 2004;109(1):120–4.
30. Zhang YH, Popovic ZB, Bibevski S, Fakhry I, Sica DA, Van Wagoner DR, et al. Chronic vagus nerve stimulation improves autonomic control and attenuates systemic inflammation and heart failure progression in a Canine High-Rate Pacing Model. Circ-Heart Fail. 2009;2(6):692–9.
31. Schwartz PJ, De Ferrari GM, Sanzo A, Landolina M, Rordorf R, Raineri C, et al. Long term vagal stimulation in patients with advanced heart failure first experience in man. Eur J Heart Fail. 2008;10(9):884–91.
32. Agnew WF, Mccreery DB. Considerations for Safety with Chronically Implanted Nerve Electrodes. Epilepsia. 1990;31:S27–32.
33. Sabbah HN, Wang M, Jiang A, Ruble SB, Hamann JJ. Right vagus nerve stimulation improves left ventricular function in dogs with heart failure. J Am Coll Cardiol. 2010;55(10 suppl): A16–E151.
34. Hamann JJ, Ruble SB, Stolen C, Wang MJ, Gupta RC, Rastogi S, et al. Vagus nerve stimulation improves left ventricular function in a canine model of chronic heart failure. Eur J Heart Fail. 2013;15(12):1319–26.
35. Hasenfuss G. Animal models of human cardiovascular disease, heart failure and hypertrophy. Cardiovasc Res. 1998;39(1):60–76.
36. Lompre AM, Mercadier JJ, Wisnewsky C, Bouveret P, Pantaloni C, Dalbis A, et al. Species-dependent and age-dependent changes in the relative amounts of cardiac myosin isoenzymes in mammals. Dev Biol. 1981;84(2):286–90.
37. Englot DJ, Chang EF, Auguste KI. Vagus nerve stimulation for epilepsy: a meta-analysis of efficacy and predictors of response a review. J Neurosurg. 2011;115(6):1248–55.
38. Shuchman M. Approving the vagus-nerve stimulator for depression. N Engl J Med. 2007;356(16):1604–7.
39. De Ferrari GM, Crijns HJGM, Borggrefe M, Milasinovic G, Smid J, Zabel M, et al. Chronic vagus nerve stimulation: a new and promising therapeutic approach for chronic heart failure. Eur Heart J. 2011;32(7):847–55.
40. Hauptman PJ, Schwartz PJ, Gold MR, Borggrefe M, Van Veldhuisen DJ, Starling RC, et al. Rationale and study design of the Increase of vagal tone in heart failure study: INOVATE-HF. Am Heart J. 2012;163(6):954.
41. Dicarlo L, Libbus I, Amurthur B, Kenknight BH, Anand IS. Autonomic regulation therapy for the improvement of left ventricular function and heart failure symptoms: the ANTHEM-HF study. J Card Fail. 2013;19(9):655–60.
42. De Ferrari GM, Tuinenburg AE, Ruble S, Brugada J, Klein H, Butter C, et al. Rationale and study design of the NEuroCardiac TherApy foR Heart Failure Study: NECTAR-HF. Eur J Heart Fail. 2014;16(6):692–9.
43. Zannad F, De Ferrari GM, Tuinenburg AE, Wright D, Brugada J, Butter C, et al. Chronic vagal stimulation for the treatment of low ejection fraction heart failure: results of the neural cardiac therapy for heart failure (NECTAR-HF) randomized controlled trial. Eur Heart J. 2014; Epub 2014/09/02
44. La Rovere MT, Pinna GD, Raczak G. Baroreflex sensitivity: measurement and clinical implications. Ann Noninvasive Electrocardiol. 2008;13(2):191–207.
45. Berntson GG, Bigger JT, Eckberg DL, Grossman P, Kaufmann PG, Malik M, et al. Heart rate variability: origins, methods, and interpretive caveats. Psychophysiology. 1997;34(6):623–48.
46. Casolo G, Balli E, Taddei T, Amuhasi J, Gori C. Decreased spontaneous heart-rate variability in congestive heart-failure. Am J Cardiol. 1989;64(18):1162–7.
47. Tsuji H, Larson MG, Venditti FJ, Manders ES, Evans JC, Feldman CL, et al. Impact of reduced heart rate variability on risk for cardiac events - The Framingham Heart Study. Circulation. 1996;94(11):2850–5.

48. Nolan J, Batin PD, Andrews R, Lindsay SJ, Brooksby P, Mullen H, et al. Prospective study of heart rate variability and mortality in chronic heart failure - results of the United Kingdom heart failure evaluation and assessment of risk trial (UK-Heart). Circulation. 1998;98(15):1510–6.
49. Monfredi O, Lyashkov AE, Johnsen AB, Inada S, Schneider H, Wang R, et al. Biophysical characterization of the underappreciated and important relationship between heart rate variability and heart rate. Hypertension. 2014;64(6):1334–43. Epub 2014/09/17
50. Hille B. Ionic channels of excitable membranes. Sunderland: Sinauer Associates, INC; 1992.
51. Levy MN, Yang T, Wallick DW. Assessment of beat-by-beat control of heart-rate by the autonomic nervous-system - molecular-biology techniques are necessary, but not sufficient. J Cardiovasc Electrophysiol. 1993;4(2):183–93.
52. Sabbah HN, Imai M, Zaretsky A, Rastogi S, Wang M, Jiang A, et al. Therapy with vagus nerve electrical stimulation combined with beta-blockade improves left ventricular systolic function in dogs with heart failure beyond that seen with beta-blockade alone. Eur J Heart Fail. 2007;6:114.
53. Bohm M, Borer J, Ford I, Gonzalez-Juanatey JR, Komajda M, Lopez-Sendon J, et al. Heart rate at baseline influences the effect of ivabradine on cardiovascular outcomes in chronic heart failure: analysis from the SHIFT study. Clin Res Cardiol. 2013;102(1):11–22.
54. Levine B, Kalman J, Mayer L, Fillit HM, Packer M. Elevated circulating levels of tumor-necrosis-factor in severe chronic heart-failure. N Engl J Med. 1990;323(4):236–41.
55. TorreAmione G, Kapadia S, Benedict C, Oral H, Young JB, Mann DL. Proinflammatory cytokine levels in patients with depressed left ventricular ejection fraction: a report from the studies of left ventricular dysfunction (SOLVD). J Am Coll Cardiol. 1996;27(5):1201–6.
56. Testa M, Yeh M, Lee P, Fanelli R, Loperfido F, Berman JW, et al. Circulating levels of cytokines and their endogenous modulators in patients with mild to severe congestive heart failure due to coronary artery disease or hypertension. J Am Coll Cardiol. 1996;28(4):964–71.
57. Aukrust P, Ueland T, Lien E, Bendtzen K, Muller F, Andreassen AK, et al. Cytokine network in congestive heart failure secondary to ischemic or idiopathic dilated cardiomyopathy. Am J Cardiol. 1999;83(3):376–82.
58. TorreAmione G, Kapadia S, Lee J, Durand JB, Bies RD, Young JB, et al. Tumor necrosis factor-alpha and tumor necrosis factor receptors in the failing human heart. Circulation. 1996;93(4):704–11.
59. Yndestad A, Damas JK, Oie E, Ueland T, Gullestad L, Aukrust P. Systemic inflammation in heart failure - the whys and wherefores. Heart Fail Rev. 2006;11(1):83–92.
60. Tsutamoto T, Wada A, Ohnishi M, Tsutsui T, Ishii C, Ohno K, et al. Transcardiac increase in tumor necrosis factor-alpha and left ventricular end-diastolic volume in patients with dilated cardiomyopathy. Eur J Heart Fail. 2004;6(2):173–80.
61. Sabbah HN, Ilsar I, Zaretsky A, Rastogi S, Wang MJ, Gupta RC. Vagus nerve stimulation in experimental heart failure. Heart Fail Rev. 2011;16(2):171–8.
62. Borovikova LV, Ivanova S, Zhang MH, Yang H, Botchkina GI, Watkins LR, et al. Vagus nerve stimulation attenuates the systemic inflammatory response to endotoxin. Nature. 2000;405(6785):458–62.
63. Wang H, Yu M, Ochani M, Amella CA, Tanovic M, Susarla S, et al. Nicotinic acetylcholine receptor alpha 7 subunit is an essential regulator of inflammation. Nature. 2003;421(6921):384–8.
64. Chung ES, Packer M, Lo KH, Fasanmade AA, Willerson JT, Investigators A. Randomized, double-blind, placebo-controlled, pilot trial of infliximab, a chimeric monoclonal antibody to tumor necrosis factor-alpha, in patients with moderate-to-severe heart failure - results of the anti-TNF Therapy Against Congestive Heart Failure (ATTACH) trial. Circulation. 2003;107(25):3133–40.
65. Mann DL, McMurray JJV, Packer M, Swedberg K, Borer JS, Colucci WS, et al. Targeted anticytokine therapy in patients with chronic heart failure - results of the Randomized Etanercept Worldwide evALuation (RENEWAL). Circulation. 2004;109(13):1594–602.
66. Calvillo L, Vanoli E, Andreoli E, Besana A, Omodeo E, Gnecchi M, et al. Vagal stimulation, through its nicotinic action, limits infarct size and the inflammatory response to myocardial ischemia and reperfusion. J Cardiovasc Pharmacol. 2011;58(5):500–7.

67. Kjekshus J. Arrhythmias and mortality in congestive heart-failure. Am J Cardiol. 1990; 65(19):I42–I8.
68. Harris AL, Locke D. Connexins: a guide. New York: Springer Science & Buisness Media; 2008.
69. Jongsma HJ, Wilders R. Gap junctions in cardiovascular disease. Circ Res. 2000;86(12): 1193–7.
70. Wang XJ, Gerdes AM. Chronic pressure overload cardiac hypertrophy and failure in guinea pigs: III. Intercalated rise remodeling. J Mol Cell Cardiol. 1999;31(2):333–43.
71. Dupont E, Matsushita T, Kaba RA, Vozzi C, Coppen SR, Khan N, et al. Altered connexin expression in human congestive heart failure. J Mol Cell Cardiol. 2001;33(2):359–71.
72. Poelzing S, Rosenbaum DS. Altered connexin43 expression produces arrhythmia substrate in heart failure. Am J Physiol-Heart Circ Physiol. 2004;287(4):H1762–H70.
73. Tomaselli GF, Zipes DP. What causes sudden death in heart failure? Circ Res. 2004;95(8): 754–63.
74. Rastogi S, Mishra S, Ilsar I, Zaretsky A, Sabbah HN. Chronic therapy with electric vagus nerve stimulation normalizes mRNA and protein expression of connexin-40,-43 and-45 in left ventricular myocardium of dogs with heart failure. Circulation. 2007;116(16):218.
75. Sears CE, Ashley EA, Casadei B. Nitric oxide control of cardiac function: is neuronal nitric oxide synthase a key component? Philos Trans R Soc Lond B Biol sci. 2004;359(1446):1021–44.
76. Patten RD, DeNofrio D, El-Zaru M, Kakkar R, Saunders J, Celestin F, et al. Ventricular assist device therapy normalizes inducible nitric oxide synthase expression and reduces cardiomyocyte apoptosis in the failing human heart. J Am Coll Cardiol. 2005;45(9):1419–24.
77. Mungrue IN, Gros R, You XM, Pirani A, Azad A, Csont T, et al. Cardiomyocyte overexpression of iNOS in mice results in peroxynitrite generation, heart block, and sudden death. J Clin Invest. 2002;109(6):735–43.
78. Damy T, Ratajczak P, Robidel E, Bendall JK, Oliviero P, Boczkowski J, et al. Up-regulation of cardiac nitric oxide synthase 1-derived nitric oxide after myocardial infarction in senescent rats. FASEB J. 2003;17(11):1934.
79. Brack KE, Patel VH, Mantravardi R, Coote JH, Ng GA. Direct evidence of nitric oxide release from neuronal nitric oxide synthase activation in the left ventricle as a result of cervical vagus nerve stimulation. J Physiol. 2009;587(12):3045–54.
80. Balligand JL, Kobzik L, Han XQ, Kaye DM, Belhassen L, Ohara DS, et al. Nitric oxide-dependent parasympathetic signaling is due to activation of constitutive endothelial (Type-III) nitric-oxide synthase in cardiac myocytes. J Biol Chem. 1995;270(24):14582–6.
81. Brahmajothi MV, Campbell DL. Heterogeneous basal expression of nitric oxide synthase and superoxide dismutase isoforms in mammalian heart - implications for mechanisms governing indirect and direct nitric oxide-related effects. Circ Res. 1999;85(7):575–87.
82. Barouch LA, Harrison RW, Skaf MW, Rosas GO, Cappola TP, Kobeissi ZA, et al. Nitric oxide regulates the heart by spatial confinement of nitric oxide synthase isoforms. Nature. 2002;416(6878):337–40.
83. Xu KY, Huso DL, Dawson TM, Bredt DS, Becker LC. Nitric oxide synthase in cardiac sarcoplasmic reticulum. Proc Natl Acad Sci USA. 1999;96(2):657–62.
84. Bers DM. Cardiac excitation-contraction coupling. Nature. 2002;415(6868):198–205.
85. Tamargo J, Caballero R, Gomez R, Delpon E. Cardiac electrophysiological effects of nitric oxide. Cardiovasc Res. 2010;87(4):593–600.
86. Ziolo MT. The fork in the nitric oxide road: Cyclic GMP or nitrosylation? Nitric Oxide. 2008;18(3):153–6.

Chapter 8
VNS Therapy for the Treatment of Epilepsy

Clinton W. Wright, Lu Bu, April Jones, and Natasha Calder Green

Abstract Vagus nerve stimulation (VNS Therapy) for the treatment of drug resistant epilepsy was CE marked in 1994 and approved in the US in 1997. This chapter will review the history of the treatment, mechanisms of action, and the technology involved, including programming. Efficacy, selection of candidates, initiation of therapy, and maintenance therapy will also be covered. Finally, complications and adverse events, strengths and limitations, and other vagus nerve stimulation devices will be discussed.

Keywords Therapy of epilepsy • Pharmacoresistant epilepsy • Drug resistant epilepsy • Refractory epilepsy • VNS • Vagus nerve stimulation • Vagal nerve stimulation

VNS Therapy for the Treatment of Epilepsy

Around 70 million people worldwide have epilepsy, and annually, there are between 34 and 76 new cases diagnosed per 100,000 people in the general population [1].

Epilepsy responds to treatment about 70% of the time. Although antiepileptic drugs (AEDs) are the primary form of treatment, outcomes reveal only mixed success rates, even with the new AEDs, some of which have unique mechanisms of action [2, 3]. Approximately one third of patients have seizures that are unresponsive

C.W. Wright, PharmD, BCPP (✉)
Cyberonics, Inc., 100 Cyberonics Blvd, Houston, TX 77058, USA
e-mail: clinton.wright@cyberonics.com

L. Bu, BS, MBA
Department of Clinical and Medical Affairs, Cyberonics, Inc., Houston, TX, USA
e-mail: lu.bu@cyberonics.com

A. Jones, BS
Cyberonics, New Products and Clinical Engineering, Houston, TX, USA
e-mail: april.jones@cyberonics.com

N. Calder Green, MA, ELS
Department of Global Medical Affairs, Cyberonics, Houston, TX, USA
e-mail: natasha.green@cyberonics.com

A. Majid (ed.), *Electroceuticals*, DOI 10.1007/978-3-319-28612-9_8

to pharmacologic therapy [4–6]. In addition, safety and tolerability issues associated with both the acute and chronic side effects and toxicity complications further diminish the effectiveness of AEDs [7–13]. Nonadherence to AEDs, which is highly prevalent in the epilepsy population, also diminishes treatment effectiveness and further increases mortality as well as significantly increases health care utilization [14]. Other treatment options are available for select subgroups of patients, including the ketogenic diet, which provides benefit to some children [15, 16], and epilepsy surgery, which may manage or lessen poorly controlled seizures. However, children and adults with uncontrolled seizures continue to carry a burden of higher mortality rates, higher rates of accidents and injuries, greater incidence of cognitive and psychiatric impairment, poor self-esteem, higher levels of anxiety and depression, and social stigmatization or isolation compared with the general population [17–19]. The shortcomings of AEDs, dietary therapy, and epilepsy surgery in improving overall outcome highlight the need for other treatments, one of which is vagus nerve stimulation therapy (VNS Therapy).

History of the Treatment

In 1883, Corning [20] proposed that vagus nerve stimulation could control seizures via a decrease in heart rate and cerebral blood flow. Bailey and Bremer [21] found that repetitive electrical stimulation of the central end of the vagus nerve of the cat leads to increased amplitude and frequency of the spontaneous potentials of the orbital surface of the frontal lobes of the cerebral cortex. Schweitzer and Wright [22] reported inhibition of motor activity by activation of visceral vagal afferents, later confirmed by Paintal [23]. Dell and Olsen [24] reported that vagus stimulation affected slow wave activity in awake cats.

In the mid-1980s, Jacob Zabara, a biophysicist at Temple University, again suggested that electrical stimulation of the vagus nerve might prevent seizures. Zabara [25] stimulated the cervical vagus nerve in a strychnine dog model of status epilepsy (N = 20). He reported that vagus stimulation would interrupt the strychnine-induced seizure. In 1987 Cyberonics, Inc. (Houston, TX) was founded to develop VNS therapy, which would be delivered by a patented method using a generator device modeled after a cardiac pacemaker.

Pre-clinical Mechanisms of Actions

The vagus nerve comprises approximately 80% afferent fibers. These fibers enter the nucleus tractus solitaries and branch bi-laterally into both sides of the brain. For the most part, both the right and left vagus seem to have very similar projections into neural networks. Both project equally into the right and left sides of the brain.

The mechanisms by which VNS reduces seizure activity in humans were not known at the time VNS therapy was approved by the FDA. However, considerable progress in mechanistic VNS research has been made over the last 15 years. Electrical stimulation of the peripheral vagus nerve requires polysynaptic transmission to mediate the anti-seizure effect. The anatomical distribution of vagal projections underlies the therapeutic actions of VNS therapy. Vagal visceral afferents have a diffuse CNS projection, with activation of these pathways broadly affecting neuronal excitability [26–28]. Another review [27] examined the vagus nerve projections and CNS connections, as well as the current animal and human imaging studies, which indicate that VNS exerts both acute and long-term antiepileptic effects.

The first studies of the anticonvulsant effects of VNS were conducted in 1937 [28]. Subsequent experiments in cats showed that vagal stimulation produced EEG desynchronization [29] or synchronization, depending on the parameters used [30, 31]. Stimulation of the slow-conducting fibers most effectively resulted in EEG desynchronization. Hypersynchronized cortical and thalamocortical neuronal interactions characterize seizures; therefore, it was postulated that desynchronizing these activities would lead to anticonvulsant effects of VNS.

Initial work in cats and later studies of strychnine-induced seizures in the dog, maximal electroshock and pentylenetetrazol-induced seizures in the rat, and the alumina-gel monkey model [25, 29, 32–35] showed that cervical vagal stimulation decreased interictal epileptiform discharges (IEDs) and shortened or aborted seizures; the antiepileptic effects outlasted the stimulus [25, 32, 35, 36] and depended on its frequency and cumulative duration [32–34, 36]. These effects are now known to be mediated by activation of myelinated A and B fibers [37–39]. Most central projections of the vagus nerve terminate in the nucleus of the solitary tract, with extensions to brain stem nuclei, thalamus, amygdala, and hypothalamus. Increased release of α-aminobutyric acid (GABA) and glycine by brain stem and subcortical nuclei was proposed as the antiepileptic mechanism of VNS therapy [33, 34]. Brain stem nuclei are known to influence seizure susceptibility [40–44]; based on animal studies, the nucleus of the tractus solitarius is likely the key brain stem structure involved in transmitting and modulating VNS antiseizure effects.

Also unknown are the processes that mediate the sustained anticonvulsant effect of VNS therapy, but this effect, which outlasts the stimulation, suggests long-term changes in neural activity. Expression of *fos* immunoreactivity was induced by VNS in regions of the rat brain important in epileptogenesis [45]; *fos* immunolabeling in the locus ceruleus suggested VNS modulation of norepinephrine release. Increased norepinephrine release by the locus ceruleus is antiepileptogenic. In rats with chronic or acute locus ceruleus lesions, VNS-induced seizure suppression was attenuated, supporting a noradrenergic mechanism [40]. This first evidence of a structure mediating the anticonvulsant action of VNS may have pharmacologic implications for clinical practice. Drugs that activate the locus ceruleus or potentiate norepinephrine effects may enhance the efficacy of VNS. Pending the results of further animal testing, it is likely that the antiepileptic action of VNS is mediated through neuronal networks that project from brain stem to forebrain structures.

Vagal projections to noradrenergic and serotonergic neuromodulatory systems of the brain may also explain the positive effects of VNS in improving mood disorders.

In summary, animal studies have established three distinct temporal patterns for the anticonvulsant effects of VNS: (i) acute abortive effects, in which an ongoing seizure is attenuated by VNS; (ii) acute prophylactic effects, in which seizure-inducing agents are less effective in provoking seizures when applied at the end of VNS; and (iii) chronic progressive prophylactic effects, in which total seizure counts are reduced more following chronic VNS stimulation. In addition, animal studies have shown that VNS can antagonize the development of epilepsy in the kindling model of epileptogenesis [46]. Based on these studies, the mechanism of action of VNS therapy appears to be largely distinct from that of AED therapies [27].

Clinical Mechanisms of Actions

Initial scalp recording performed in a small number of adults did not demonstrate a significant effect of VNS on EEG total power, median frequency, power in any of the conventional frequency bands [47], interictal epileptiform activity, or the waking or sleep background rhythms [47–50]. At seizure onset, however, VNS terminated both the clinical and the EEG seizure activity [49]. Studies that are more recent have suggested that some patients may have a change in interictal epileptiform discharges with VNS. In a study of 15 adults with refractory partial-onset seizure disorders and with VNS treatment for $\geq$ 6 months, all showed a significant reduction in interictal epileptiform discharges during stimulation and the interstimulation period immediately following stimulation, compared with baseline, with the reduction in interical epileptiform discharges greater among patients whose seizures decreased by more than 50% on VNS. Additionally, the patients who had a significant decrease in interical epileptiform discharges experienced the positive effect of magnetic activation, resulting in extra stimulation, abolishing seizures [51]. Another case study of a single adult patient undergoing presurgical evaluation with intrahippocampal depth electrodes showed alteration of interictal epileptiform discharges by VNS (increased spikes at 5 Hz, decreased at 30 Hz) [52]. Chronic VNS in another study was reported to reduce interictal epileptiform discharges [53]. However, this population was quite different from that in the earlier adult series. Included were patients with generalized and partial-onset seizures, greater frequency of interictal epileptiform discharges, and younger age. During 12 months of VNS therapy, both generalized and focal spikes were diminished; however, this did not correlate well with seizure reduction. Pattern-reversal visual-evoked potentials, brain stem auditory-evoked potentials, and cognitive (P300) potentials were all unaffected by VNS [54].

Release of anticonvulsant neurotransmitters at the projection sites of vagus nerve afferent fibers was hypothesized as a mechanism of action [54, 55]. Cerebrospinal fluid samples assayed for amino acid and neurotransmitter metabolites in 16 patients before and after 3 months of VNS therapy showed a treatment-induced increase in GABA (an inhibitory amino acid), a decrease in aspartate (an excitatory amino acid), and an increase in ethanolamine (a membrane lipid precursor) [55].

Positron emission tomography (PET) $H_2{}^{15}O$ cerebral blood flow (CBF) imaging identifies the neuroanatomical structures recruited by VNS in humans. A pilot study of three adults showed activation of the right thalamus, right posterotemporal cortex, left putamen, and left inferior cerebellum [56]. Localization to the thalamus may explain the therapeutic benefit of VNS and is consistent with the role of that structure as a generator and modulator of cerebral activity. Moreover, anatomic and physiologic evidence from both animal and human data further support the role of the thalamus in epilepsy [57], with stimulation of either the anterior thalamic nucleus or centromedian thalamic nucleus in animals being associated with anticonvulsant effects [58]. In a study of high and low stimulation [59], PET demonstrated CBF alterations at sites that receive vagal afferents and projections, including dorsal medulla, right postcentral gyrus, thalamus, cerebellum bilaterally, and limbic structures (bilateral hippocampus and amygdala). The high-stimulation group had more activation and deactivation sites, although the anatomical patterns during VNS were similar in both groups. Finally, acute CBF alterations were correlated with long-term therapeutic response, in an attempt to exclude those regions that show changes in VNS-induced synaptic activity but may not participate in VNS-related anticonvulsant actions [60]. Decreased seizure frequency was associated with increased CBF only in the right and left thalami. Studies of chronic VNS therapy have shown the same anatomical distribution of CBF [56, 61]. Demonstration of these acute regional alterations does not clarify the mechanism of action of long term, intermittent VNS, which may involve neurotransmitters or neurochemicals at those sites that outlast the stimulation.

Functional magnetic resonance imaging (fMRI) evaluating the time course of regional CBF alterations during VNS therapy can be performed safely in patients implanted with a vagal nerve stimulator [62]. Preliminary fMRI studies have agreed with the PET studies, with the most robust activation observed in the thalami and insular cortices, with some activation also seen in ipsilateral basal ganglia, anterior parietal cortex, and other cortical areas [62, 63].

Maximal stimulation of the myelinated A and B fibers of the vagus nerve to achieve a therapeutic effect is the key component of treatment of seizures. To help understand how to achieve maximal stimulation of the A and B fibers, a digital model of the vagus nerve was constructed to explore the effects of combinations of output current and pulse width. The combination of these two parameter settings defines the amount of charge delivered to the nerve fibers and reflects the probability of achieving effective activation of the vagus nerve. The computer model showed that for optimal stimulation, output current settings may range between 0.75 and 1.75 mA with pulse width settings of 250 or 500 μs. Such settings will likely provide sufficient vagal activation in adults and in children over 12 years of age, with minimal side effects. These settings may not apply to children under the age of 12 years. Other studies have shown children 10 years and younger require higher output currents to achieve activation of the vagus nerve, which may be due to the level of nerve maturation during development. There are other factors not considered in this model that may also influence the effectiveness of VNS therapy: signal frequency, duty cycle, virtual anodes, virtual cathodes, conduction blocking, and fibrotic tissue of varying thickness. The contribution of signal frequency and duty cycle are not fully understood [64].

Technology and Programming

The VNS Therapy System consists of implantable and external components. The implantable components include the VNS pulse generator and bipolar lead (Fig. 8.1), which work together to deliver mild electrical pulses to the vagus nerve. The pulse generator is typically implanted in the left chest, in a subcutaneous pocket below the clavicle. The lead electrodes are wrapped around the left vagus nerve in the neck, near the carotid artery, and subcutaneously connected to the pulse generator.

The external components of the VNS Therapy System include the programming system (Fig. 8.2a) and the VNS Therapy magnet (Fig. 8.2b). The programming system consists of programming software on a compatible computer and a programming wand. It allows healthcare professionals to adjust dosing (i.e., the timing and amount of the VNS Therapy), perform device diagnostics, and review programming history. The VNS Therapy magnet allows the patient to activate additional stimulation or to temporarily stop stimulation at any time.

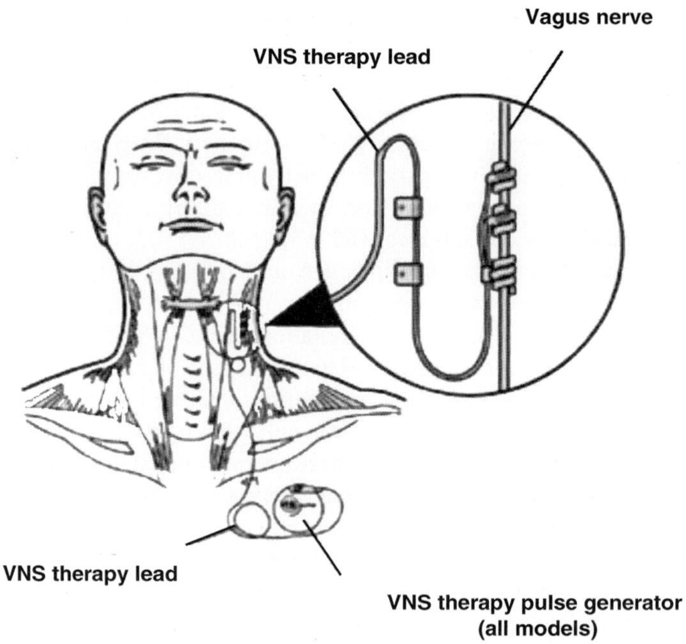

Fig. 8.1 Implantable components of VNS therapy

The pulse generator operates in two modes of stimulation, normal mode and magnet mode. The normal mode stimulation is delivered automatically according to a pre-programmed schedule. The magnet mode, if enabled, is only delivered when the patient briefly passes the magnet over the pulse generator. This mode allows the patient to activate additional stimulation as needed, typically right before or during a seizure, to help abort the seizure or reduce its intensity.

There are eight VNS Therapy parameters that can be adjusted with the external programming system. They include five stimulation parameters in Normal Mode and three stimulation parameters in Magnet Mode. Table 8.1 lists the different VNS Therapy parameters and available settings within each parameter. Each stimulation period is preceded by 2 s of ramp-up time and followed by 2 s of ramp-down time.

Four models of the VNS therapy generators are currently available: the Pulse Model 102/Pulse Duo Model 102R, the Demipulse Model 103/Demipulse Duo Model 104, the AspireHC Model 105, and the AspireSR Model 106.

PulseDuo and Demipulse Duo are dual-pin while all other generators are single-pin. Demipulse, AspireHC and AspireSR are second-generation devices

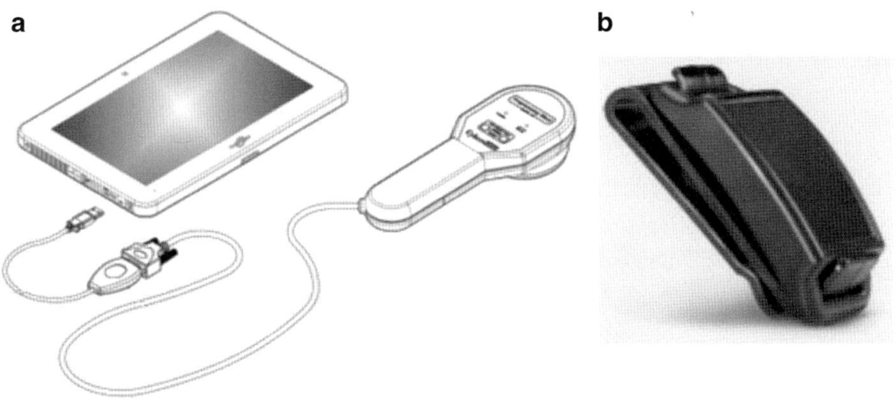

Fig. 8.2 (**a**) VNS programming system. (**b**) VNS therapy magnet

Table 8.1 VNS therapy programmable parameters

Stimulation mode	Parameter name	Available parameter settings
Normal	Output current	0–3.5 mA in 0.25 mA steps
	Signal frequency	1, 2, 5, 10, 15, 20, 25, 30 Hz
	Pulse width	130, 250, 500, 750, 1000 μs
	On time	7, 14, 21, 30, 60 s
	Off time	0.2, 0.3, 0.5, 0.8, 1.1, 1.8, 3 min, and 5–180 min (5–60 in 5-min steps; 60–180 in 30-min steps)
Magnet	Magnet output current	0–3.5 mA in 0.25 mA steps

compared to Pulse generators and offer improved diagnostics and faster communication with the programming system. Due to its smaller size, Demipulse generators may have shorter battery life at higher duty cycles than the Pulse generators (Fig. 8.3).

The Perennia Model 303 and PerenniaFLEX Model 304 leads are widely available. In some markets, the older Model 302 lead is also available. All current lead models are single pin and come in two sizes to accommodate to various sizes of the vagus nerve: 2.0 or 3.0 mm (inner diameters of the helical coil). Dual-pin leads are no longer manufactured. Therefore, the dual-pin generators (Model 102R and Model 104) are only used for replacement procedures in patients with the previous dual-pin lead models. The Demipulse, AspireHC, AspireSR generators and Perennia model leads are not yet available in all countries.

Safety and effectiveness was established for left vagal nerve stimulation in the VNS Therapy pivotal clinical trials. There have been limited studies conducted for right vagal nerve stimulation. Primate studies by Lockard [65] did not note any effects on heart rate or gastric function via stimulation of the right vagus nerve. Several other reports regarding right-sided vagal nerve stimulation also have not mentioned cardiac effects [66–71]. In a pilot study of right vagus nerve stimulation for congestive heart failure, a positive clinical result was noted [71]. Although right-sided VNS may be safe, it should be used cautiously as its safety has not been established in clinical studies.

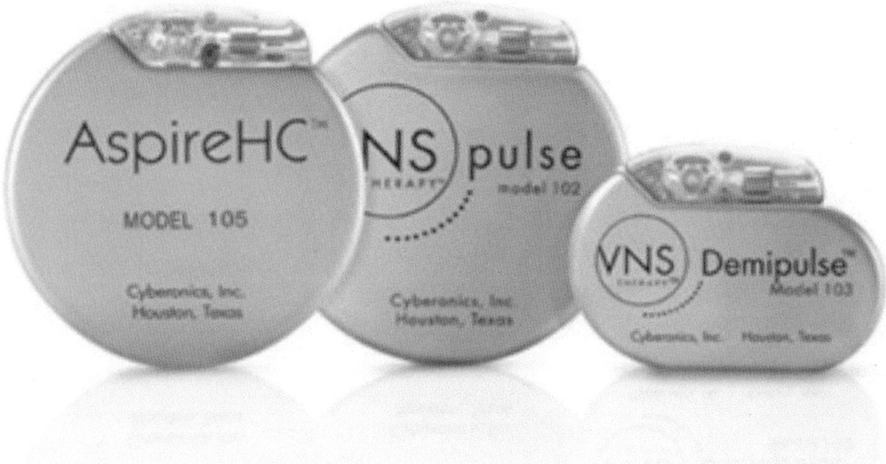

Fig. 8.3 PulseDuo and Demipulse Duo are dual-pin while all other generators are single-pin. Demipulse, AspireHC and AspireSR are second-generation devices compared to Pulse generators and offer improved diagnostics and faster communication with the programming system. Due to its smaller size, Demipulse generators may have shorter battery life at higher duty cycles than the Pulse generators

Efficacy

Five trials were conducted to support the approval of VNS Therapy (E-01–E-05). Morris et al. [72] reported on the long-term results from these pilot and pivotal trials. A total of 440 patients were included in the analysis. Patients were followed until approval so not all patient data were available at all time points. The responder rate (≥ 50% reduction in seizures improved over time (Fig. 8.4). Continuation rates were 96.7% (426/444) at year 1, 84.7% (254/300) at year 2, and 72.1% (124/172) at year 3. These studies led to approval of VNS therapy by the U.S. Food and Drug Administration (FDA) in July 1997 for the adjunctive treatment of refractory partial-onset seizures among patients 12 years of age or older. VNS therapy is also approved for the treatment of epilepsy without age or seizure type restrictions (in most countries in more than 70 countries around the world, including member nations of the European Union, Japan, Canada, Australia, and China. As of May 2015, more than 80,000 patients have received VNS Therapy worldwide.

In addition to the clinical trial data, post-approval outcome studies show that VNS therapy is an effective treatment with increasing or sustained response rates over time. Response rates from the literature for studies reporting on at least 100 patients with a minimum of 12 months to more than 5 years of follow-up range from 50% to 64% (Fig. 8.5) [73–77].

The Elliott et al. study was a retrospective review of a prospectively created database of 436 consecutive patients, both adults and children, at a single center. In addition to the 64% response rate, it showed a significant reduction in mean seizure frequency (mean reduction of 55.8%; P < 0.0001) at a mean follow-up of 4.94 years

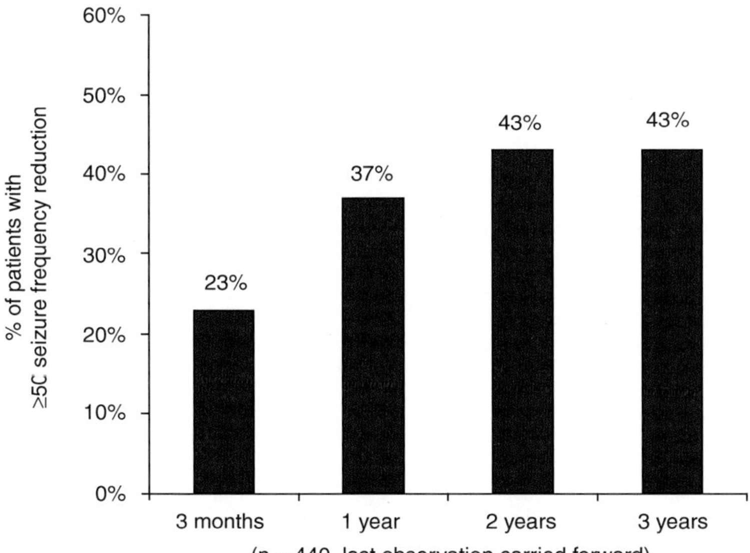

Fig. 8.4 Results from open-label, long-term efficacy and safety trial (E-01- E-05 Extension)

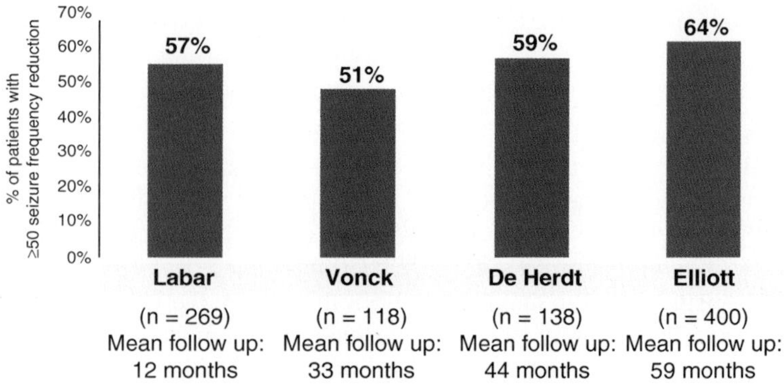

Fig. 8.5 Response rates in post-approval outcome studies with VNS therapy

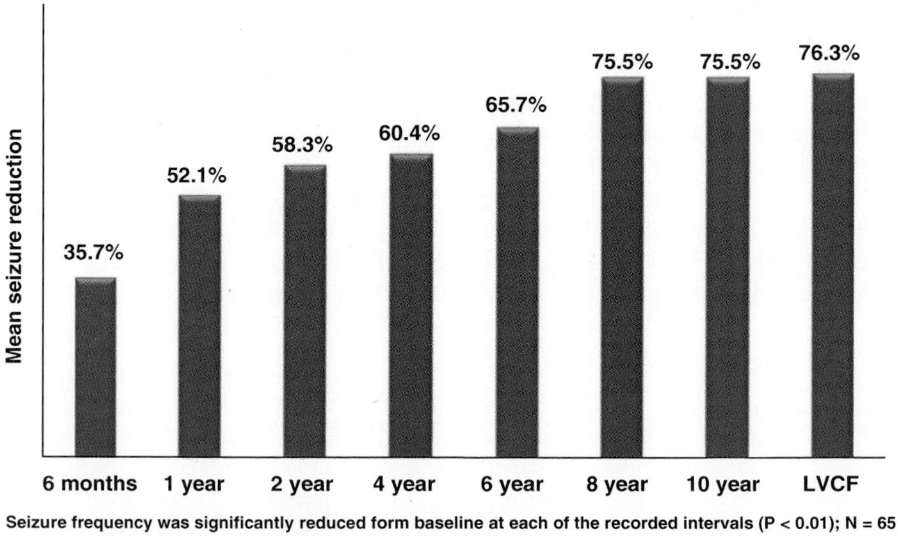

Fig. 8.6 Mean seizure reduction of 65 patients treated with VNS therapy >10 years

[77]. A subset of this group that had at least 10 years of follow-up (n = 65) showed continued improvement over time, with a mean reduction in seizure frequency of 75% at 10 years (LOCF, 76%) [78]. At each recorded interval at 6 months and at years 1, 2, 4, 6, 8, and 10, seizure frequency was significantly reduced from baseline ($P < 0.001$; Fig. 8.6) [78]. The overall responder rate at last follow-up was 91%, with 10 patients seizure free for at least 2 years before their last follow-up visit.

VNS therapy patients with a history of intracranial epilepsy surgery (IES) were compared to those without, and was reported in an additional article [78]. Of the 436 total patients, 376 has data for at least 1 year of therapy. The mean duration of VNS Therapy was 5.1 years. The difference in mean percentage seizure reduction between the groups was not significant (59.1% for patients with prior IES and 56.5% for patients without prior IES; P=0.42).

Elliott et al. [79] looked at a subset of 141 children 18 years of age and younger with treatment-resistant epilepsy and at least 1 year of follow up from his data set, seizure frequency significantly improved with VNS therapy (mean reduction 58.9%, $p < 0.0001$). The mean age at initiation of VNS therapy was 11.1 years (range, 1–18); 86 (61%) were under age 12 years when they received VNS therapy. The mean duration of VNS therapy was 5.2 years (range, 25 days to 11.4 years). The overall responder rate for this population was 65%, with 41% experiencing 75% or greater reduction in seizure frequency. Comparisons between those older than 12 years of age with those younger than 12 years of age showed no differences in efficacy or safety between the groups.

Selection of Candidates

VNS Therapy is indicated as an adjunctive treatment for patients 12 years of age or older with refractory partial-onset seizures in the US [80] and as an adjunctive treatment for patients with partial- or generalized-onset seizures without an age limitation in the EU. There are no known predictors of response to VNS Therapy (e.g. age, sex, seizure type, etiology, frequency of seizures, type or number of co-administered antiepileptic drugs, etc.) as the indications for use were derived from clinical experience rather than an understanding of the underlying mechanism of action. Favorable outcomes have been in reported in many studies, although complete seizure freedom is rarely achieved [81]. One recent study indicated that VNS therapy should be considered in patients with posttraumatic epilepsy, which is often resistant to AED therapy and not resectable [82].

Although optimal use parameters for VNS Therapy continue to be defined, candidates should meet the following criteria: (i) medically refractory seizures, (ii) adequate trials of at least two antiepileptic drugs, (iii) exclusion of non-epileptic events, and (iv) ineligibility for epilepsy surgery. Recent open studies suggest that VNS therapy may be used among patients considered for corpus callosotomy, producing lower rates of morbidity [60–63, 82–91]. Earlier use (within 2 years of seizure onset or after failure of two or three AEDs) of VNS Therapy may also produce a higher response rate, as well as reduce the negative side effects associated with long-term epilepsy and AED therapy, which hinder development [78, 92–94]. Patients with a history of nonadherence to their AED regimens, particularly those on polypharmacy, may also be good candidates for VNS therapy because of the assured compliance and lack of further drug–drug interactions with VNS therapy [95, 96].

Patients who have had a prior bilateral or left cervical vagotomy are contraindicated for VNS. As mentioned earlier, safety and efficacy have not been established for stimulation of the right vagus nerve. Patients with existing pulmonary or cardiac disease should be evaluated carefully before implantation, as chronic obstructive pulmonary disease may increase the risk for dyspnea, and patients with cardiac conduction disorders were not studied in the controlled trials. A cardiologist's evaluation

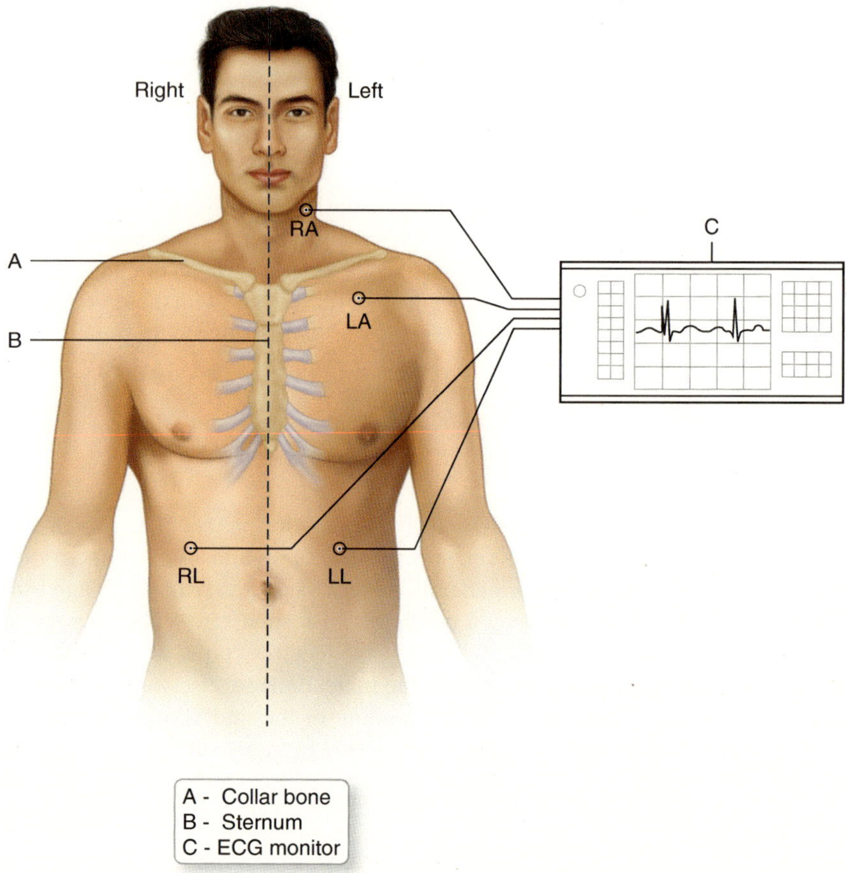

Fig. 8.7 AspireSR generator may properly detect heartbeats. In this procedure, surface ECG electrodes are placed on to the subject

should precede implantation, with post-procedural Holter monitoring performed if clinically indicated. Patients with a history of obstructive sleep apnea should be treated with care, as an increase in apneic events during stimulation is possible [97, 98]. Lowering stimulation frequency (i.e., pulse width and signal frequency to 250 μsec and 20 Hz, respectively) may prevent exacerbation of this condition [97]. However, most studies showing a decrease in airflow during sleep with VNS therapy reported this condition to be clinically insignificant [98]. Moreover, beneficial effects on sleep and increases in slow wave sleep also have been reported with VNS therapy, which may play a role in the antiepileptic mechanisms of VNS [99, 100].

For the AspireSR pulse generator, other patient selection criteria apply in addition to considerations mentioned above. Patients who experience seizures that are associated with cardiac rhythm increases known as ictal tachycardia may benefit from using the AutoStim feature of the AspireSR generator. For screening purposes,

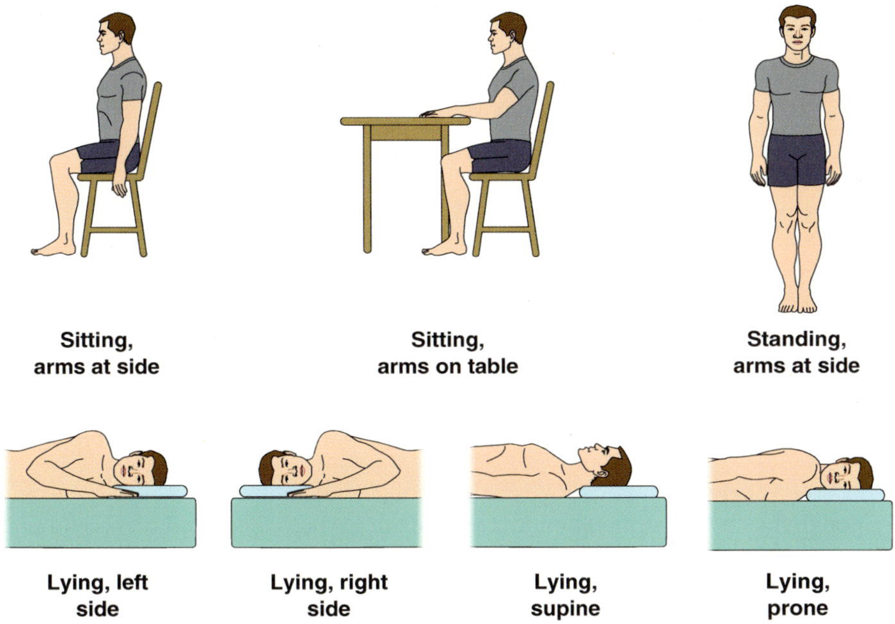

Fig. 8.8 The measurements are then taken according to the positions

this is defined as an increase in heart rate during a seizure, specifically from a baseline heart rate to a rate that is greater than 100 bpm and is at least a 55% increase or 35 bpm increase from baseline. The screening of ictal tachycardia should be performed with objective data, such as hospital vital sign recordings, telemetry data, ECG rhythm strip recordings, Holter recordings, and/or video EEG/ECG recordings.

In addition to screening for ictal tachycardia, a screening process for implant position must also be performed for the AspireSR generator. This procedure utilizes surface ECG measurements from seven body positions to identify a suitable implant position, so that once implanted, the AspireSR generator may properly detect heart beats. In this procedure, surface ECG electrodes are placed on to the subject as per Fig. 8.7 below. The measurements are then taken according to the positions in Fig. 8.8. For a desired implant location for the AspireSR generator, the peak-to-peak R-wave amplitude must be greater or equal to 0.4 mV in all body positions.

Initiation and Maintenance of Therapy

Hospitalization for implantation of the device is preceded by evaluations by a neurologist and by a surgeon with experience in the carotid sheath. With the patient typically under general anesthesia (although local or regional anesthesia has been used successfully as well) [101], the lead electrodes are placed on the left cervical vagus nerve and the generator is placed in a subcutaneous pocket in the left upper chest. The lead body is routed subcutaneously from the neck to the chest. [102, 103] (see VNS Therapy surgical implant video). Intraoperative electrical impedance testing ensures integrity of the system. The anesthesiologist should be notified immediately before this test as there have been rare cases of bradycardia, asystole, or both during the intraoperative test [80, 104, 105]. Stimulation following intraoperative bradycardia has been shown to be safe, with no reports of change in cardiac rhythm upon initiation of postoperative VNS, even under ECG monitoring [106]. Correct placement of the lead electrodes around the vagus nerve is critical. If there is concern about the lead placement, two methods have been utilized to help confirm correct placement of the electrodes intraoperatively [107], depending on the type of anesthesia used for the procedure. For patients receiving general anesthesia, the larynx and vocal cords can be monitored by fiberoptic endoscopy for contraction of the left lateral larynx wall and vocal cord tightening. For patients being implanted under local and regional anesthesia, stimulation intensities can be increased until a voice alteration is noticed. Neither procedure is harmful to the patient nor greatly extends the length of the surgery.

Prophylactic antibiotics may be administered both in the operating room and postoperatively. The patient can be discharged after the procedure, which usually lasts for 1–2 h, or can be observed overnight. Discharge education should include care of the incisions and use of the magnet. In clinical studies, the generator's output current was kept at 0 mA for the first 2 weeks; however, programmed stimulation is now being initiated at 0.25 mA in many operating rooms [108]. Dosages of antiepileptic drugs are generally kept stable for the first 3–6 months of stimulation unless an early response is noted [109].

A few weeks after implantation, the patient is examined to confirm wound healing and proper generator operation either to begin or to continue programming. Output current is increased in 0.25-mA increments until stimulation is comfortable (Table 8.1). The subsequent stimulation schedule is determined by patient response. Standard parameter settings range from a frequency of 20–30 Hz at a pulse width of 250–500 μsec for 30 s "on" time and 5 min "off" time [53]. The magnet stimulation is typically set slightly higher to an output current at 0.25 mA greater than the normal mode output current (physician training slides). For an adult, to generate an action potential in the nerve (a therapeutic effect), research shows that optimal output current settings may range from 0.75 mA to 1.75 mA and pulse width from 250 to 500 μsec [64]. At each visit, the generator's battery is assessed for end of service, and proper operation of the system is checked through diagnostic testing. The battery's life expectancy of 3–8 years depends on the programmed stimulation parameters. If VNS therapy is to be continued after battery depletion, the generator can be replaced at the appropriate time in less than 1 h. If diagnostics shows the system is not operating properly, surgery to troubleshoot and/or replace the lead and potentially generator is necessary to continue VNS Therapy.

VNS may be continued indefinitely and without damage to the vagus nerve as long as the stimulation is less than 50 Hz and the on time remains less than the off time [80, 110, 111]. Two safety features that protect patients from continuous stimulation or uncomfortable side effects are the magnet and the watchdog timer. The magnet can act as an "off" switch when held or taped over the generator. The watchdog timer is an internal monitor that limits the number of pulses to be delivered without an "off" time to prevent excess stimulation.

Complications and Adverse Effects

Surgical complications and difficulties are rare. Incisional infections are unusual and generally respond to antibiotic therapy. Fluid accumulation at the generator site with or without infection occurs in 1–2% of implantations and resolves with aspiration and antibiotics; the rare cases of refractory infection require removal of the generator. However, one case of deep wound infection associated with implantation of the generator was reported to be managed successfully with open wound treatment without removal of the device, an alternative option if removal of the device appears hazardous [112]. Unilateral vocal cord paralysis, which accompanies approximately 1% of implants, may be caused by excess manipulation of the vagus nerve, and subsequent damage to the vagal artery and its reinforcing arterioles [113]; in most cases, it remits completely over several weeks.

Common side effects, which occur primarily when the stimulator is actually delivering a pulse, are dose dependent and usually mild or absent when VNS parameters are appropriately programmed [114–116]; many patients become accustomed to them with time. Most patients experience hoarseness or a change in vocal quality and tingling over the left cervical region on delivery of the electrical pulse. Subjective dyspnea or a sensation of muscle tightening in the neck may occur, without changes on pulmonary function testing [115]. Cough or throat pain during stimulus delivery sometimes necessitates a reduction in current or pulse width [117].

Despite the widespread visceral efferent projections of the vagus nerve, systemic effects are rare. Pulmonary function does not change significantly in patients without concomitant lung disease [115, 118], but may deteriorate in the face of intense stimulation and obstructive lung disease [118]. Inhalation of ipratropium bromide or lowering of the stimulus frequency or current is recommended. No substantial effects on cardiac function were reported during clinical studies [80, 114–116, 119]. An analysis of total mortality and sudden death in epileptic patients (to August 1996) revealed the expected rate in individuals with severe, intractable epilepsy [120, 121]. The clinical studies demonstrated no clinically relevant effects on the gastrointestinal system, serum chemistries, AED concentrations, vital signs, or weight.

Rare reported side effects associated with VNS therapy include diarrhea [122], sternocleidomastoid muscle spasm [123], phrenic nerve stimulation [124], tonsillar pain [125], emergent psychiatric disorders [126, 127], and prominent drooling and vomiting [128]. Of seven patients treated with VNS therapy who developed a major psychiatric disorder [126], all had a history of a dysphoric disorder and most had daily seizures before treatment with VNS. The severe dysphoric or psychotic conditions emerged once seizure frequency was reduced by 75% or more, but remitted or improved satisfactorily with psychotropic medication, with two patients also requiring a decrease or interruption of VNS therapy. Children with a history of dysphagia may experience swallowing difficulties during VNS therapy [128–130]; adjusting the device settings or using a magnet to turn off the stimulator during mealtime may help. The majority of side effects, including many of the rare incidents reported, are amenable to stimulus modifications, which could include changes in output current and/or pulse width.

Strengths and Limitations

Many patients maintained on VNS therapy can decrease their total AED burden, which consequently can improve patient alertness and lessen the cognitive or systemic side effects typically associated with multiple therapies. Therefore, use of AED monotherapy with VNS therapy may produce a better risk to benefit ratio than that with multiple AEDs. VNS therapy may alleviate seizures with no risk of toxic organ reactions, drug interactions or failures, allergies, rashes, and other systemic adverse effects or cognitive side effects, even in cases where AEDs cannot be substantially decreased or withdrawn [131, 132]. In some patients, memory, alertness, mood, and communication have been shown to improve [48, 133–137]. Improvements in QoL independent of treatment effect on seizure frequency, as well as increased daytime vigilance, have also been reported [138–140]. In addition, VNS therapy may be an ideal treatment for the partially compliant as it does not require active patient participation [95, 96]. Teratogenesis is not expected with VNS therapy. Although no controlled studies of VNS therapy in pregnancy have been conducted, a study in rabbits showed no harm to fertility or to the fetus [141]. Cases also have been reported in the literature of patients who became pregnant while treated with VNS therapy and gave birth to healthy babies [142, 143]. Finally, VNS therapy can both prevent and abort seizures. The ability to activate on-demand stimulation with the magnet empowers the patient and provides a sense of control over epilepsy.

On the other hand, VNS is an empiric therapy, with no way to predict response except by trial. The initial cost (often between $15,000 and $25,000) can be prohibitive without coverage by a third-party payer. Over the life of the system, however, this cost approximates that of many of the new AEDs [144]. Moreover, although weeks to months may elapse before seizure frequency decreases, cost-effectiveness studies indicate that VNS therapy provides a substantial cost-savings benefit to hospitals over the long-term course of treatment [145, 146]. These cost benefits are sustained over time and are sufficient to cover or exceed the cost of the device. Further savings can be seen in significant reductions in health care utilization and time spent on epilepsy-related matters with VNS therapy over time. A Kaiser study, which looked at health care utilization of 138 patients with refractory epilepsy comparing 1 year of baseline data followed by 4 years of quarterly follow-up data with VNS therapy, showed significant reductions in the numbers of emergency department visits (decreased by 99%), hospitalizations (70% decrease), and hospital lengths of stay (67% decrease) beginning with the first quarter after implantation with VNS Therapy ($P < 0.05$ for all post-implantation quarters) [147]. A 91% decrease was also seen in outpatient visits post-VNS therapy, and significant decreases were seen for average number of days on which patients could not work because of health-related concerns ($P = 0.002$) and average time spent caring for health problems ($P < 0.001$). These metrics reflect the positive changes in the QoL of both patients and their caregivers, as well as health care utilization savings as a result of VNS therapy. In a US study evaluating the long-term medical and economic benefits of VNS therapy using Medicaid data from five states (n = 1655), VNS therapy was associated with lower average healthcare costs and epilepsy-related clinical events [95]. Hospitalizations, emergency room visits, and outpatient visits all were significantly reduced during the post-VNS period compared with the pre-VNS period (P < 0.0001). Serious events such as grand mal status, fractures, and traumatic head injuries also were reduced in the post-VNS period. Despite the initial expense of VNS therapy, the reductions in healthcare utilization and epilepsy events resulted in a net cost savings for VNS therapy after 1.5 years of treatment.

According to the manufacturer of the device, a transmit-and-receive head coil MRI should be used for head and extremity scans rather than a full-body MRI, with the generator programmed to 0 mA for the procedure and returned to the original settings thereafter [80]. MRI scans following these procedures are safe in 1.5 T and 3 T scanners [80]. However, successful head coil MRIs have been performed among patients both with and without the device turned off [148]. If the device was accidentally left on during the MRI, the device should be interrogated post-procedure to ensure that the magnetic field did not deactivate the device or change the pre-MRI settings. If a full-body scan is required using RF coil, surgical removal of the VNS therapy system is required. Although not recommended by the manufacturer, successful body coil MRIs with the use of an ice pack over the area of the device leads have been reported among three patients [149]. Diathermy, which could heat the system above safe levels and thereby cause either temporary or permanent tissue or nerve damage, should be avoided in patients receiving VNS therapy.

Other VNS Devices

Stefan et al. described the use of the Cerbomed NEMOS device in a pilot study among ten patients [150]. Electrical stimulation was applied transcutaneously three times per day to the auricular branch of the vagus nerve (ABVN) of the left ear for 9 months. Seven of the 10 patients were able to complete the study. Of the 7 patients, 5 experienced an overall seizure reduction after treatment with t-VNS, although a 50% response rate was not reached [150].

Electrocore Medical manufactures the gammaCore battery-powered device that is held against the neck and provides a single 180 s burst of vagus nerve stimulation. A number of presentations and publications of pilot studies have reported encouraging results for migraine, cluster headaches, asthma, and bronchial COPD. Electrocore Medical has a CE Mark for epilepsy, but no epilepsy studies have been reported as of February 2014.

Conclusions

VNS Therapy has demonstrated to be an effective non-pharmacologic treatment for drug resistant epilepsy. This has sparked interest in the role of neurostimulation in treating epilepsy. As the mechanisms are further explored beyond its effect on the norepinephrine and serotonin system, treatment of other chronic illnesses are being considered and tested. Its place in therapy should be considered earlier in the course of the disease in those patients for whom surgery is not an option and that are drug resistant. Several other opportunities still exist to optimize the therapy and therefore improve patient outcomes. These include optimizing the dose based on seizure type, syndromes, age groups and concomitant medications; developing an algorithm for dose titration and ideal parameter settings; characterizing the impact of VNS Therapy on factors other than seizure count; and providing a closed-loop responsive device to name a few. Meeting these opportunities will expand the role of VNS Therapy in drug resistant epilepsy.

References

1. Ngugi AK, Kariuki SM, Bottomly C, Kleinschmidt I, Sander JW, Newton CR. Incidence of epilepsy: a systematic review and meta-analysis. Neurology. 2011;77:1005–12.
2. Brodie MJ. Road to refractory epilepsy: The Glasgow story. Epilepsia. 2013;54:5–8.
3. Schmidt D. The clinical impact of new antiepileptic drugs after a decade of use in epilepsy. Epilepsy Res. 2002;50:21–32.
4. Kwan P, Brodie MJ. Early identification of refractory epilepsy. N Engl J Med. 2000;342: 314–9.
5. Mohanraj R, Brodie MJ. Diagnosing refractory epilepsy: response to sequential treatment schedules. Eur J Neurol. 2006;13:277–82.
6. Hitiris N, Mohanraj R, Norrie J, et al. Predictors of pharmacoresistant epilepsy. Epilepsy Res. 2007;75:192–6.
7. Jallon P. The problem of intractability: the continuing need for new medical therapies in epilepsy. Epilepsia. 1997;38(Suppl 9):S37–42.
8. Patsalos PN, Duncan JS. Antiepileptic drugs. A review of clinically significant drug interactions. Drug Saf. 1993;9:156–84.
9. Pellock JM, Pippenger CE. Adverse effects of antiepileptic drugs. In: Dodson WE, Pellock JM, editors. Pediatric epilepsy: diagnosis and therapy. New York: Demos; 1993. p. 253–64.
10. Schmidt D. Adverse Effects of Antiepileptic Drugs. New York: Raven Press; 1982.
11. Pellock JM. Antiepileptic drug therapy in the United States: a review of clinical studies and unmet needs. Neurology. 1995;45:S17–24.

12. Kwan P, Brodie MJ. Effectiveness of first antiepileptic drug. Epilepsia. 2001;42:1255–60.
13. Camfield P, Camfield C. Acute and chronic toxicity of antiepileptic medications: a selective review. Can J Neurol Sci. 1994;21:S7–S11.
14. Faught E, Duh MS, Weiner JR, et al. Nonadherence to antiepileptic drugs and increased mortality: findings from the RANSOM Study. Neurology. 2008;71:1572–8.
15. Wheless JW, Ashwal S. The ketogenic diet. In: Swaiman KF, Ashwal S, editors. Pediatric neurology: principles and practice. Philadelphia: CV Mosby Co; 1999. p. 719–28.
16. Vining EP, Freeman JM, Ballaban-Gil K, et al. A multicenter study of the efficacy of the ketogenic diet. Arch Neurol. 1998;55:1433–7.
17. Epilepsy Foundation of America. Epilepsy: A Report to the Nation. Landover: Epilepsy Foundation of America; 1999.
18. Fisher RS, Parks-Trusz SL, Lehman C. Social issues in epilepsy. In: Shorvon S, Dreifus F, Fish D, et al., editors. The treatment of epilepsy. Cambridge: Blackwell Science; 1996. p. 357–69.
19. Wheless JW. Intractable epilepsy: a survey of patients and caregivers. Epilepsy Behav. 2006; 8:756–64.
20. Corning J. Considerations on pathology and therapeutics of epilepsy. J Nerv Ment Dis. 1883;10:243–8.
21. Bailey P, Bremer F. A sensory cortical representation of the vagus nerve with a note on the effects of low blood pressure on the cortical electrograms. J Neurophysiol. 1938:405–12.
22. Schweitzer A, Wright S. Effects on the knee jerk of stimulation of the central end of the vagus and of various changes in the circulation and respiration. J Physiol. 1937;515:459–75.
23. Paintal AS. Vagal sensory receptors and their reflex effects. Physiol Rev. 1973;53(1):159–227.
24. Dell P, Olson R. Secondary mesencephalic, diencephalic and amygdalian projections of vagal visceral afferences. C R Seances Soc Biol Fil. 1951;145(13–14):1088–91.
25. Zabara J. Inhibition of experimental seizures in canines by repetitive vagal stimulation. Epilepsia. 1992;33:1005–12.
26. Schachter SC, Saper CB. Vagus nerve stimulation. Epilepsia. 1998;39:677–86.
27. Henry TR. Therapeutic mechanisms of vagus nerve stimulation. Neurology. 2002;59:S3–S14.
28. Rutecki P. Anatomical, physiological, and theoretical basis for the antiepileptic effect of vagus nerve stimulation. Epilepsia. 1990;31(Suppl 2):S1–6.
29. Zanchetti A, Wang SC, Moruzzi G. The effect of vagal afferent stimulation on the EEG pattern of the cat. Electroencephalogr Clin Neurophysiol. 1952;4:357–61.
30. Chase MH, Nakamura Y, Clemente CD, et al. Afferent vagal stimulation: neurographic correlates of induced EEG synchronization and desynchronization. Brain Res. 1967;5:236–49.
31. Chase MH, Sterman MB, Clemente CD. Cortical and subcortical patterns of response to afferent vagal stimulation. Exp Neurol. 1966;16:36–49.
32. Takaya M, Terry WJ, Naritoku DK. Vagus nerve stimulation induces a sustained anticonvulsant effect. Epilepsia. 1996;37:1111–6.
33. Woodbury JW, Woodbury DM. Vagal stimulation reduces the severity of maximal electroshock seizures in intact rats: use of a cuff electrode for stimulating and recording. Pacing Clin Electrophysiol. 1991;14:94–107.
34. Woodbury DM, Woodbury JW. Effects of vagal stimulation on experimentally induced seizures in rats. Epilepsia. 1990;31(Suppl 2):S7–S19.
35. Lockard JS, Congdon WC, DuCharme LL. Feasibility and safety of vagal stimulation in monkey model. Epilepsia. 1990;31(Suppl 2):S20–6.
36. McLachlan RS. Suppression of interictal spikes and seizures by stimulation of the vagus nerve. Epilepsia. 1993;34:918–23.
37. Krahl SE, Senanayake SS, Handforth A. Destruction of peripheral C-fibers does not alter subsequent vagus nerve stimulation-induced seizure suppression in rats. Epilepsia. 2001;42:586–9.
38. Zagon A, Kemeny AA. Slow hyperpolarization in cortical neurons: a possible mechanism behind vagus nerve simulation therapy for refractory epilepsy? Epilepsia. 2000;41:1382–9.
39. Banzett RB, Guz A, Paydarfar D, et al. Cardiorespiratory variables and sensation during stimulation of the left vagus in patients with epilepsy. Epilepsy Res. 1999;35:1–11.

40. Krahl SE, Clark KB, Smith DC, et al. Locus coeruleus lesions suppress the seizure-attenuating effects of vagus nerve stimulation. Epilepsia. 1998;39:709–14.
41. Walker BR, Easton A, Gale K. Regulation of limbic motor seizures by GABA and glutamate transmission in nucleus tractus solitarius. Epilepsia. 1999;40:1051–7.
42. Depaulis A, Vergnes M, Liu Z, et al. Involvement of the nigral output pathways in the inhibitory control of the substantia nigra over generalized non-convulsive seizures in the rat. Neuroscience. 1990;39:339–49.
43. Miller JW. The role of mesencephalic and thalamic arousal systems in experimental seizures. Prog Neurobiol. 1992;39:155–78.
44. Magdaleno-Madrigal VM, Valdes-Cruz A, Martinez-Vargas D, et al. Effect of electrical stimulation of the nucleus of the solitary tract on the development of electrical amygdaloid kindling in the cat. Epilepsia. 2002;43:964–9.
45. Naritoku DK, Terry WJ, Helfert RH. Regional induction of fos immunoreactivity in the brain by anticonvulsant stimulation of the vagus nerve. Epilepsy Res. 1995;22:53–62.
46. Fernandez-Guardiola A, Martinez A, Valdes-Cruz A, et al. Vagus nerve prolonged stimulation in cats: effects on epileptogenesis (amygdala electrical kindling): behavioral and electrographic changes. Epilepsia. 1999;40:822–9.
47. Salinsky MC, Burchiel KJ. Vagus nerve stimulation has no effect on awake EEG rhythms in humans. Epilepsia. 1993;34:299–304.
48. Hammond EJ, Uthman BM, Reid SA, et al. Electrophysiological studies of cervical vagus nerve stimulation in humans: I. EEG effects. Epilepsia. 1992;33:1013–20.
49. Hammond EJ, Uthman BM, Reid SA, et al. Vagus nerve stimulation in humans: neurophysiological studies and electrophysiological monitoring. Epilepsia. 1990;31(Suppl 2):S51–9.
50. Penry JK, Dean JC. Prevention of intractable partial seizures by intermittent vagal stimulation in humans: preliminary results. Epilepsia. 1990;31(Suppl 2):S40–3.
51. Kuba R, Guzaninova M, Brazdil M, et al. Effect of vagal nerve stimulation on interictal epileptiform discharges: a scalp EEG study. Epilepsia. 2002;43:1181–8.
52. Olejniczak PW, Fisch BJ, Carey M, et al. The effect of vagus nerve stimulation on epileptiform activity recorded from hippocampal depth electrodes. Epilepsia. 2001;42:423–9.
53. Koo B. EEG changes with vagus nerve stimulation. J Clin Neurophysiol. 2001;18:434–41.
54. Hammond EJ, Uthman BM, Wilder BJ, et al. Neurochemical effects of vagus nerve stimulation in humans. Brain Res. 1992;583:300–3.
55. Ben-Menachem E, Hamberger A, Hedner T, et al. Effects of vagus nerve stimulation on amino acids and other metabolites in the CSF of patients with partial seizures. Epilepsy Res. 1995;20:221–7.
56. Ko D, Heck C, Grafton S, et al. Vagus nerve stimulation activates central nervous system structures in epileptic patients during PET H2(15)O blood flow imaging. Neurosurgery. 1996;39:426–30. discussion 430–431
57. Salanova V, Worth R. Neurostimulators in epilepsy. Curr Neurol Neurosci Rep. 2007;7: 315–9.
58. Krauss GL, Koubeissi MZ. Cerebellar and thalamic stimulation treatment for epilepsy. Acta Neurochir Suppl. 2007;97:347–56.
59. Henry TR, Bakay RA, Votaw JR, et al. Brain blood flow alterations induced by therapeutic vagus nerve stimulation in partial epilepsy: I. Acute effects at high and low levels of stimulation. Epilepsia. 1998;39:983–90.
60. Henry TR, Votaw JR, Pennell PB, et al. Acute blood flow changes and efficacy of vagus nerve stimulation in partial epilepsy. Neurology. 1999;52:1166–73.
61. Henry TR, Votaw JR, Bakay RAE, et al. Vagus nerve stimulation-indcued cerebral blood flow changes differ in acute and chornic therapy of complex partial seizures. Epilepsia. 1998;39:92.
62. Sucholeiki R, Alsaadi TM, Morris 3rd GL, et al. fMRI in patients implanted with a vagal nerve stimulator. Seizure. 2002;11:157–62.
63. Narayanan JT, Watts R, Haddad N, et al. Cerebral activation during vagus nerve stimulation: a functional MR study. Epilepsia. 2002;43:1509–14.

64. Helmers SL, Begnaud J, Cowley A, et al. Application of a computational model of vagus nerve stimulation. Acta Neurol Scand. 2012;126:336–43.
65. Lockard JS, Congdon WC. Feasibility and safety of vagal stimulation in monkey model. Epilepsia. 1990;31(Suppl 2):S20–6.
66. Navas M, Navarrete EG. Treatment of refractory epilepsy in adult patients with rightsided vagus nerve stimulation. Epilepsy Res. 2010;90(1–2):1–7.
67. Spuck S, Nowak G. Right-sided vagus nerve stimulation in humans: an effective therapy? Epilepsy Res. 2008;82(2–3):232–4.
68. Tubbs RS, Salter EG. Right-sided vagus nerve stimulation inhibits induced spinal cord seizures. Clin Anat. 2007;20(1):23–6.
69. McGregor A, Wheless J. Right-sided vagus nerve stimulation as a treatment for refractory epilepsy in humans. Epilepsia. 2005;46(1):91–6.
70. Krahl SE, Senanayake SS. Right-sided vagus nerve stimulation reduces generalized seizure severity in rats as effectively as left-sided. Epilepsy Res. 2003;56(1):1–4.
71. De Ferrari GC. Chronic vagus nerve stimulation: a new and promising therapeutic approach for chronic heart failure. Eur Heart J. 2011;32(7):847–55.
72. Morris III GL, Mueller WM. Long-term treatment with vagus nerve stimulation in patients with refractory epilepsy. The Vagus Nerve Stimulation Study Group E01-E05. Neurology. 1999;53:1731–5.
73. Labar D. Vagus nerve stimulation for 1 year in 269 patients on unchanged antiepileptic drugs. Seizure. 2004;13:392–8.
74. Vonck K, Thadani V, Gilbert K, et al. Vagus nerve stimulation for refractory epilepsy: a transatlantic experience. J Clin Neurophysiol. 2004;21:283–9.
75. De Herdt V, Boon P, Ceulemans B, et al. Vagus nerve stimulation for refractory epilepsy: a Belgian multicenter study. Eur J Paediatr Neurol. 2007;11:261–9.
76. Elliott RE, Morsi A, Kalhorn SP, et al. Vagus nerve stimulation in 436 consecutive patients with treatment-resistant epilepsy: long-term outcomes and predictors of response. Epilepsy Behav. 2011;20:57–63.
77. Elliott RE, Morsi A, Tanweer O, et al. Efficacy of vagus nerve stimulation over time: review of 65 consecutive patients with treatment-resistant epilepsy treated with VNS > 10 years. Epilepsy Behav. 2011;20:478–83.
78. Elliott RE, Rodgers SD, Bassani L, et al. Vagus nerve stimulation for children with treatment-resistant epilepsy: a consecutive series of 141 cases. J Neurosurg Pediatr. 2011;7:491–500.
79. Elliott RE, Morsi A, Geller EB, et al. Impact of failed intracranial epilepsy surgery on the effectiveness of subsequent vagus nerve stimulation. Neurosurgery. 2011;69:1210–7.
80. Cyberonics, Inc. VNS therapy physician's manual. Houston: Cyberonics, Inc; 2006. Available at: http://www.vnstherapy.com/epilepsy/hcp/manuals/default.aspx.
81. Englot DJ, Chang EF, Auguste KI. Vagus nerve stimulation for epilepsy: a meta-analysis of efficacy and predictors of response. J Neurosurg. 2011;115:1248–55.
82. Englot DJ, Rolston JD, Wang DD, et al. Efficacy of vagus nerve stimulation in posttraumatic versus nontraumatic epilepsy. J Neurosurg. 2012;117:970–7.
83. Labar DR. Antiepileptic drug use during the first 12 months of vagus nerve stimulation therapy: a registry study. Neurology. 2002;59(Suppl 4):S38–43.
84. Morris 3rd GL, Gloss D, Buchhalter J, et al. Evidence-based guideline update: vagus nerve stimulation for the treatment of epilepsy: report of the Guideline Development Subcommittee of the American Academy of Neurology. Neurology. 2013;81:1453–9.
85. Van Ness PC. Surgical outcome for neocortical (extrahippocampal) focal epilepsy. In: Luders HO, editor. Epilepsy surgery. New York: Raven Press; 1992. p. 613–24.
86. Sperling MR, O'Connor MF, Saykin AJ, et al. Temporal lobectomy for refractory epilepsy. JAMA. 1996;276:470–5.
87. Fisher RS, Handforth A. Reassessment: vagus nerve stimulation for epilepsy: a report of the therapeutics and technology assessment subcommittee of the american academy of neurology. Neurology. 1999;53:666–9.

88. Baumgartner JE, Clifton GL, Wheless JW, et al. Corpus callosotomy. Tech Neurosurg. 1995;1:45–51.
89. Sorenson JM, Wheless JW, Baumgartner JE, et al. Corpus callosotomy for medically intractable seizures. Pediatr Neurosurg. 1997;27:260–7.
90. Camfield PR, Camfield CS. Vagal nerve stimulation for treatment of children with epilepsy. J Pediatr. 1999;134:532–3.
91. Lancman G, Virk M, Shao H, et al. Vagus nerve stimulation vs. corpus callosotomy in the treatment of Lennox-Gastaut syndrome: a meta-analysis. Seizure. 2013;22:3–8.
92. Renfroe JB, Wheless JW. Earlier use of adjunctive vagus nerve stimulation therapy for refractory epilepsy. Neurology. 2002;59:S26–30.
93. Scherrmann J, Hoppe C, Kral T, et al. Vagus nerve stimulation: clinical experience in a large patient series. J Clin Neurophysiol. 2001;18:408–14.
94. Helmers SL, Griesemer DA, Dean JC, et al. Observations on the use of vagus nerve stimulation earlier in the course of pharmacoresistant epilepsy: patients with seizures for six years or less. Neurologist. 2003;9:160–4.
95. Helmers SL, Duh MS, Guérin A, et al. Clinical and economic impact of vagus nerve stimulation therapy in patients with drug-resistant epilepsy. Epilepsy Behav. 2011;22:370–5.
96. Helmers SL, Duh MS, Guérin A, et al. Clinical outcomes, quality of life, and costs associated with implantation of vagus nerve stimulation therapy in pediatric patients with drug-resistant epilepsy. Eur J Paediatr Neurol. 2012;16:449–58.
97. Malow BA, Edwards J, Marzec M, et al. Effects of vagus nerve stimulation on respiration during sleep: a pilot study. Neurology. 2000;55:1450–4.
98. Hsieh T, Chen M, McAfee A, et al. Sleep-related breathing disorder in children with vagal nerve stimulators. Pediatr Neurol. 2008;38:99–103.
99. Hallbook T, Lundgren J, Kohler S, et al. Beneficial effects on sleep of vagus nerve stimulation in children with therapy resistant epilepsy. Eur J Paediatr Neurol. 2005;9:399–407.
100. Kotagal P, Yardi N. The relationship between sleep and epilepsy. Semin Pediatr Neurol. 2008;15:42–9.
101. Bernard EJ, Passannante AN, Mann B, et al. Insertion of vagal nerve stimulator using local and regional anesthesia. Surg Neurol. 2002;57:94–8.
102. Reid SA. Surgical technique for implantation of the neurocybernetic prosthesis. Epilepsia. 1990;31(Suppl 2):S38–9.
103. Amar AP, Heck CN, Levy ML, et al. An institutional experience with cervical vagus nerve trunk stimulation for medically refractory epilepsy: rationale, technique, and outcome. Neurosurgery. 1998;43:1265–76. discussion 1276–1280
104. Tatum 4th WO, Moore DB, Stecker MM, et al. Ventricular asystole during vagus nerve stimulation for epilepsy in humans. Neurology. 1999;52:1267–9.
105. Asconape JJ, Moore DD, Zipes DP, et al. Early experience with vagus nerve stimulation for the treatment of epilepsy: cardiac complications. Epilepsia. 1998;39:193.
106. Ardesch JJ, Buschman HP, van der Burgh PH, et al. Cardiac responses of vagus nerve stimulation: intraoperative bradycardia and subsequent chronic stimulation. Clin Neurol Neurosurg. 2007;109:849–52.
107. Vaughn BV, Bernard E, Lannon S, et al. Intraoperative methods for confirmation of correct placement of the vagus nerve stimulator. Epileptic Disord. 2001;3:75–8.
108. Helmers SL, Wheless JW, Frost M, et al. Vagus nerve stimulation therapy in pediatric patients with refractory epilepsy: retrospective study. J Child Neurol. 2001;16:843–8.
109. Heck C, Helmers SL, DeGiorgio CM. Vagus nerve stimulation therapy, epilepsy, and device parameters: scientific basis and recommendations for use. Neurology. 2002;59:S31–7.
110. Agnew WF, McCreery DB. Considerations for safety with chronically implanted nerve electrodes. Epilepsia. 1990;31(Suppl 2):S27–32.
111. Agnew WF, McCreery DB, Yuen TG, et al. Histologic and physiologic evaluation of electrically stimulated peripheral nerve: considerations for the selection of parameters. Ann Biomed Eng. 1989;17:39–60.

112. Ortler M, Luef G, Kofler A, et al. Deep wound infection after vagus nerve stimulator implantation: treatment without removal of the device. Epilepsia. 2001;42:133–5.
113. Fernando DA, Lord RS. The blood supply of vagus nerve in the human: its implication in carotid endarterectomy, thyroidectomy and carotid arch aneurectomy. Anat Anz. 1994;176:333–7.
114. Ramsay RE, Uthman BM, Augustinsson LE, et al. Vagus nerve stimulation for treatment of partial seizures: 2. Safety, side effects, and tolerability First International Vagus Nerve Stimulation Study Group. Epilepsia. 1994;35:627–36.
115. Handforth A, DeGiorgio CM, Schachter SC, et al. Vagus nerve stimulation therapy for partial-onset seizures: a randomized active-control trial. Neurology. 1998;51:48–55.
116. A randomized controlled trial of chronic vagus nerve stimulation for treatment of medically intractable seizures: The Vagus Nerve Stimulation Study Group. Neurology. 1995;45:224–30.
117. Liporace J, Hucko D, Morrow R, et al. Vagal nerve stimulation: adjustments to reduce painful side effects. Neurology. 2001;57:885–6.
118. Lotvall J, Lunde H, Augustinson LE, et al. Airway effects of direct left-sided cervical vagal stimulation in patients with complex partial seizures. Epilepsy Res. 1994;18:149–54.
119. Setty AB, Vaughn BV, Quint SR, et al. Heart period variability during vagal nerve stimulation. Seizure. 1998;7:213–7.
120. Annegers JF, Coan SP, Hauser WA, et al. Epilepsy, vagal nerve stimulation by the NCP system, all-cause mortality, and sudden, unexpected, unexplained death. Epilepsia. 2000;41: 549–53.
121. Annegers JF, Coan SP, Hauser WA, et al. Epilepsy, vagal nerve stimulation by the NCP system, mortality, and sudden, unexpected, unexplained death. Epilepsia. 1998;39:206–12.
122. Sanossian N, Haut S. Chronic diarrhea associated with vagal nerve stimulation. Neurology. 2002;58:330.
123. Iriarte J, Artieda J, Alegre M, et al. Spasm of the sternocleidomastoid muscle induced by vagal nerve stimulation. Neurology. 2001;57:2319–20.
124. Leijten FS, Van Rijen PC. Stimulation of the phrenic nerve as a complication of vagus nerve pacing in a patient with epilepsy. Neurology. 1998;51:1224–5.
125. Duhaime AC, Melamed S, Clancy RR. Tonsillar pain mimicking glossopharyngeal neuralgia as a complication of vagus nerve stimulation: case report. Epilepsia. 2000;41:903–5.
126. Blumer D, Davies K, Alexander A, et al. Major psychiatric disorders subsequent to treating epilepsy by vagus nerve stimulation. Epilepsy Behav. 2001;2:466–72.
127. Klein JP, Jean-Baptiste M, Thompson JL, et al. A case report of hypomania following vagus nerve stimulation for refractory epilepsy. J Clin Psychiatry. 2003;64:485.
128. Pearl PL, Conry JA, Yaun A, et al. Misidentification of vagus nerve stimulator for intravenous access and other major adverse events. Pediatr Neurol. 2008;38:248–51.
129. Schallert G, Foster J, Lindquist N, et al. Chronic stimulation of the left vagal nerve in children: effect on swallowing. Epilepsia. 1998;39:1113–4.
130. Lundgren J, Ekberg O, Olsson R. Aspiration: a potential complication to vagus nerve stimulation. Epilepsia. 1998;39:998–1000.
131. Ben-Menachem E. Vagus-nerve stimulation for the treatment of epilepsy. Lancet Neurol. 2002;1:477–82.
132. Hoppe C, Helmstaedter C, Scherrmann J, et al. No evidence for cognitive side effects after 6 months of vagus nerve stimulation in epilepsy patients. Epilepsy Behav. 2001;2:351–6.
133. Clarke BM, Upton AR, Griffin H, et al. Chronic stimulation of the left vagus nerve in epilepsy: balance effects. Can J Neurol Sci. 1997;24:230–4.
134. Clarke BM, Upton AR, Griffin H, et al. Chronic stimulation of the left vagus nerve: cognitive motor effects. Can J Neurol Sci. 1997;24:226–9.
135. Harden CL. Mood changes in epilepsy patients treated with vagus nerve stimulation. Epilepsy Behav. 2001;2:S17–20.
136. Clark KB, Naritoku DK, Smith DC, et al. Enhanced recognition memory following vagus nerve stimulation in human subjects. Nat Neurosci. 1999;2:94–8.

137. Ghacibeh GA, Shenker JI, Shenal B, et al. The influence of vagus nerve stimulation on memory. Cogn Behav Neurol. 2006;19:119–22.
138. Cramer JA. Exploration of changes in health-related quality of life after 3 months of vagus nerve stimulation. Epilepsy Behav. 2001;2:460–5.
139. Malow BA, Edwards J, Marzec M, et al. Vagus nerve stimulation reduces daytime sleepiness in epilepsy patients. Neurology. 2001;57:879–84.
140. Galli R, Bonanni E, Pizzanelli C, et al. Daytime vigilance and quality of life in epileptic patients treated with vagus nerve stimulation. Epilepsy Behav. 2003;4:185–91.
141. Danielsson I, Lister L. A pilot study of the teratogenicity of vagus nerve stimulation in a rabbit model. Brain Stimul. 2009;2:41–9.
142. Husain MM, Stegman D, Trevino K. Pregnancy and delivery while receiving vagus nerve stimulation for the treatment of major depression: a case report. Ann Gen Psychiatry. 2005;4:16.
143. Ben-Menachem E, Hellstrom K, Waldton C, et al. Evaluation of refractory epilepsy treated with vagus nerve stimulation for up to 5 years. Neurology. 1999;52:1265–7.
144. Graves N. Anticonvulsants: choices and costs. Am J Manag Care. 1998;49:S463–74.
145. Boon P, D'Have M, Van Walleghem P, et al. Direct medical costs of refractory epilepsy incurred by three different treatment modalities: a prospective assessment. Epilepsia. 2002;43:96–102.
146. Ben-Menachem E, Hellstrom K, Verstappen D. Analysis of direct hospital costs before and 18 months after treatment with vagus nerve stimulation therapy in 43 patients. Neurology. 2002;59(6 Suppl 4):S44–7.
147. Bernstein AL, Barkan H, Hess T. Vagus nerve stimulation therapy for pharmacoresistant epilepsy: effect on health care utilization. Epilepsy Behav. 2007;10:134–7.
148. Benbadis SR, Nyhenhuis J, Tatum 4th WO, et al. MRI of the brain is safe in patients implanted with the vagus nerve stimulator. Seizure. 2001;10:512–5.
149. Wilfong AA. Body MRI and vagus nerve stimulation. Epilepsia. 2002;43(Suppl 7):347.
150. Stefan H, Kreiselmeyer G. Transcutaneous vagus nerve stimulation (t-VNS) in pharmacoresistant epilepsies: a proof of concept trial. Epilepsia. 2012;53(7):e115–8.

Chapter 9
VNS for the Treatment of Inflammatory Disorders of the Gastrointestinal Tract

Bruno Bonaz, Valérie Sinniger, Sonia Pellissier, and Didier Clarençon

Abstract The brain and the gut communicate bi-directionally through the autonomic nervous system of which the vagus nerve is a major component. The vagus nerve has a well-documented anti-inflammatory activity through its afferents and the hypothalamic-pituitary-adrenal axis. More recently, an anti-inflammatory role of vagal efferents has also been discovered through the cholinergic anti-inflammatory pathway. Vagus nerve stimulation, used in the treatment of drug resistant epilepsy and depression, could be an effective tool to treat inflammatory disorders of the gastro-intestinal tract, such as inflammatory bowel disease, irritable bowel syndrome, as well as postoperative ileus which are characterized by an autonomic imbalance with a low vagal tone.

Keywords Autonomic nervous system • Brain-gut axis • Cholinergic anti-inflammatory pathway • Gastro-intestinal tract • Iinflammation • Inflammatory bowel diseases • Irritable bowel syndrome • Postoperative ileus • Vagus nerve • Vagus nerve stimulation

---

B. Bonaz, MD, PhD (✉)
Clinique Universitaire d'Hépato-Gastroentérologie, CHU Grenoble,
CS-10217, 38043 Grenoble Cedex 09, France

University Grenoble Alpes, Grenoble Institut des Neurosciences, Grenoble, France
e-mail: BBonaz@chu-grenoble.fr

V. Sinniger, PhD
University Hospital, Grenoble Alpes, Department of Hepatogastroenterology,
Institute of Neurosciences, Grenoble, France
e-mail: valerie.sinniger@ujf-grenoble.fr

S. Pellissier, PhD
Universite Savoie Mont-Blanc, Laboratoire Interuniversitaire de Pschologie,
Personnalite, Cognition, et Changement Social, Grenoble Institute of Neurosciences,
Chambéry, France
e-mail: sonia.pellissier@univ-savoie.fr

D. Clarençon, PhD
University Grenoble Alpes, Grenoble Institut des Neurosciences, Grenoble, France

Institut de Recherche Biomedicale des Armees, Paris, France
e-mail: didierclarencon@free.fr

A. Majid (ed.), *Electroceuticals*, DOI 10.1007/978-3-319-28612-9_9

Abbreviations

α7nAChR	Alpha7 nicotinic Ach receptors
Ach	Acetylcholine
ANS	Autonomic nervous system
CAP	Cholinergic anti-inflammatory pathway
CD	Crohn's disease
CRF	Corticotrophin-releasing factor
DMNV	Dorsal motor nucleus of the vagus
FDA	Food and drug administration
HPA axis	Hypothalamic pituitary adrenal axis
HRV	Heart rate variability
IBD	Inflammatory bowel disease
IBS	Irritable bowel syndrome
IL	Interleukin
LC	Locus coeruleus
LPS	Lipopolysaccharides
NTS	Nucleus tractus solitarius
PB	Parabrachial nucleus
POI	Postoperative ileus
PVH	Paraventricular nucleus of the hypothalamus
TNF	Tumor necrosis factor
UC	Ulcerative colitis
VN	Vagus nerve
VNS	Vagus nerve stimulation

Introduction

There is bidirectional communication, between the brain and the gut through the autonomic nervous system (ANS). Dysfunction of this axis may underlie the pathogenesis of disorders of the gastrointestinal tract such as irritable bowel syndrome (IBS) and inflammatory bowel diseases (IBD) [1, 2]. An imbalance of the ANS is observed in IBS and IBD [3].

The vagus nerve (VN) is a key element of the ANS and is emerging as a therapeutic target in IBS and IBD based on its role in inflammation through its afferent and efferent pathways [4]. VN stimulation (VNS) is used in the treatment of drug refractory epilepsy and depression and could be a therapeutic tool in the management of inflammatory disorders of the digestive tract [4].

Rationale for Using Vagus Nerve Stimulation for the Treatment of Gastrointestinal Disorders

Neuro-anatomical Basis

The VN, historically cited as the pneumogastric nerve, is the tenth cranial nerve. It is the longest nerve in the body and innervates a number of organs including most of the GI tract. The VN are paired but they are normally referred to in the singular. The VN is the principal component of the parasympathetic nervous system, and with the sympathetic nervous system is a part of the ANS. The vagi enter the abdomen as two trunks coursing over the esophagus (dorsal and ventral) and then dividing into four or five distinct primary branches at the subdiaphragmatic esophageal level. The gastric branches control stomach acid secretion; the hepatic branch has been shown to influence the motility of the gall bladder and biliary tract, and the celiac branches mediate the motility of the distal intestine and colon [5]. The VN is a mixed nerve composed mainly of unmyelinated fibers, with 80% afferent fibers that convey visceral, somatic and taste sensations and 20% efferent fibers, which are involved in the control of gastro-intestinal motility and secretion.

Vagal efferents, are preganglionic neurons and originate in the dorsal motor nucleus of the vagus (DMNV) located in the dorsal part of the brainstem, in the medulla, below the nucleus tractus solitarius (NTS) which receives vagal afferents. Vagal efferents innervate the digestive tract from the esophagus to the splenic flexure while the rest of the digestive tract, i.e. the left colon and rectum, is innervated by the sacral parasympathetic nucleus, the other part of the parasympathetic nervous system, which originates in the sacral (S2-S4) spinal cord. Within the DMNV, the preganglionic neurons are organized into longitudinal columns, corresponding to a different abdominal branch. Indeed, there is a viscerotopic organization of vagal efferents in the DMNV. Neurons that reach the stomach are concentrated in the medial part of the DMNV while those innervating the colon except the rectum are located in the lateral part [6]. In the rat, the VN innervates all the digestive tract with the exception of the rectum [6] while in human it provides the innervation of the GI tract until the splenic flexure [7]. Some anatomists believe that the VN innervates all the digestive tract in human [8].

In the digestive tract, preganglionic neurons originating suppress in from the DMNV connect to the second neurons (i.e. post-ganglionic neurons). The latters are a part of the enteric nervous system sometimes referred to as the little brain of the gut or the "gut brain" and provides autonomous functioning of the digestive tract.

The neuromediator of the VN is acetylcholine (Ach) which is released both at the end of the VN where it acts on nicotinic receptors, and at the end of the post-ganglionic neuron in the enteric nervous system, where it acts on nicotinic or muscarinic receptors. Vagal efferents do not directly reach the intestinal lamina propria

[9]. Indeed, they form cholinergic synapses onto enteric neurons that innervate the lamina propria. Enteric neurons respond to locally released inflammatory stimuli [10]. Anatomical and physiological evidence clearly suggests that these neurons contribute to the regulation of gut immunity, independently of the VN although under its influence [11].

Vagal afferents originate from all layers of the digestive tract, i.e. from the mucosa to the muscle layers. The sensory afferent cell bodies reside in the nodose ganglia and relay information to the NTS, according to a rostro-caudal viscerotopy, and to the area postrema which is located in the medulla, above and in close proximity to the DMNV to form the dorsal vagal complex. The NTS is divided into various subnuclei, partly correlated with the areas of projection of peripheral afferent endings. Altschuller et al. have described a viscerotopic representation of the digestive tract in the NTS in rats [12]. Indeed, esophageal and stomach afferents terminate in the subnucleus centralis and subnucleus gelatinosus respectively while colonic afferents terminate in the medial and commissural part of the NTS [6, 12]. The vagal afferent system is well positioned to detect immune-related events in the periphery and generate appropriate autonomic, endocrine, and behavioral responses via central reflex pathways. The NTS sends viscero-sensory information to the DMNV, which is positioned downstream to vagal afferents. Indeed, there are integrated vago-vagal reflexes where vagal afferents ending in the NTS are connected with dendrites of vagal motoneurons located in the DMNV thus influencing the functioning of vagal efferents [13].

Vagal sensory inputs arriving in the NTS are transmitted to widespread areas of the central nervous system [14–16]. From the NTS, there is an ascending system through the brainstem, distributing fibers to both diencephalic and telencephalic structures. Most project to the parabrachial (PB) region but also to the locus coeruleus (LC), the periventricular nucleus of the thalamus, the central nucleus of the amygdala, the dorsomedial and paraventricular nucleus of the hypothalamus (PVH), the medial preoptic area and the arcuate nucleus of the hypothalamus, ventrolateral medulla (A1 noradrenergic nucleus). These projections suggest that there is an integration of visceral information with an autonomic, behavioral, and endocrine response. NTS neurons may directly modulate the activity of LC neurons and may serve to integrate autonomic responses in the brain by influencing the widespread noradrenergic projections of the LC [17]. Neurons of the rostral ventrolateral medulla oblongata provide one of two major sources of afferent inputs to the LC [18], which in turn has projections to widespread areas of the cortex that are associated with stress-related behaviors and affective disorders [19]. The PVH projects to the bed nucleus of the stria terminalis, the dorsomedial and arcuate hypothalamic nuclei, the medial preoptic area, the periventricular nucleus of the thalamus, the PB region, and the nucleus tegmenti dorsalis lateralis [20]. The PB nucleus in turn projects to the central nucleus of the amygdala, the bed nucleus of the stria terminalis and the PVH [21]. The PVH projects directly to the NTS [20, 22], thereby establishing a feedback loop between the NTS and the forebrain. Thus visceral information vehiculated by the VN is integrated in the central autonomic network which is composed by a central network roughly divided into executive structures, mainly hypothalamic, coordinating structures, mainly included in the limbic system, and high level control structures, mainly the frontal cortex. This central autonomic network is able to modify the ANS, i.e. the VN, sacral parasympathetic nucleus and sympathetic nucleus, and the endocrine response i.e. the hypothalamic pituitary adrenal (HPA) axis. The VN could mediate the sixth sense [22], based on the hypothesis that sensory inputs originating from the internal environment, such as gut feelings, act to alter –heighten or dull – the perception of the outside world and influence the elicited behavioural response.

Anti-inflammatory Properties of the Vagus Nerve

The VN has a dual anti-inflammatory role both through its afferents and efferents. The peripheral release of pro-inflammatory cytokines such as interleukin (IL)-1, Il-6 and tumor necrosis factor α (TNF), following administration of lipopolysaccharides (LPS), is able to activate vagal afferents through the linkage of cytokine to glomus cells of most paraganglia of the VN [23], which express IL-1 receptors. This effect is disrupted by subdiaphragmatic vagotomy [24]. Toll-like receptor 4, the principal endotoxin receptor of LPS, is expressed by neurons in the nodose ganglia [25], thus LPS can activate the afferent VN at the level of nodose ganglion. Then neurons activated in the NTS, particularly in the A2 noradrenergic group, send projections to the hypothalamus, to corticotrophin-releasing factor (CRF)-containing neurons of the parvo-cellular part of the PVH. The release of CRF by these neurons will then activate the release of adrenocorticotropin hormone by the pituitary thus stimulating the release of glucocorticoids by the adrenal glands i.e. the HPA axis. This anti-inflammatory pathway has been described by Hans Selye as a key component of the brain-gut stress response [26].

More recently, in 2000, a parasympathetic anti-inflammatory pathway involving vagal efferents has been described by KJ Tracey and colleagues [27]. These authors showed that VNS, in vagotomized animals, on the distal end of the left cervical VN trunk, was able to prevent a septic shock induced in rats by LPS. Additional studies showed that vagal efferents are involved in a *cholinergic anti-inflammatory pathway (CAP)* through which the brain modulates systemic inflammatory responses to endotoxin (Fig. 9.1) [28]. These authors showed that Ach, the principle neuromediator of the VN, significantly decreased the release of pro-inflammatory cytokines such TNFα, IL-1beta, IL-6 and IL-18, but not the anti-inflammatory cytokine IL-10, in LPS-stimulated human macrophage cultures. Thus ACh released by efferent VN inhibits macrophage activation. VNS of the left cervical VN performed on the distal end of vagotomized rats *in vivo* during lethal endotoxaemia inhibited TNF synthesis in liver, attenuated peak serum TNF amounts, and prevented the development of shock. This group also demonstrated that the CAP was mediated through the link of Ach with alpha7 nicotinic Ach receptors (α7nAChR) of macrophages since this effect was not observed in α7 knock-out animals [29]. De Jonge et al. [30] have shown that the CAP acts through α7 subunit-mediated Jak2-STAT3 activation.

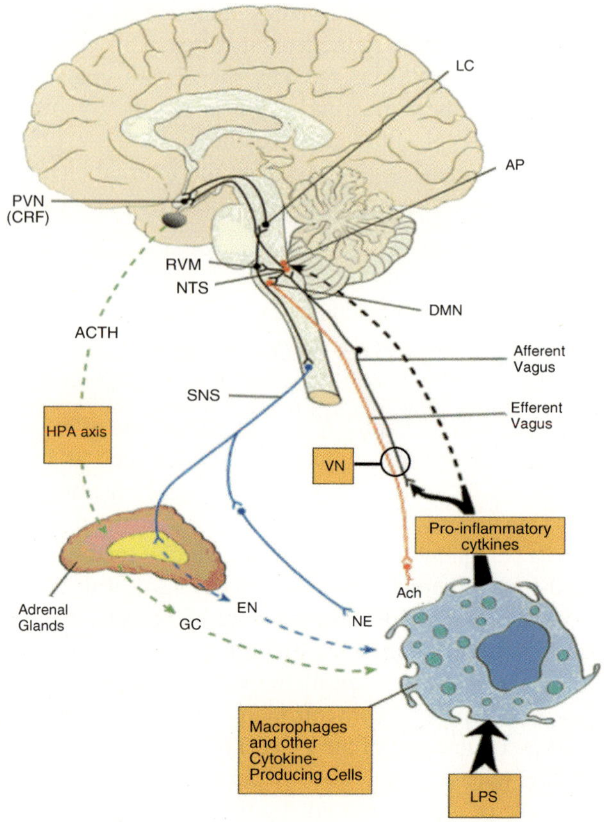

Fig. 9.1 The neuro-endocrine-immune axis. *ACh* acetylcholine, *ACTH* adrenocorticotropin hormone, *AP* area postrema, *CRF* corticotrophin-releasing factor, *DMN* dorsal motor nucleus of the vagus, *EN* epinephrine, *GC* glucocorticoids, *HPA* hypothalamic pituitary adrenal, *LC* locus coeruleus, *LPS* lipopolysaccharides, *NE* norepinephrine, *NTS* nucleus tractus solitarius, *PVN* paraventricular nucleus of the hypothalamus, *RVM* rostral ventrolateral medulla, *SNS* sympathetic nervous system, *VN* vagus nerve [28]

These authors also showed that, stimulation of the VN improved surgery-induced inflammation and postoperative ileus (POI) in a mouse model of intestinal manipulation by activating STAT3 in intestinal macrophages. Alpha-7nAChRs also mediate potent anti-inflammatory effects in macrophages by inducing the synthesis of miRNA-124, which inhibits the synthesis and release of TNF and IL-6 [31].

Another pathway through which the CAP could act is through the spleen, which is known to be a source of TNFα. Huston et al. [32] showed that VNS fails to inhibit TNF production in splenectomized animals during lethal endotoxemia. Selective lesioning of the common celiac nerve abolished TNF suppression by VNS, suggesting that the CAP is functionally hard wired to the spleen via this branch of the VN. Huston et al. [33] have also shown that administration of nicotine significantly reduced levels of CD11b, a β2-integrin involved in cell adhesion and leukocyte chemotaxis, on the surface of neutrophils in a dose-dependent manner and that this function requires the spleen. Moreover, they showed that VNS attenuated neutrophil surface CD11b levels required an intact and innervated spleen. The effects of the CAP on the spleen are thought to involve an interaction of the VN, which synapses with sympathetic neurons at the celiac/superior mesenteric ganglia [34] with the splenic sympathetic nerve through a vago-sympathetic activating pathway. Ach released at the distal end of the VN activates the splenic nerve through an interaction with α7nAChR activating the release of norepinephrine by the splenic nerve, which could then either:

(i) inhibit the release of TNF by spleen macrophages through an interaction with β2adrenergic receptors

or

(ii) activate the release of Ach by spleen lymphocytes through a link to β2adrenergic receptor. (Here ACh-synthesizing T lymphocytes provide an essential non-neural link of ACh which then inhibits the release of TNF by spleen macrophages through an effect on α7nAChR) [35].

Downs et al. [36] have recently shown that α7 nAChR mRNA and protein are highly expressed in the celiac/superior mesenteric ganglia. This provides a site for the action of ACh or nicotinic agonists to induce norepinephrine release in the spleen. Alpha-7nAChRs are also present prejunctionally on noradrenergic nerve fibers within the spleen, and these receptors may enhance the release of norepinephrine through a positive feedback mechanism with lymphocyte-derived ACh. The involvement of the spleen has also been described by Ghia and colleagues who showed that central cholinergic activation induced by the acetylcholinesterase inhibitor galantamine or a muscarinic acetylcholine receptor agonist improved colitis in mice and that the CAP was abolished in mice with vagotomy, splenic neurectomy, or splenectomy [37]. Xue et al. [38] also showed that VNS fails to protect against septic shock in rats subjected to splenectomy or common celiac branch vagotomy, indicating that the spleen may be a vital target of the CAP. In addition, we have shown that VNS is able to modify splenocyte activation [39]. However, the anatomical relationships between the peripheral cholinergic system and immune cells located in these lymphoid tissues remain unclear due to inherent technical difficulties with currently available neuroanatomical methods. Indeed, Martelli et al. [40] have shown that VNS does not drive action potentials in the splenic nerve and for these authors the anti-inflammatory effect of VNS in the intestine is independent of the spleen and T cells. They showed that the efferent arm of the inflammatory reflex is in the splanchnic sympathetic nerves, not the vagi as previously proposed.

Gautron et al. [41], using a new neural tract tracing methodology have recently identified cholinergic neuronal and non-neuronal cells in a position to modulate gastrointestinal and splenic immunity in the mouse. They found only a sparse innervation in the spleen mostly consisting of neuronal fibers of spinal origin around arterioles and in lymphocyte-containing areas of the white pulp while the spleen itself contained a novel population of cholinergic B-cells, fewer T-cells. The

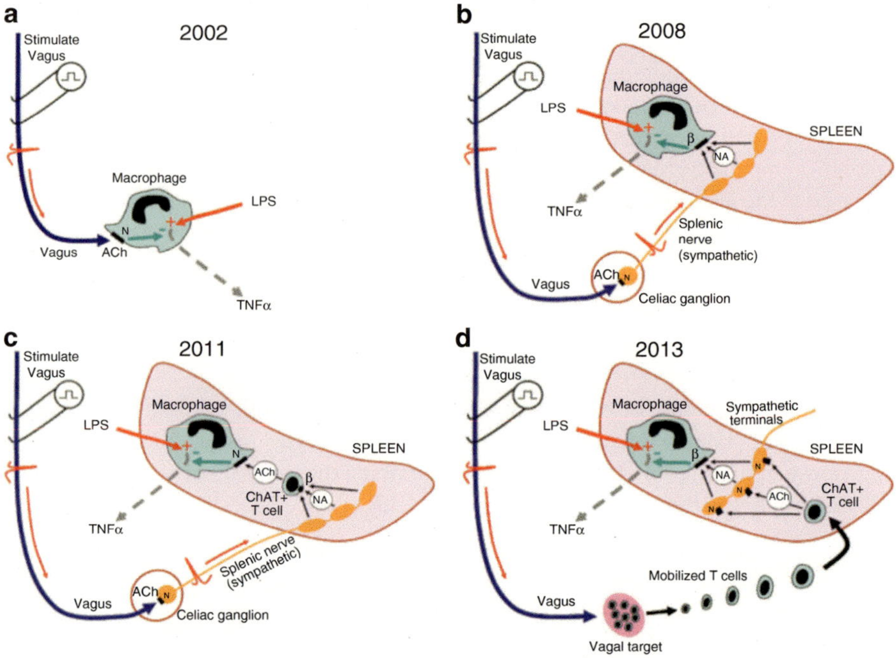

Fig. 9.2 The evolution of the cholinergic anti-inflammatory pathway [45]. (**a**) The original formulation in which vagal efferent fibers are proposed to act directly on immune cells (principally macrophages) to suppress their production of TNFα and other inflammatory mediators. (**b**) The discovery of the importance of the spleen and the splenic nerves and the lack of direct vagal innervation of the spleen prompted this revision. Here, the preganglionic vagal fibers are postulated to synapse with postganglionic splenic (sympathetic) neurons in the celiac ganglion. One suggested site for the essential α7-containing nicotinic receptor was on the postganglionic splenic neuron. (**c**) This version incorporates the recognition of the essential role of acetylcholine-synthesizing T-cells. Here, the essential α7-containing nicotinic receptor is placed in the spleen, on splenic macrophages. (**d**) The model proposed here recognizes that the link from the vagus to the spleen is non-neural. In this version the essential α7-containing nicotinic receptor is placed not on the cell bodies but on the peripheral terminals of the splenic sympathetic nerves. When stimulated by acetylcholine from incoming T-cells, they release noradrenaline, which then acts on beta adrenergic receptors on splenic macrophages to suppress their production of TNFα. No action potentials are required. If, on the other hand, action potentials are generated in the splenic nerve by direct stimulation, the anti-inflammatory action bypasses the need for α7-containing nicotinic receptors. Abbreviations: *ACh* acetylcholine, *β* beta adrenergic receptor, *ChAT+* choline acetyl transferase positive, i.e., ACh-synthesizing, T-cell, *LPS* lipopolysaccharide, *N* nicotinic cholinergic receptor, *NA* noradrenaline, *TNF-α* tumor necrosis factor alpha

cholinergic fibers found in the spleen were found to come from cholinergic postganglionic sympathetic neurons located in the para- and/or prevertebral chains.

ACh can be released by epithelial and immune cells, in addition to nerve endings [42]. The ultimate role of immune-derived ACh appears to be the suppression of proinflammatory cytokines released from macrophages. This evidence suggests that the gut-associated lymphoid tissue may play an underestimated role in the immunodulatory actions of peripheral acetylcholine and VNS.

In summary, it remains difficult to explain how this assembly of cholinergic structures is recruited by the electric stimulation of the efferent VN, primarily because vagal efferents do not project to the spleen and do not contact spleen-projecting sympathetic neurons [43, 44]. One possibility, as proposed by Martelli et al. [45], is a non-neuronal link between the VN and the spleen. In that case, the essential α7-containing nicotinic receptor is placed not on the cell bodies but on the peripheral terminals of the splenic sympathetic nerves. When stimulated by ACh from incoming T-cells, they release noradrenaline, which then acts on β-adrenergic receptors on splenic macrophages to suppress their production of TNFα (Fig. 9.2). No action potentials are required for this activity. If, on the other hand, action potentials are generated in the splenic nerve by direct stimulation, the anti-inflammatory action bypasses the need for α7-containing nicotinic receptors [46]. Cailotto et al. [47] have recently shown that the VN does not directly interact with resident macrophages in the gut or spleen. Instead, the VN preferentially interacts with nNOS, VIP and ChAT enteric neurons located within the gut muscularis with nerve endings in close proximity of the resident macrophages.

Vagus Nerve Stimulation

The use of VNS for suppression of seizures was first performed by JL Corning, in the early 1880s [48], using an electrocompressor for transcutaneous VNS of the VN cervical trunk based on the idea that seizures may be due to alterations in cerebral blood flow. It was not until 1938 that Bailey and Bremer [49] reported that VNS in the cat elicited synchronized activity in the orbital cortex. The first device implanted into a human for treatment of drug-resistant epilepsy was reported in 1988 [50]. VNS has been approved by the US Food and Drug Administration (FDA) for treatment of refractory epilepsy since 1997 while the approval in Europe was in 1994. Over 100,000 VNS devices have been implanted in more than 75,000 patients worldwide as of August 2014 [Cyberonics Inc. 2013 Annual Report. http://ir.cyberonics.com/annuals.cfm (accessed 03/05/2014)]. VNS was also approved in 2005 by the FDA for the adjunctive, long-term treatment of chronic or recurrent depression in patients who are experiencing an episode of major depression and have not had an adequate response to four or more antidepressant treatments [VNS Therapy System Physician's Manual. Houston, TX: Cyberonics Inc., 2013. http://dynamic.cyberonics.com/manuals/ (accessed 01/05/2015)]. The use of VNS in depression was based on improvements in well-being, mood, alertness, memory and thinking skills, independent of seizure activity, These outcomes were observed in patients who received implantable VNS for refractory epilepsy followed by a 1-year open-label extension on 205 patients of a negative sham-controlled study performed during 10 weeks [51, 52].

The massive central projections of the VN are likely to be responsible for the antiepileptic and antidepressive properties of afferent vagal stimulation in humans although the neuronal mechanisms by which such stimulation exerts therapeutic effects are not well understood. There are several possible loci for influence through a polysynaptic pathway from the NTS such as the neocortex and hippocampus, the

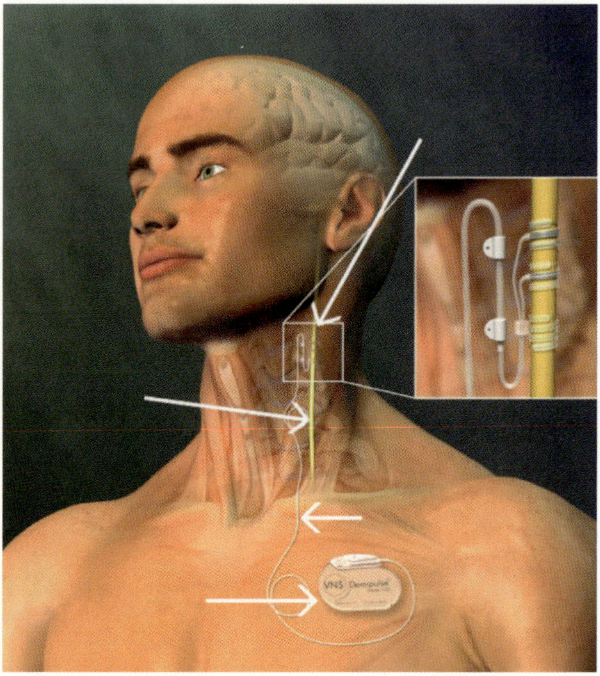

Fig. 9.3 The Vagus nerve stimulation device with the pulse generator, placed in a subcutaneous pocket in the left chest wall, and a spiral electrode wrapped around the left vagus nerve in the neck (With permission © Cyberonics, Inc)

thalamus, the LC. The excitability of epileptogenic tissue may decrease due to neuroplastic changes in relevant structures [53]. The anti-epileptic effect of VNS is not attributed to vagal C-fibers, as their destruction does not alter subsequent VNS-induced seizure suppression in rats. This suggests that seizure suppression results from activation of vagal A- and B-fibers [54].

Five different parameters (i.e. intensity, frequency, pulse width, on-time, and off-time) of stimulation are used for VNS in epilepsy/depression. For example: intensity 0.5–3.5 mA, frequency 20–30 Hz, pulse width 500 micros, and stimulation on-time of 30–90 s followed by off-time of 5 min. A large range of frequency (2–300 Hz) of VNS produced electroencephalographic desynchronization of the "encéphale isolé" cat that was abolished by a tight ligature of the proximal end of the vagal trunk [55], thus suggesting that vagal afferent fibers are involved in such effect. High frequency VNS is over 50% more effective than low frequency VNS [56]. However, frequencies of 50 Hz and above caused major irreversible damage to the VN [57]. VNS at antiepileptic parameters induces *c-fos* expression in rats in brain nuclei involved in the genesis and regulation of seizures such as the amygdala, cingulate cortex, locus coeruleus, and hypothalamus [58]. By comparison, brain imaging studies in humans have shown modifications in regions targeted by VN afferents such as the thalamus, cerebellum, orbitofrontal cortex, limbic system, hypothalamus, and medulla [59]. A 50% seizure reduction is observed in patients after 2 and 3 years of VNS [60].

VNS is successful in 20% of treatment-resistant depression patients [61]. VNS for 9 months or 12 months (for those that initially received sham treatment) produced an increase in the efficacy of VNS over time with response and remission rates of 27.2% and 15.8% respectively [52]. Studies looking at the 2-year outcome of VNS reported response rates of 53% and remission rates of 39% [62].

VNS is classically applied through a spiral electrode wrapped around the left cervical VN in the neck [63]. The connected cable is tunneled subcutaneously to and connected with a pulse generator located in the left chest wall (Fig. 9.3). The implantation (~1 h duration) is performed under general anesthesia generally by neurosurgeons because of the familiarity with epilepsy. Because the right VN innervates the sinoatrial node (involved in the pace-maker function of the heart) while the left VN innervates the atrioventricular node (regulating the force of contraction of the heart muscle with less influence over heart rate) [64], VNS is performed on the left VN with no major cardiac adverse events. The VNS device is manufactured by Cyberonics (Houston, TX, USA) and includes a pair of helical electrodes (2 or 3 mm diameter), a battery-powered generator, a tunneling tool, software and programming tools, and supplies for the patient (http://us.cyberonics.com/en/). The price of the generator pulse (model 102) plus the electrode (model 302) is ~9000 euros. The battery for the stimulator lasts approximately 5–10 years, depending on the settings used. Implantable VNS is safe and well tolerated as withdrawals are rare [56], with minor adverse events which are classically voice alteration, cough, dyspnea, paresthesia, nausea, headache and pain that decline with continued treatment and easy to control by reducing the stimulation intensity [65].

The concept of the CAP is based on the activation of vagal efferents (see above). In those studies, VNS was used at low frequency (1–5-10 Hz) stimulation. Indeed, in the referent work of Borovikova et al. [27], VNS was performed in rats with cervical vagotomy and applied at low frequency of stimulation of the distal end (thus stimulating vagal efferents) of the VN using the following parameters: 5 V, 2 ms, 1 Hz. Bernik et al. [66] performed VNS to either the left or right VN, in anesthetized rats with intact vagi, with constant voltage of either 1 V (2 ms, 5 Hz) or 5 V (2 ms, 5 Hz) for 10 min intervals before and after LPS injection, for a total of 20 continuous minutes. They showed that intact VNS protected against endotoxin-induced hypotension and endotoxin-induced shock; this effect was prevented by surgical or chemical vagotomy. de Jonge et al. [30] performed VNS in a mouse model of POI following intestinal manipulation by stimulating the distal part of the ligated left VN trunk or of the distal part of the VN after vagotomy thus activating vagal efferents. Voltage stimuli (5 Hz for 2 ms at 1 or 5 V) were applied for 5 min before and for 15 min after intestinal manipulation; VNS improved surgery-induced inflammation and POI through $\alpha7$ subunit-mediated Jak2-STAT3 activation. Costantini al. [67] performed VNS of the intact right VN at 1 Hz (2 mA) in anesthetized male BALB/c mice and showed an increased activation of enteric glia cells resulting in attenuation of burn-induced intestinal barrier injury. The protective effect of VNS was prevented by abdominal vagotomy at the gastroesophageal junction, thus confirming that VN efferent signaling modulates gut barrier integrity following injury. VNS performed at 10 Hz recommended to activate vagal efferents did not induce deleterious side effects [59, 68] and no significant difference was found in withdrawal rates between high and low stimulation groups in an updated version of a Cochrane review [56]. If theoretically, low frequency (5–10 Hz) VNS activates vagal efferents, we have shown that low frequency VNS performed in anesthetized animals with intact vagi also activates vagal afferents [69].

Disorders of the Digestive Tract That May Benefit from VNS

Based on the anti-inflammatory properties of the VN, disorders of the GI tract like IBD, (Crohn's disease, CD and ulcerative colitis, UC), IBS, as well as POI may be amenable to treatment using VNS.

Inflammatory Bowel Diseases

IBDs are organic diseases classically divided in CD and UC involving the digestive tract, particularly the colon and small-bowel (CD) starting early in life (between 15 and 30 years), and involve alternating periods of flares and remissions of variable duration. Symptoms are characterized by abdominal pain, diarrhea, fever, weight loss, and extra-intestinal manifestations. IBD affects an estimated 1.5 million Americans and 2.2 million people in Europe. The rising incidence of IBD in Western countries supports the hypothesis that "Westernization" of our lifestyle has led to the increased incidence and prevalence of IBD. The highest annual incidence of UC is 24.3 per 100,000 person-years in Europe and 19.2 per 100,000 person-years in North America. The highest annual incidence of CD is 12.7 per 100,000 person-years in Europe and 20.2 per 100,000 person-years in North America. The highest reported prevalence values for IBD were in Europe (UC, 505 per 100,000 persons; CD, 322 per 100,000 persons) and North America (UC, 249 per 100,000 persons; CD, 319 per 100,000 persons) [70].

The pathophysiology of IBD is multifactorial involving immunologic, genetic, infectious and environmental factors [71]. Stress, through brain-gut interactions, as well as environmental factors, based on experimental and clinical data [2] have been proposed as contributors. An imbalance of the ANS is observed in IBD - sympathetic dysfunction in CD [72] and a vagal dysfunction in UC [73]. We have recently shown that this dysautonomia may be dependent on psychological adjustment. Indeed, the equilibrium of the ANS is differentially adapted according to the disease. This equilibrium is conjugated with positive affective and cognitive adjustment in IBD [3]. Currently, there is no 1 treatment that will cure IBD. Current treatments suppress disease activity and there is generally a relapse of the disease after discontinuation of the treatment. TNF is a key cytokine which is involved in IBD and anti-TNF therapies are presently the gold standard in the treatment of IBD [74]. However, anti-TNF therapies are not devoid of adverse events [75] and patients are often hesitant to take such treatment. In addition, 20% to 40% of IBD patients are not compliant with their treatment [76]. Thus, a treatment targeting TNF using an intrinsic anti-TNF pathway, with few side effects, devoid of problem of compliance, and cheaper than biologicals (i.e. anti-TNF) would be of great value. In this context, VNS, as a non-drug therapy could serve as an alternative to classical biological therapy. We have shown recently that there is a specific homeostatic link between vagal tone and TNF-alpha in CD patients since a low vagal tone was associated with a high plasma TNF levels [77]. In addition, since stress is classically known to stimulate the sympathetic nervous system, which has a pro-inflammatory effect, and to inhibit the VN [78], and thus the CAP, VNS may help to restore equilibrium of the sympatho-vagal balance.

Irritable Bowel Syndrome

IBS is the most common functional digestive disorder, with a prevalence rate in the general population of 10–15% in industrialized countries [79]. IBS is characterized by abdominal pain, bloating and altered bowel habits without any organic cause with a higher prevalence of symptoms in women [1]. IBS accounts for up to 12% of visits to primary care doctors and 28% of visits to gastroenterologists [80]. IBS is associated with a significant impairment in quality of life, a high rate of absence from work and a significant increase in health care costs. Extra-intestinal manifestations are frequently associated with digestive symptoms such as headache, arthralgia, urinary problems, insomnia, and fatigue. Fibromyalgia is often observed in IBS [81]. Psychiatric comorbidity, mainly major depression, anxiety, and somatoform disorders are observed in 20 to 50% of IBS patients [82]. Numerous data argue for a role of stress in the pathophysiology of IBS [1]. A history of emotional, sexual, or physical abuse is found in 30%–50% of IBS patients [83]. A majority of patients with IBS have a visceral hypersensitivity as represented by lower pain thresholds to intestinal distension compared to healthy controls [84]. Among the peripheral mechanisms of this visceral hypersensitivity, low-grade inflammation in the GI tract could favor modifications of neuronal plasticity [85, 86] and mast cells could also be involved in the sensitization of visceral afferent terminals [87]. A post-infectious IBS has been observed in 4–30% following bacterial gastroenteritis [88]; perceived stress, anxiety, somatisation and negative illness beliefs at the time of infection in favor of a cognitive-behavioral model of IBS were predictors of post-infectious IBS [89]. Immune activation with an increased number of T lymphocytes and mast cells associated with mucosa as well as an increased level of pro-inflammatory cytokines (IL-10 and IL-12, suggesting Th1 polarization) has been described [90] so that some authors have compared IBS to an IBD "a minima". Modifications in central sensory processing are described in IBS [91], which is similar to a central sensitization syndrome [92].

Globally, IBS can be described by a biopsychosocial model with the concept that it is due to a brain-gut axis dysfunction consistent with an up-regulation in neural processing between the gut and the brain. There is a hypervigilance state that explains the visceral hypersensitivity observed in IBS patients. A dysautonomia, with a high sympathetic and a low parasympathetic tone, whatever the positive or negative affective adjustment has been described [3]. Because of the complexity of the pathophysiology of IBS, its medical treatment is limited, primarily to target symptoms. Non-medical treatments, like cognitive behavioral therapy or hypnosis, known to improve vagal tone [93, 94], are of interest [95].

In this context, based on its peripheral anti-inflammatory effect but also through its effect on the central nervous system, as an anti-depressive treatment, VNS would be of interest in the treatment of IBS. In addition, VNS has been shown to modify central pain processing. Indeed, VNS increases the pain threshold in visceral pain models in rats [96] and modulates visceral pain-related affective memory [97]. Modification of pain by VNS has been reported in epileptic patients and VNS might affect peripheral nociceptor function in humans [98]. We are starting a clinical trial to evaluate the effect of VNS in IBS (ClinicalTrials.gov Identifier: NCT02420158).

Post-operative Ileus

POI can develop after abdominal surgery irrespective of the site of surgery and is characterized by a delay in gastric emptying and a prolongation of intestinal transit. In most cases, the functions of the stomach and small intestine recover within 24–48 h while the colon can take up to 72 h. POI can lead to longer hospitalization times and higher healthcare costs. Recent research has led to a better understanding of the pathophysiology of POI. Sympathoadrenergic as well as vagal nonadrenergic-noncholinergic inhibitory efferent pathways are involved in the mechanisms mediating POI while capsaicin-sensitive afferent neurons have been implicated in the afferent limb of the reflex [99]. Brain transmitters and pathways that may be part of supra-spinal reflex circuitry have also been described such as *c-fos* expression of specific hypothalamic and pontine-medullary neurons [100]. CRF in the PVH plays a role in the central mechanism of stress-induced delay in gastric emptying and this effect is reduced by central injection of the CRF antagonist a-helical CRF-(9–41) [101]. This effect is mediated through CRF1 receptors since CRF1-deficient mice do not develop POI [102].

More recently, a role for the CAP has also been demonstrated in POI. Indeed, gentle manipulation of the small bowel during abdominal surgery induces inflammation of the muscularis propria [103, 104]. VNS reduced the inflammatory response to mechanical manipulation of the intestine during surgery, thereby preventing surgery-induced delayed gastric emptying [30]; systemic administration of selective nACh agonists has the same effect [105]. This anti-inflammatory effect is mediated by a reduction in macrophage activation and cytokine production through the CAP. Semapimod, a tetravalent guanyl hydrazone, also known as CNI-1493, prevents macrophage activation via inhibition of mitogen-activated protein kinase signaling [106]. This effect is mediated through central activation of the CAP [107] as observed with galantamine, a drug used in the treatment of Alzheimer disease that crosses the blood-brain barrier and activates the CAP [37]. Gum chewing reduces POI by stimulating vagal activity [108]. Peptides are involved in gastric emptying; ghrelin has a prokinetic effect thus stimulating gastric emptying [109] and abdominal surgery inhibits circulating ghrelin level in rats [110]. Somatostatin and its somatostatin receptor 2 (sst2) are highly expressed in the stomach and sst2 is involved in abdominal surgery-induced POI since sst2 antagonists prevent surgery-induced reduction of circulating ghrelin in rats [110]. Through its anti-inflammatory role, VNS is a potential treatment to reduce POI and a clinical trial is running to evaluate the anti-inflammatory effect of peroperative VNS to shorten POI in human (ClinicalTrials.gov Identifier: NCT01572155).

Science, Technique and Data That Underpins the Use of VNS for the Treatment of Inflammatory Disorders of the Gastrointestinal Tract

Based on the inflammatory reflex described by Tracey and colleagues, most of the studies using VNS to activate the CAP were performed in vagotomized, anesthetized animals with VNS performed at the distal end of the cut VN or in animals with stimulation of the distal part of the ligated VN trunk, thus stimulating selectively vagal efferent fibers without any effect on afferents. When performed in intact vagi, VNS was generally performed in anesthetized animals but anesthesia can change the threshold for activation of different types of fibers in the vagal bundle [111]. In addition, isoflurane commonly used in studies where long-term anesthesia is necessary because of different positive aspects has anti-inflammatory properties which can be sources of interferences in studies concerning inflammation [39, 112]. Lidocaine is also reported to reduce inflammatory markers, including cytokines and chemokines [113]. Most of these studies were also performed under acute but not chronic VNS. One might expect that VNS chronically performed in awakened animals would be of interest to extrapolate experimental data on inflammation to clinical data. As observed for VNS in epilepsy or depression, such a translational therapeutic approach is necessary to address inflammatory digestive disorders as well as extra-digestive disorders in human.

For this purpose, we have developed a chronic low frequency VNS of the left cervical VN in non-anesthetized freely moving rats with colitis, which shares features of Crohn's disease, for 3 h per day for five consecutive days, with stimulation parameters (1 mA, 5 Hz, pulse width of 500 ls; 10 s ON, 90 s OFF; continuous cycle) adapted from previous studies [58, 66]. We have used a global multivariate index of colitis (including body weight, myeloperoxidase quantification, telemetric data, and areas of lesions, cytokine and cytokine-related mRNAs) for a better characterization of colonic inflammation. We have shown that VNS has an anti-inflammatory effect as demonstrated by an improvement of this multivariate index of colitis [114]. Neurons of the DMNV that project to the digestive tract exhibit slow (1–2 Hz) spontaneous pacemaker-like activity in vitro as well as in vivo [115, 116] the rate of which can be modulated by synaptic inputs. Consequently, stimulation at a frequency of 5 Hz, generally used in experimental VNS of vagal efferents, is in the range of normal nerve traffic in the VN. In contrast, the majority of NTS neurons do not possess pacemaker activity; their inputs onto DMV neurons must be driven and are modulated by synaptic activity, either from the afferent VN, from other areas of the central nervous system, or via circulating hormones [117]. Lomarev et al. [68] showed a frequency/dose-effect of VNS on acute blood flow changes looking at fMRI modifications in the brain of depressed patients under low (5 HZ) or high (20 Hz) VNS; 5 Hz stimulation was associated with reduced brain activation by comparison to 20 Hz. In the same way, Osharina et al. [118] performed VNS of the central cut left VN and showed a gradual increase in *c-fos* expression in the brain of animals with VNS from 1 to 10 Hz; 1 Hz VNS only discretely affected the level of *c-fos* expression in the NTS, compared to sham-operation, while in contrast, *c-fos* expression was markedly above sham-operation levels in the NTS following 10 Hz stimulation. We have recently shown that low-frequency (5 Hz) VNS, known to activate vagal efferents, with anti-inflammatory properties in a model of colitis in rats [114] is also able to activate the central nervous system. Indeed, we have shown for the first time, using fMRI, that a 1-h VNS in anesthetized rodents induced highly significant VNS-related deactivations in the NTS and connected structures [69] such as the PB, the LC and the hippocampus as well as the prefrontal cortex and retrosplenial cortex, regions that express *c-fos* after continuous 30 Hz VNS [58]. Most of the deactivated structures observed in this study belong to the central ANS [119]. When VNS was performed on the distal end cut of the VN (i.e. disrupted vagal afferents), no brain activation was observed while brain activations remained unchanged when stimulation was performed on the proximal end of the VN (i.e. disrupted vagal afferents). Thus, even low-frequency stimulation at 5 Hz, that theoretically activate vagal efferents, also activate vagal afferents to the brain thus suggesting that the anti-inflammatory effect of low frequency VNS of the intact VN involve both a peripheral (i.e. the CAP) and central effect (through the vago-vagal inflammatory reflex and/or a stimulation of the HPA axis and/or a modification of the central ANS). This was corroborated by an electroencephalographic study that we have performed in a CD patient with chronic low frequency (10 Hz) VNS. Electroencephalographic (EEG) and electrocardiographic recordings were performed 1 week before, at week 6 and months 6, 9 and 12 post VNS implantation. VNS induced significant ($P < 0.05$) changes in resting EEG in all frequency bands with shared spatial pattern. In particular, activations were observed over the mediofrontal electrodes for both low and high frequency bands with the most important activation for the theta band. An additional activation was found in the occipital electrodes for the gamma band. We observed significant correlations between EEG and the high frequency component of heart rate variability (HRV) for delta, theta, beta, and gamma frequency bands. We can hypothesize that the increase in mediofrontal theta could reflect an activation of the anterior cingulate cortex, part of the central autonomic network that modulates the parasympathetic nervous system. The changes in theta and gamma bands observed in this study provide evidence that forebrain areas could be involved in the mediation of VNS effect on HRV. In parallel, the hypotonicity of vagal tone observed in this patient before VNS was regularly corrected during the 1-year of VNS and the patient was in deep (clinical and endoscopical) remission [120]. We are presently performing a pilot study of VNS in patients with CD (clinical trial.gov identifier NCT01569503) where VNS is positioned as an alternative treatment to classical anti-TNF. We have presently implanted 7 patients with moderate to severe CD, with a neurostimulator (model 102) and an electrode (model 302) from Cyberonics, using the following stimulation parameters: intensity 0.5–1.5 mA, frequency 10 Hz, pulse width 500 micros, and stimulation on-time of 30 s followed by off-time of 5 min. The first patient was implanted in April 2012 and the last patient in December 2014. After a 6-month follow-up, 5/7 have responded to VNS with clinical, biological and endoscopic improvement/healing. One patient switched to surgery (ileo-cecal resection) and another to a combotherapy with azathioprine and infliximab. Among the five patients in remission at 6 months still under VNS only one of them is under immunosuppressant (azathioprine) [121]. These preliminary data are of interest and justify a controlled study on more patients.

Advances in Technology and Future Directions

Non-invasive VNS (nVNS) that eliminates the need for surgical implantation, thus improving the safety and tolerability of VNS, is of interest. However, these devices rely on patient adherence for treatment.

The VN includes a sensory “auricular” branch that innervates the external ear. The cymba conchae of the external ear is innervated exclusively by this branch [122]. A direct projection of the auricular branch of the VN to the NTS has been shown in cats [123] and rats [124]. Transcutaneous auricular VNS (ta-VNS) produces cognitive and behavioral effects that are also produced by VNS [125]. A very recent fMRI study, performed in healthy adults, has shown that non-invasive electrical stimulation (continuous 0.25 ms pulses at 25 Hz, mean intensity 0.43 mA) of the auricular branch of the VN via the left cymba conchae significantly affects the central projections of the VN, compared to earlobe (control) stimulation [126]. This non-invasive electrical stimulation of the “somatic” (i.e., external ear) afferent branch of the VN activates both “visceral” and “somatic” vagal projections in the brain, thus providing a point of reference for understanding the mechanisms underlying the anti-convulsive, antidepressive, and antinociceptive effects of ta-VNS and VNS. There is a close connection between auricular concha, NTS, DMNV, and VN, which constructs the pathway of the auricular-vagal reflex, thus a connection between the auricular concha and vagal efferents. Consequently, such an anti-inflammatory reflex could be activated through ta-VNS. Experimental data support this hypothesis since ta-VNS has been shown to suppress LPS-induced inflammatory responses via α7nAChR-mediated CAP in rats [127]. In this study the authors used VNS or ta-VNS. Similar to the effect of VNS, ta-VNS suppressed the serum proinflammatory cytokines levels, such as TNF-α, IL-1β, and IL-6 as well as NF-kappa B p65 expressions of lung tissues. ta-VNS could not suppress LPS-induced TNF-α and NF-κB after vagotomy or with α7nAChR antagonist injection.

We detail below the non-invasive devices that are able to activate the inflammatory reflex although they are not presently used for this indication but for epilepsy, depression, and headache. However, one can extrapolate these devices to their use in inflammatory digestive disorders such as IBD, IBS and POI as well as others.

NEMOS (Cerbomed, Erlangen, Germany) is an external device that provides ta-VNS by using a dedicated intra-auricular electrode (like an earphone), which stimulates the auricular branch of the VN [128]. The device has received the European clearance (CE mark) in 2010 for epilepsy and is available in Germany, Austria, Switzerland, and Italy. The patient controls VNS stimulation intensity according to his individual sensitivity, which can vary from day to day or even over the period of the therapy. For optimal stimulation, they should choose the intensity so they feel a prickling or tingling sensation but not painful or uncomfortable, within a defined range and self-treatment sessions lasting 1–4 h, three to four times daily and as necessary (e.g. before a seizure) [128]. The treatment is carried out autonomously by the patients. The recommended daily stimulation dose is 4 h and should be reached daily. An overall reduction of seizure frequency was observed in five out of seven patients after 9 months of ta-VNS [128]. Aihua et al. [129] showed that after 12 months of ta-VNS, the monthly seizure frequency was significantly lower in the treatment group than in the control group. Rong et al. [130] also observed that after 8 weeks' treatment, the percentages of average seizure frequency in ta-VNS and tn-VNS were significantly reduced by 42.6% and 11.5% respectively. ta-VNS is able to increase HRV and reduce sympathetic nerve outflow in healthy controls [131], ta-VNS can therefore influence human physiology and provide a simple and inexpensive alternative to invasive VNS.

GammaCore (electroCore LLC, Basking Ridge, NJ, USA) is a non-invasive VNS that uses proprietary electrical signals to treat primary headache. It consists of a portable stimulator with a battery, signal-generating and -amplifying electronics and a digital control user interface that controls signal amplitude. Two stainless steel round discs function as skin contact surfaces that deliver a proprietary, low-voltage electrical signal to the cervical VN. The device delivers a programmable number of stimulation cycles, each lasting 120 s. In an open-label observational cohort study, fifteen patients with cluster headache reported an overall improvement with 4 reporting no change, providing a mean overall estimated improvement of 48%. About 47% of attacks were aborted within an average of 11 ± 1 min after stimulation. Ten patients reduced their acute use of high-flow oxygen by 55% with 9 reducing triptan use by 48%. Prophylactic use of the device resulted in a substantial reduction in estimated mean attack frequency from 4.5/24 to 2.6/24 h ($p < 0.0005$) posttreatment [132]. In another study performed in 73 patients with chronic migraine, mean visual analog scale pain scores were significantly reduced at 2 h from baseline; nine of 19 patients were pain free, six had reduced pain and four remained unchanged. Adverse events included two reports of brief paresthesia, which resolved within a few minutes [133]. GammaCore is now evaluated in four multicenter, randomized, controlled trials in the EU and North America in primary headache disorders. No significant serious device-related adverse events have been reported. Such a device could be applied, by comparaison to NEMOS, to inflammatory digestive disorders.

VNS coupled to the detection of HRV modification such as the neurostimulator could be activated when a low vagal tone is observed would be of interest, particularly in patients with vagal dysautonomia i.e. vagal hypotonia as observed in IBD and IBS [3]. *CardioFit* (BioControl Medical Ltd., Yehud, Israel) is an implantable VNS device being investigated in heart failure acting by preferential activation of vagal efferent fibers [134]. The stimulation is designed to correct the autonomic imbalance (sustained sympathetic overdrive and parasympathetic withdrawal) that is maladaptive in heart failure. The CardioFit system consists of a stimulator, a sensor lead and a stimulation lead, which are implanted under the skin of the chest. The sensor lead is extended from the stimulator to the right ventricle of the heart, and the stimulation lead is extended from the stimulator to the VN on the right side of the neck. Once activated, the stimulator's electrical pulses are transferred via the stimulation lead to the VN. At the same time, the sensor lead monitors changes in heart activity and turns stimulation on or off accordingly. Like a pacemaker, the CardioFit System can be programmed on and off via external communication with the device. However, Cardiofit is an implantable device for heart failure that is not applicable, in its present form, to inflammatory digestive disorders and one can hope that such a device or better an external device as described for ta-VNS coupled to the monitoring of HRV would be of interest to stimulate vagal efferents when necessary i.e. in case of low vagal tone.

Conclusion

The use of VNS in the treatment of GI inflammatory disorders, with a special interest to IBD and IBS, is relevant because it is a safe technique that uses an intrinsic physiological antiinflammatory pathway and is able to restore an equilibrated sympatho-vagal balance. The development of non-invasive VNS, such as ta-VNS is of interest. VNS could be extrapolated to other inflammatory disorders such as rheumatoid arthritis.

References

1. Mulak A, Bonaz B. Irritable bowel syndrome: a model of the brain-gut interactions. Med Sci Monit. 2004;10(4):RA55–62.
2. Bonaz BL, Bernstein CN. Brain-gut interactions in inflammatory bowel disease. Gastroenterology. 2013;144(1):36–49.
3. Pellissier S, Dantzer C, Canini F, Mathieu N, Bonaz B. Psychological adjustment and autonomic disturbances in inflammatory bowel diseases and irritable bowel syndrome. Psychoneuroendocrinology. 2010;35(5):653–62.
4. Bonaz B, Picq C, Sinniger V, Mayol JF, Clarençon D. Vagus nerve stimulation: from epilepsy to the cholinergic anti-inflammatory pathway. Neurogastroenterol Motil. 2013;25(3):208–21.
5. Prechtl JC, Powley TL. The fiber composition of the abdominal vagus of the rat. Anat Embryol (Berl). 1990;181(2):101–15.

6. Altschuler SM, Escardo J, Lynn RB, Miselis RR. The central organization of the vagus nerve innervating the colon of the rat. Gastroenterology. 1993;104(2):502–9.
7. Netter FH. Atlas of human anatomy. Ardsley: Ciba-Geigy Corporation; 1989.
8. Delmas et Laux. Anatomie médico-chirurgicale du système nerveux végétatif. Masson, 1933.
9. Berthoud HR, Carlson NR, Powley TL. Topography of efferent vagal innervation of the rat gastrointestinal tract. Am J Physiol. 1991;260(1 Pt 2):R200–7.
10. Sharkey KA, Kroese AB. Consequences of intestinal inflammation on the enteric nervous system: neuronal activation induced by inflammatory mediators. Anat Rec. 2001;262(1):79–90.
11. Margolis KG, Stevanovic K, Karamooz N, Li ZS, Ahuja A, D'Autréaux F, Saurman V, Chalazonitis A, Gershon MD. Enteric neuronal density contributes to the severity of intestinal inflammation. Gastroenterology. 2011;141(2):588–98. 598.e1–2.
12. Altschuler SM, Bao XM, Bieger D, Hopkins DA, Miselis RR. Viscerotopic representation of the upper alimentary tract in the rat: sensory ganglia and nuclei of the solitary and spinal trigeminal tracts. J Comp Neurol. 1989;283(2):248–68.
13. Rinaman L, Card JP, Schwaber JS, Miselis RR. Ultrastructural demonstration of a gastric monosynaptic vagal circuit in the nucleus of the solitary tract in rat. J Neurosci. 1989; 9(6):1985–96.
14. Ricardo JA, Koh ET. Anatomical evidence of direct projections from the nucleus of the solitary tract to the hypothalamus, amygdala, and other forebrain structures in the rat. Brain Res. 1978;153(1):1–26.
15. Sawchenko PE. Central connections of the sensory and motor nuclei of the vagus nerve. J Auton Nerv Syst. 1983;9(1):13–26.
16. Ruggiero DA, Underwood MD, Mann JJ, Anwar M, Arango V. The human nucleus of the solitary tract: visceral pathways revealed with an "in vitro" postmortem tracing method. J Auton Nerv Syst. 2000;79(2–3):181–90.
17. Van Bockstaele EJ, Peoples J, Telegan P. Efferent projections of the nucleus of the solitary tract to peri-locus coeruleus dendrites in rat brain: evidence for a monosynaptic pathway. J Comp Neurol. 1999;412(3):410–28.
18. Aston-Jones G, Ennis M, Pieribone VA, Nickell WT, Shipley MT. The brain nucleus locus coeruleus: restricted afferent control of a broad efferent network. Science. 1986;234(4777): 734–7.
19. Zagon A, Hughes DI. Gating of vagal inputs by sciatic afferents in nonspinally projecting neurons in the rat rostral ventrolateral medulla oblongata. Eur J Neurosci. 2001;13(4): 781–92.
20. Conrad LC, Pfaff DW. Efferents from medial basal forebrain and hypothalamus in the rat. II. An autoradiographic study of the anterior hypothalamus. J Comp Neurol. 1976;169(2): 221–61.
21. Norgren R. Taste pathways to hypothalamus and amygdala. J Comp Neurol. 1976;166(1): 17–30.
22. Zagon A. Does the vagus nerve mediate the sixth sense? Trends Neurosci. 2001;24(11):671–3.
23. Goehler LE, Relton JK, Dripps D, Kiechle R, Tartaglia N, Maier SF, Watkins LR. Vagal paraganglia bind biotinylated interleukin-1 receptor antagonist: a possible mechanism for immune-to-brain communication. Brain Res Bull. 1997;43(3):357–64.
24. Watkins LR, Goehler LE, Relton JK, Tartaglia N, Silbert L, Martin D, Maier SF. Blockade of interleukin-1 induced hyperthermia by subdiaphragmatic vagotomy: evidence for vagal mediation of immune-brain communication. Neurosci Lett. 1995;183(1–2):27–31.
25. Hosoi T, Okuma Y, Matsuda T, Nomura Y. Novel pathway for LPS-induced afferent vagus nerve activation: possible role of nodose ganglion. Auton Neurosci. 2005;120(1–2):104–7.
26. Taché Y, Brunnhuber S. From Hans Selye's discovery of biological stress to the identification of corticotropin-releasing factor signaling pathways: implication in stress-related functional bowel diseases. Ann N Y Acad Sci. 2008;1148:29–41.
27. Borovikova LV, Ivanova S, Zhang M, Yang H, Botchkina GI, Watkins LR, Wang H, Abumrad N, Eaton JW, Tracey KJ. Vagus nerve stimulation attenuates the systemic inflammatory response to endotoxin. Nature. 2000;405(6785):458–62.

28. Pavlov VA, Wang H, Czura CJ, Friedman SG, Tracey KJ. The cholinergic anti-inflammatory pathway: a missing link in neuroimmunomodulation. Mol Med. 2003;9(5–8):125–34.
29. Wang H, Yu M, Ochani M, Amella CA, Tanovic M, Susarla S, Li JH, Wang H, Yang H, Ulloa L, Al-Abed Y, Czura CJ, Tracey KJ. Nicotinic acetylcholine receptor alpha7 subunit is an essential regulator of inflammation. Nature. 2003;421(6921):384–8.
30. de Jonge WJ, van der Zanden EP, The FO, Bijlsma MF, van Westerloo DJ, Bennink RJ, Berthoud HR, Uematsu S, Akira S, van den Wijngaard RM, Boeckxstaens GE. Stimulation of the vagus nerve attenuates macrophage activation by activating the Jak2-STAT3 signaling pathway. Nat Immunol. 2005;6(8):844–51.
31. Sun Y, Li Q, Gui H, Xu DP, Yang YL, Su DF, Liu X. MicroRNA-124 mediates the cholinergic anti-inflammatory action through inhibiting the production of pro-inflammatory cytokines. Cell Res. 2013;23(11):1270–83.
32. Huston JM, Ochani M, Rosas-Ballina M, Liao H, Ochani K, Pavlov VA, Gallowitsch-Puerta M, Ashok M, Czura CJ, Foxwell B, Tracey KJ, Ulloa L. Splenectomy inactivates the cholinergic antiinflammatory pathway during lethal endotoxemia and polymicrobial sepsis. J Exp Med. 2006;203(7):1623–8.
33. Huston JM, Rosas-Ballina M, Xue X, Dowling O, Ochani K, Ochani M, Yeboah MM, Chatterjee PK, Tracey KJ, Metz CN. Cholinergic neural signals to the spleen down-regulate leukocyte trafficking via CD11b. J Immunol. 2009;183(1):552–9.
34. Berthoud HR, Powley TL. Interaction between parasympathetic and sympathetic nerves in prevertebral ganglia: morphological evidence for vagal efferent innervation of ganglion cells in the rat. Microsc Res Tech. 1996;35(1):80–6.
35. Rosas-Ballina M, Tracey KJ. The neurology of the immune system: neural reflexes regulate immunity. Neuron. 2009;64(1):28–32.
36. Downs AM. Bond CE1, Hoover DB2. Localization of α7 nicotinic acetylcholine receptor mRNA and protein within the cholinergic anti-inflammatory pathway. Neuroscience. 2014;266:178–85.
37. Ji H, Rabbi MF, Labis B, Pavlov VA, Tracey KJ, Ghia JE. Central cholinergic activation of a vagus nerve-to-spleen circuit alleviates experimental colitis. Mucosal Immunol. 2014;7(2):335–47.
38. Xue N, Liang H, Yao H, Song XM, Li JG. The role of spleen in vagus nerve stimulation for treatment against septic shock in rats. Zhongguo Wei Zhong Bing Ji Jiu Yi Xue. 2011;23(5):263–6.
39. Picq CA, Clarençon D, Sinniger VE, Bonaz BL, Mayol JF. Impact of Anesthetics on Immune Functions in a Rat Model of Vagus Nerve Stimulation. PLoS One. 2013;8(6):e67086.
40. Martelli D, Yao ST, McKinley MJ, McAllen RM. Reflex control of inflammation by sympathetic nerves, not the vagus. J Physiol. 2014;592(Pt 7):1677–86.
41. Gautron L, Rutkowski JM, Burton MD, Wei W, Wan Y, Elmquist JK. Neuronal and nonneuronal cholinergic structures in the mouse gastrointestinal tract and spleen. J Comp Neurol. 2013;521(16):3741–67.
42. Wessler I, Kirkpatrick CJ, Racké K. Non-neuronal acetylcholine, a locally acting molecule, widely distributed in biological systems: expression and function in humans. Pharmacol Ther. 1998;77(1):59–79.
43. Cano G, Sved AF, Rinaman L, Rabin BS, Card JP. Characterization of the central nervous system innervation of the rat spleen using viral transneuronal tracing. J Comp Neurol. 2001;439(1):1–18.
44. Bratton BO, Martelli D, McKinley MJ, Trevaks D, Anderson CR, McAllen RM. Neural regulation of inflammation: no neural connection from the vagus to splenic sympathetic neurons. Exp Physiol. 2012;97(11):1180–5.
45. Martelli D, McKinley MJ, McAllen RM. The cholinergic anti-inflammatory pathway: a critical review. Auton Neurosci. 2014;182:65–9.
46. Vida G, Peña G, Kanashiro A, Thompson-Bonilla Mdel R, Palange D, Deitch EA, Ulloa L. β2-Adrenoreceptors of regulatory lymphocytes are essential for vagal neuromodulation of the innate immune system. FASEB J. 2011;25(12):4476–85.
47. Cailotto C, Gomez-Pinilla PJ, Costes LM, van der Vliet J, Di Giovangiulio M, Némethova A, Matteoli G, Boeckxstaens GE. Neuro-anatomical evidence indicating indirect modulation of

macrophages by vagal efferents in the intestine but not in the spleen. PLoS One. 2014;9(1):e87785.
48. Lanska DJ. J.L. Corning and vagal nerve stimulation for seizures in the 1880s. Neurology. 2002;58(3):452–9.
49. Bailey H, Bremer FA. Sensory cortical representation of the vagus nerve. J Neurophysiol. 1938;1:405–12.
50. Penry JK, Dean JC. Prevention of intractable partial seizures by intermittent vagal stimulation in humans: preliminary results. Epilepsia. 1990;31(Suppl 2):S40–3.
51. Rush AJ, Marangell LB, Sackeim HA, George MS, Brannan SK, Davis SM, Howland R, Kling MA, Rittberg BR, Burke WJ, Rapaport MH, Zajecka J, Nierenberg AA, Husain MM, Ginsberg D, Cooke RG. Vagus nerve stimulation for treatment-resistant depression: a randomized, controlled acute phase trial. Biol Psychiatry. 2005;58(5):347–54.
52. Rush AJ, Sackeim HA, Marangell LB, George MS, Brannan SK, Davis SM, Lavori P, Howland R, Kling MA, Rittberg B, Carpenter L, Ninan P, Moreno F, Schwartz T, Conway C, Burke M, Barry JJ. Effects of 12 months of vagus nerve stimulation in treatment-resistant depression: a naturalistic study. Biol Psychiatry. 2005;58(5):355–63.
53. Fanselow EE. Central mechanisms of cranial nerve stimulation for epilepsy. Surg Neurol Int. 2012;3(Suppl 4):S247–54.
54. Krahl SE, Senanayake SS, Handforth A. Destruction of peripheral C-fibers does not alter subsequent vagus nerve stimulation-induced seizure suppression in rats. Epilepsia. 2001; 42(5):586–9.
55. Zanchetti A, Wang SC, Moruzzi G. Effect of afferent vagal stimulation on the electroencephalogram of the cat in cerebral isolation. Boll Soc Ital Biol Sper. 1952;28(4):627–8.
56. Panebianco M, Rigby A, Weston J, Marson AG. Vagus nerve stimulation for partial seizures. Cochrane Database Syst Rev. 2015;4:CD002896.
57. Groves DA, Brown VJ. Vagal nerve stimulation: a review of its applications and potential mechanisms that mediate its clinical effects. Neurosci Biobehav Rev. 2005;29(3):493–500.
58. Naritoku DK, Terry WJ, Helfert RH. Regional induction of fos immunoreactivity in the brain by anticonvulsant stimulation of the vagus nerve. Epilepsy Res. 1995;22(1):53–62.
59. Chae JH, Nahas Z, Lomarev M, Denslow S, Lorberbaum JP, Bohning DE, George MS. A review of functional neuroimaging studies of vagus nerve stimulation (VNS). J Psychiatr Res. 2003;37(6):443–55.
60. Morris 3rd GL, Mueller WM. Long-term treatment with vagus nerve stimulation in patients with refractory epilepsy. The Vagus Nerve Stimulation Study Group E01-E05. Neurology. 1999;53(8):1731–5.
61. Tisi G, Franzini A, Messina G, Savino M, Gambini O. Vagus nerve stimulation therapy in treatment-resistant depression: a series report. Psychiatry Clin Neurosci. 2014;68(8): 606–11.
62. Bajbouj M, Merkl A, Schlaepfer TE, Frick C, Zobel A, Maier W, O'Keane V, Corcoran C, Adolfsson R, Trimble M, Rau H, Hoff HJ, Padberg F, Müller-Siecheneder F, Audenaert K, van den Abbeele D, Matthews K, Christmas D, Eljamel S, Heuser I. Two-year outcome of vagus nerve stimulation in treatment-resistant depression. J Clin Psychopharmacol. 2010;30(3):273–81.
63. Reid SA. Surgical technique for implantation of the neurocybernetic prosthesis. Epilepsia. 1990;31(Suppl 2):S38–9.
64. Hamlin RL, Smith CR. Effects of vagal stimulation on S-A and A-V nodes. Am J Physiol. 1968;215(3):560–8.
65. Ben-Menachem E. Vagus nerve stimulation, side effects, and long-term safety. J Clin Neurophysiol. 2001;18(5):415–8.
66. Bernik TR, Friedman SG, Ochani M, DiRaimo R, Ulloa L, Yang H, Sudan S, Czura CJ, Ivanova SM, Tracey KJ. Pharmacological stimulation of the cholinergic antiinflammatory pathway. J Exp Med. 2002;195(6):781–8.
67. Costantini TW, Bansal V, Krzyzaniak M, Putnam JG, Peterson CY, Loomis WH, Wolf P, Baird A, Eliceiri BP, Coimbra R. Vagal nerve stimulation protects against burn-induced intes-

tinal injury through activation of enteric glia cells. Am J Physiol Gastrointest Liver Physiol. 2010;299(6):G1308–18.
68. Lomarev M, Denslow S, Nahas Z, Chae JH, George MS, Bohning DE. Vagus nerve stimulation (VNS) synchronized BOLD fMRI suggests that VNS in depressed adults has frequency/dose dependent effects. J Psychiatr Res. 2002;36(4):219–27.
69. Reyt S, Picq C, Sinniger V, Clarençon D, Bonaz B, David O. Dynamic Causal Modelling and physiological confounds: a functional MRI study of vagus nerve stimulation. Neuroimage. 2010;52(4):1456–64.
70. Molodecky NA, Soon IS, Rabi DM, Ghali WA, Ferris M, Chernoff G, Benchimol EI, Panaccione R, Ghosh S, Barkema HW, Kaplan GG. Increasing incidence and prevalence of the inflammatory bowel diseases with time, based on systematic review. Gastroenterology. 2012;142(1):46–54.
71. Danese S, Fiocchi C. Etiopathogenesis of inflammatory bowel diseases. World J Gastroenterol. 2006;12(30):4807–12.
72. Lindgren S, Lilja B, Rosén I, Sundkvist G. Disturbed autonomic nerve function in patients with Crohn's disease. Scand J Gastroenterol. 1991;26(4):361–6.
73. Lindgren S, Stewenius J, Sjölund K, Lilja B, Sundkvist G. Autonomic vagal nerve dysfunction in patients with ulcerative colitis. Scand J Gastroenterol. 1993;28(7):638–42.
74. Billiet T, Rutgeerts P, Ferrante M, Van Assche G, Vermeire S. Targeting TNF-α for the treatment of inflammatory bowel disease. Expert Opin Biol Ther. 2014;14(1):75–101.
75. McLean LP, Cross RK. Adverse events in IBD: to stop or continue immune suppressant and biologic treatment. Expert Rev Gastroenterol Hepatol. 2014;8(3):223–40.
76. Cerveny P, Bortlik M, Vlcek J, Kubena A, Lukás M. Non-adherence to treatment in inflammatory bowel disease in Czech Republic. J Crohns Colitis. 2007;1(2):77–81.
77. Pellissier S, Dantzer C, Mondillon L, Trocme C, Gauchez AS, Ducros V, Mathieu N, Toussaint B, Fournier A, Canini F, Bonaz B. Relationship between vagal tone, cortisol, TNF-alpha, epinephrine and negative affects in Crohn's disease and irritable bowel syndrome. PLoS One. 2014;9(9):e105328.
78. Taché Y, Bonaz B. Corticotropin-releasing factor receptors and stress-related alterations of gut motor function. J Clin Invest. 2007;117(1):33–40.
79. Canavan C, West J, Card T. The epidemiology of irritable bowel syndrome. Clin Epidemiol. 2014;6:71–80.
80. Camilleri M. Pathophysiology in irritable bowel syndrome. Drug News Perspect. 2001; 14(5):268–78.
81. Chang L. The association of functional gastrointestinal disorders and fibromyalgia. Eur J Surg Suppl. 1998;583:32–6.
82. Garakani A, Win T, Virk S, Gupta S, Kaplan D, Masand PS. Comorbidity of irritable bowel syndrome in psychiatric patients: a review. Am J Ther. 2003;10(1):61–7.
83. Bradford K, Shih W, Videlock EJ, Presson AP, Naliboff BD, Mayer EA, Chang L. Association between early adverse life events and irritable bowel syndrome. Clin Gastroenterol Hepatol. 2012 Apr;10(4):385–90.e1–3.
84. Ritchie J. Pain from distension of the pelvic colon by inflating a balloon in the irritable colon syndrome. Gut. 1973;14(2):125–32.
85. Mayer EA, Gebhart GF. Basic and clinical aspects of visceral hyperalgesia. Gastroenterology. 1994;107(1):271–93.
86. Brierley SM, Linden DR. Neuroplasticity and dysfunction after gastrointestinal inflammation. Nat Rev Gastroenterol Hepatol. 2014;11(10):611–27.
87. Barbara G, Stanghellini V, De Giorgio R, Cremon C, Cottrell GS, Santini D, Pasquinelli G, Morselli-Labate AM, Grady EF, Bunnett NW, Collins SM, Corinaldesi R. Activated mast cells in proximity to colonic nerves correlate with abdominal pain in irritable bowel syndrome. Gastroenterology. 2004;126(3):693–702.
88. Gwee KA, Graham JC, McKendrick MW, Collins SM, Marshall JS, Walters SJ, Read NW. Psychometric scores and persistence of irritable bowel after infectious diarrhoea. Lancet. 1996;347(8995):150–3.

89. Spence MJ, Moss-Morris R. The cognitive behavioural model of irritable bowel syndrome: a prospective investigation of patients with gastroenteritis. Gut. 2007;56(8):1066–71.
90. Catanzaro R, Occhipinti S, Calabrese F, Anzalone MG, Milazzo M, Italia A, Marotta F. Irritable bowel syndrome: new findings in pathophysiological and therapeutic field. Minerva Gastroenterol Dietol. 2014;60(2):151–63.
91. Bonaz B, Baciu M, Papillon E, Bost R, Gueddah N, Le Bas JF, Fournet J, Segebarth C. Central processing of rectal pain in patients with irritable bowel syndrome: an fMRI study. Am J Gastroenterol. 2002;97(3):654–61.
92. Yunus MB. Role of central sensitization in symptoms beyond muscle pain, and the evaluation of a patient with widespread pain. Best Pract Res Clin Rheumatol. 2007;21(3):481–97.
93. Hinton DE, Hofmann SG, Pollack MH, Otto MW. Mechanisms of efficacy of CBT for Cambodian refugees with PTSD: improvement in emotion regulation and orthostatic blood pressure response. CNS Neurosci Ther. 2009;15(3):255–63.
94. Aubert AE, Verheyden B, Beckers F, Tack J, Vandenberghe J. Cardiac autonomic regulation under hypnosis assessed by heart rate variability: spectral analysis and fractal complexity. Neuropsychobiology. 2009;60(2):104–12.
95. Ford AC, Quigley EM, Lacy BE, Lembo AJ, Saito YA, Schiller LR, Soffer EE, Spiegel BM, Moayyedi P. Effect of antidepressants and psychological therapies, including hypnotherapy, in irritable bowel syndrome: systematic review and meta-analysis. Am J Gastroenterol. 2014;109(9):1350–65.
96. Zurowski D, Nowak Ł, Wordliczek J, Dobrogowski J, Thor PJ. Effects of vagus nerve stimulation in visceral pain model. Folia Med Cracov. 2012;52(1–2):57–69.
97. Zhang X, Cao B, Yan N, Liu J, Wang J, Tung VO, Li Y. Vagus nerve stimulation modulates visceral pain-related affective memory. Behav Brain Res. 2013;236(1):8–15.
98. Kirchner A, Stefan H, Bastian K, Birklein F. Vagus nerve stimulation suppresses pain but has limited effects on neurogenic inflammation in humans. Eur J Pain. 2006;10(5):449–55.
99. Holzer P, Lippe IT, Amann R. Participation of capsaicin-sensitive afferent neurons in gastric motor inhibition caused by laparotomy and intraperitoneal acid. Neuroscience. 1992;48(3):715–22.
100. Bonaz B, Plourde V, Taché Y. Abdominal surgery induces Fos immunoreactivity in the rat brain. J Comp Neurol. 1994;349(2):212–22.
101. Barquist E, Bonaz B, Martinez V, Rivier J, Zinner MJ, Taché Y. Neuronal pathways involved in abdominal surgery-induced gastric ileus in rats. Am J Physiol. 1996;270(4 Pt 2):R888–94.
102. Luckey A, Wang L, Jamieson PM, Basa NR, Million M, Czimmer J, Vale W, Taché Y. Corticotropin-releasing factor receptor 1-deficient mice do not develop postoperative gastric ileus. Gastroenterology. 2003;125(3):654–9.
103. Kalff JC, Carlos TM, Schraut WH, Billiar TR, Simmons RL, Bauer AJ. Surgically induced leukocytic infiltrates within the rat intestinal muscularis mediate postoperative ileus. Gastroenterology. 1999;117(2):378–87.
104. de Jonge WJ, van den Wijngaard RM, The FO, ter Beek ML, Bennink RJ, Tytgat GN, Buijs RM, Reitsma PH, van Deventer SJ, Boeckxstaens GE. Postoperative ileus is maintained by intestinal immune infiltrates that activate inhibitory neural pathways in mice. Gastroenterology. 2003;125(4):1137–47.
105. The FO, Boeckxstaens GE, Snoek SA, Cash JL, Bennink R, Larosa GJ, van den Wijngaard RM, Greaves DR, de Jonge WJ. Activation of the cholinergic anti-inflammatory pathway ameliorates postoperative ileus in mice. Gastroenterology. 2007;133(4):1219–28.
106. Löwenberg M, Verhaar A, van den Blink B, ten Kate F, van Deventer S, Peppelenbosch M, Hommes D. Specific inhibition of c-Raf activity by semapimod induces clinical remission in severe Crohn's disease. J Immunol. 2005;175(4):2293–300.

107. The FO, Cailotto C, van der Vliet J, de Jonge WJ, Bennink RJ, Buijs RM, Boeckxstaens GE. Central activation of the cholinergic anti-inflammatory pathway reduces surgical inflammation in experimental post-operative ileus. Br J Pharmacol. 2011;163(5):1007–16.
108. Noble EJ, Harris R, Hosie KB, Thomas S, Lewis SJ. Gum chewing reduces postoperative ileus? A systematic review and meta-analysis. Int J Surg. 2009;7(2):100–5.
109. Levin F, Edholm T, Schmidt PT, Grybäck P, Jacobsson H, Degerblad M, Höybye C, Holst JJ, Rehfeld JF, Hellström PM, Näslund E. Ghrelin stimulates gastric emptying and hunger in normal-weight humans. J Clin Endocrinol Metab. 2006;91(9):3296–302.
110. Stengel A, Goebel-Stengel M, Wang L, Shaikh A, Lambrecht NW, Rivier J, Taché Y. Abdominal surgery inhibits circulating acyl ghrelin and ghrelin-O-acyltransferase levels in rats: role of the somatostatin receptor subtype 2. Am J Physiol Gastrointest Liver Physiol. 2011;301(2):G239–48.
111. Woodbury DM, Woodbury JW. Effects of vagal stimulation on experimentally induced seizures in rats. Epilepsia. 1990;31(Suppl 2):S7–19.
112. Chung IS, Kim JA, Kim JA, Choi HS, Lee JJ, Yang M, Ahn HJ, Lee SM. Reactive oxygen species by isoflurane mediates inhibition of nuclear factor κB activation in lipopolysaccharide-induced acute inflammation of the lung. Anesth Analg. 2013;116(2):327–35.
113. Garutti I, Rancan L, Simón C, Cusati G, Sanchez-Pedrosa G, Moraga F, Olmedilla L, Lopez-Gil MT, Vara E. Intravenous lidocaine decreases tumor necrosis factor alpha expression both locally and systemically in pigs undergoing lung resection surgery. Anesth Analg. 2014; 119(4):815–28.
114. Meregnani J, Clarençon D, Vivier M, Peinnequin A, Mouret C, Sinniger V, Picq C, Job A, Canini F, Jacquier-Sarlin M, Bonaz B. Anti-inflammatory effect of vagus nerve stimulation in a rat model of inflammatory bowel disease. Auton Neurosci. 2011;160(1–2):82–9.
115. Travagli RA, Gillis RA, Rossiter CD, Vicini S. Glutamate and GABA-mediated synaptic currents in neurons of the rat dorsal motor nucleus of the vagus. Am J Physiol. 1991;260(3 Pt 1):G531–6.
116. Fogel R, Zhang X, Renehan WE. Relationships between the morphology and function of gastric and intestinal distention-sensitive neurons in the dorsal motor nucleus of the vagus. J Comp Neurol. 1996;364(1):78–91.
117. Travagli RA, Hermann GE, Browning KN, Rogers RC. Brainstem circuits regulating gastric function. Annu Rev Physiol. 2006;68:279–305.
118. Osharina V, Bagaev V, Wallois F, Larnicol N. Autonomic response and Fos expression in the NTS following intermittent vagal stimulation: importance of pulse frequency. Auton Neurosci. 2006;126-127:72–80.
119. Saper CB. The central autonomic nervous system: conscious visceral perception and autonomic pattern generation. Annu Rev Neurosci. 2002;25:433–69.
120. Clarençon D, Pellissier S, Sinniger V, Kibleur A, Hoffman D, Vercueil L, David O, Bonaz B. Long term effects of low frequency (10 hz) vagus nerve stimulation on EEG and heart rate variability in Crohn's disease: a case report. Brain Stimul. 2014;7(6):914–6.
121. Bonaz B, Sinniger V, Hoffmann D, Clarençon D, Mathieu N, Dantzer C, Vercueil L, Picq C, Trocmé C, Faure P, Cracowski JL, Pellissier S. Chronic vagus nerve stimulation in Crohn's disease: a 6-month follow-up pilot study. Neurogastroenterol Motil. 2016;28(6):948–53.
122. Peuker ET, Filler TJ. The nerve supply of the human auricle. Clin Anat 2002;15(1):35–7.
123. Nomura S, Mizuno N. Central distribution of primary afferent fibers in the Arnold's nerve (the auricular branch of the vagus nerve): a transganglionic HRP study in the cat. Brain Res. 1984;292(2):199–205.
124. Gao XY, Rong P, Ben H, Liu K, Zhu B, Zhang S. Morphological and electrophysiological characterization of auricular branch of vagus nerve: projections to the NTS in mediating cardiovascular inhibition evoked by the acupuncture-like stimulation. Abstr Soc Neurosci. 2010;694:22/HHH45.
125. Hein E, Nowak M, Kiess O, Biermann T, Bayerlein K, Kornhuber J, Kraus T. Auricular transcutaneous electrical nerve stimulation in depressed patients: a randomized controlled pilot study. J Neural Transm. 2013;120(5):821–7.

126. Frangos E, Ellrich J, Komisaruk BR. Non-invasive access to the vagus nerve central projections via electrical stimulation of the external ear: fMRI evidence in humans. Brain Stimul. 2015;8(3):624–36.
127. Zhao YX, He W, Jing XH, Liu JL, Rong PJ, Ben H, Liu K, Zhu B. Transcutaneous auricular vagus nerve stimulation protects endotoxemic rat from lipopolysaccharide-induced inflammation. Evid Based Complement Alternat Med. 2012;2012:627023.
128. Stefan H, Kreiselmeyer G, Kerling F, Kurzbuch K, Rauch C, Heers M, Kasper BS, Hammen T, Rzonsa M, Pauli E, Ellrich J, Graf W, Hopfengärtner R. Transcutaneous vagus nerve stimulation (t-VNS) in pharmacoresistant epilepsies: a proof of concept trial. Epilepsia. 2012;53(7):e115–8.
129. Aihua L, Lu S, Liping L, Xiuru W, Hua L, Yuping W. A controlled trial of transcutaneous vagus nerve stimulation for the treatment of pharmacoresistant epilepsy. Epilepsy Behav. 2014;39:105–10.
130. Rong P, Liu A, Zhang J, Wang Y, He W, Yang A, Li L, Ben H, Li L, Liu H, Wu P, Liu R, Zhao Y, Zhang J, Huang F, Li X, Zhu B. Transcutaneous vagus nerve stimulation for refractory epilepsy: a randomized controlled trial. Clin Sci (Lond). 2014; [Epub ahead of print].
131. Clancy JA, Mary DA, Witte KK, Greenwood JP, Deuchars SA, Deuchars J. Non-invasive vagus nerve stimulation in healthy humans reduces sympathetic nerve activity. Brain Stimul. 2014;7(6):871–7.
132. Nesbitt AD. Marin JC1, Tompkins E1, Ruttledge MH1, Goadsby PJ2. Initial use of a novel noninvasive vagus nerve stimulator for cluster headache treatment. Neurology. 2015;84(12): 1249–53.
133. Moscato D, Moscato FR. Treatment of chronic migraine by means of vagal stimulator [abstract]. J Headache Pain. 2013;14(Suppl):56–7.
134. Abraham WT, Stough WG, Piña IL, Linde C, Borer JS, De Ferrari GM, Mehran R, Stein KM, Vincent A, Yadav JS, Anker SD, Zannad F. Trials of implantable monitoring devices in heart failure: which design is optimal? Nat Rev Cardiol. 2014;11(10):576–85.

Chapter 10
Electroacoustics

Simon D. Carr and Jaydip Ray

Abstract Electroacoustics is a rapidly growing field formed by the confluence of implantation otology, audiology, electronics and robotics. The currently available devices can rehabilitate numerous parts of the auditory pathway, ranging from bone anchored hearing solutions, middle ear implants, cochlear implants through to brainstem implants. The development of the cochlear implant has been deemed one of the miraculous inventions of the twentieth Century, restoring the gift of hearing and enabling patients to communicate. This chapter is an overview of the current electroacoustic implantation devices available and discusses the future direction of the technology.

Keywords Hearing aids • Cochlear implants • Bone conduction • Ossicular prosthesis, osseointegration

Background

Physiology of Hearing

Hearing involves transfer of sound across several interfaces, transforming sound energy to mechanical energy, to hydraulic energy and finally into electrical energy.

Sound is received by the pinna, which is shaped to amplify sound and to enable sound localisation. The incoming sound wave is then propagated as a series of compressions and rarefactions, which travel down the external auditory canal (EAC) to the tympanic membrane, causing it to vibrate. This vibration, in turn causes the ossicles, situated in the middle ear space to vibrate. This mechanical transfer mechanism propagates the sound energy across the three ossicles to the footplate of the ossicle stapes which sits in the oval window of the cochlea, the hearing organ. The ratio of the size of the tympanic membrane to the relatively smaller footplate of stapes acts to further amplify the sound. The footplate moves within the oval window causing a 'travelling wave' along the basilar membrane of the cochlea. It is the

S.D. Carr, MD, FRCS (ORL-HNS) • J. Ray, MS, PhD FRCS (ORL-HNS) (✉)
Department of ENT, Royal Hallamshire Hospital, Glossop Road, Sheffield S10 2JF, UK
e-mail: simoncarr15@gmail.com; jaydip.ray@sth.nhs.uk

A. Majid (ed.), *Electroceuticals*, DOI 10.1007/978-3-319-28612-9_10

distortion of the basilar membrane in relation to the tectorial membrane of the Organ of Corti, which, in turn, distorts hair cells, causing them to depolarise, causing an impulse to pass along the cochlear nerve to the auditory cortex. Although the human ear is capable of detecting between 20 and 20,000 Hz, the speech sensitive frequencies are between 500 and 4000 Hz.

Hearing Loss

There are three main types of hearing loss: conductive, sensorineural and mixed.

Conductive hearing loss occurs as a result of a problem with the sound energy being transferred from the pinna to the footplate of the stapes i.e. the conduction of sound to the cochlea. This can be due to pathology of any part of the hearing pathway from the pinna to the cochlea.

Sensorineural hearing loss occurs as a result of pathology affecting the cochlea or cochlear nerve e.g. labyrinthitis ossificans due to meningitis.

Pure tone audiometry is performed to ascertain the hearing threshold, which is graded on a biological scale, according to how that individual can hear compared to a population of normal hearing adults.

Hearing loss is graded as follows:

Mild – 20–40 dBHL
Moderate – 40–60 dBHL
Severe – 60–90 dBHL
Profound – >90 dBHL

Hearing Rehabilitation

The field of hearing rehabilitation and implants has recently expanded significantly with many devices available on the market. Given the proliferation of electrically active implantable devices, the field of electroacousticals is predicted to grow exponentially.

Bone Conduction Hearing Devices

In 1965, Branemark et al. [1] began using osseointegrated titanium implants to fit dental prostheses, a process which results in a direct structural and functional connection between ordered, living bone and the surface of a load-bearing implant. This discovery led to the development of the first bone-anchored hearing aid (BAHA) by Tjellstrom et al. [2] in Gothenburg, Sweden in 1977. The first patients were implanted in 1982. These devices can be active or passive, and percutaneous or transcutaneous.

Clinical and Audiological Indications for Bone Conduction Implants

Bone conduction hearing devices are indicated for patients with conductive hearing losses who are unable to wear acoustic hearing aids such as a chronically discharging ear or congenital malformation of the pinna and EAC and single-sided deafness (SSD).

Audiological Criteria

Conductive and Mixed Hearing Loss

In order for a bone conduction device to successfully rehabilitate hearing, the bone conduction thresholds, which represent the hearing function of the cochlea, must be above a certain level for the sound to be heard by the patient. In patients with a conductive or mixed hearing loss, the average pure tone bone conduction threshold (0.5, 1, 2 and 3 kHz) of the indicated ear must be better than or equal to 45 dB HL. Individuals with an average air-bone gap greater than 30 dB are likely to benefit from a bone conduction device compared to an acoustic aid [3]. The hearing loss should preferably be stable and their word recognition scores should allow adequate sound discrimination.

Single-Sided Deafness

In order for the bone conduction hearing aid to work in this situation, it relies upon the fact that there is hardly any attenuation of the sound when it is transmitted through the skull to the opposite cochlea. It thereby reduces the head shadow effect i.e. the attenuation of sound when it is detected by the better hearing ear, but originates from the side of the poorer hearing ear. This can help the patient to localise sound and enables improved speech intelligibility in noise [4]. In SSD, the average bone-conduction threshold (0.5, 1, 2 and 3 kHz) of the better ear should be 20 dBHL.

Current Devices

The fixation for the bone conduction device can be either percutaneous i.e. skin penetrating or transcutaneous, which relies on a magnetic connection either side of the scalp.

Percutaneous

Examples of percutaneous device are BAHA® Connect or Dermalock (Fig. 10.1a, b) or the Oticon® Ponto Plus.

The percutaneous device consists of a titanium fixture, which is placed approximately 50 mm from the tragus along the temporal line. An abutment, which is designed to penetrate the skin, is then fitted onto the fixture. The titanium fixture undergoes osseointegration, a process by which bone grows into the fixture preventing any progressive relative movement between the fixture and the skull. After a period of 2 to 6 weeks, the sound processor is loaded onto the abutment. In children, the fitting of the abutment is delayed due to the skull being thinner and the risk of fixture loss being greater if it is fitted too early.

The BAHA Dermalock abutment was introduced in 2012. It is coated with hydroxyapatite, which enables soft tissue integration to the hydroxyapatite surface and is said to be associated with fewer skin-related complications.

Both Cochlear and Oticon have introduced a more powerful sound processor with enough gain to aid those with thresholds up to 55 dB. Their devices can also increase the output in the mid- and high-frequencies range (6–9 k bandwidth) to reproduce louder sounds [5].

As the abutment penetrates the skin, it requires daily maintenance by the patient or carer and can be associated with soft tissue complications ranging from mild erythema and granulation to florid infection necessitating removal of the abutment. According to the literature, the rate of adverse skin reactions ranges from 9% to 16% [6, 7]. The other main complication associated with this device is fixture loss,

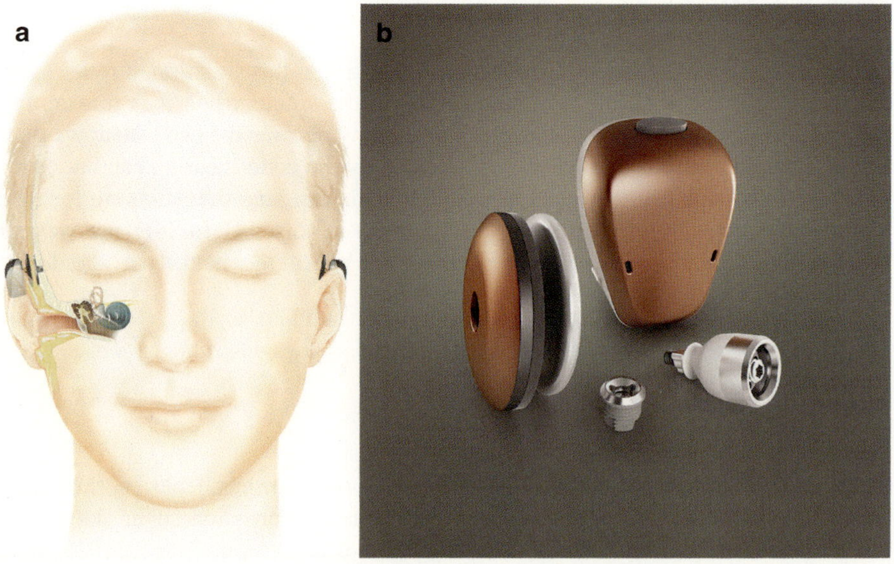

Fig. 10.1 (**a**) BAHA working principle (Cochlear); (**b**) BAHA 5 components (Cochlear)

which ranges from 2.5% to 3.8% [6] in an adult patient group. This significantly increases in children to 15.2% according to Dun et al. [8] due to thinner skull bone and the greater risk of trauma dislodging the abutment. Oticon introduced a wider implant for increased surface contact with bone.

Transcutaneous

The transcutaneous device overcomes the skin problems associated with the percutaneous device as the underlying skin is left intact.

The first transcutaneous bone conduction device, the Xomed-Audiant, was developed in 1986 by Hough et al. [9]. This consisted of a permanent magnet, covered by a thinned skin flap, which was driven by an external coil positioned on the skin above the implanted magnet and secured by a coupling magnet. The major disadvantage was the significantly reduced gain and maximum output compared to the percutaneous device [10], a consequence of the distance between the implanted magnet and the external driving coil [11]. Examples of transcutaneous devices are the BAHA Attract and the Sophono Alpha 1.

BAHA® Attract

This new transcutaneous, osseointegrated bone conduction device uses magnet retention to connect the sound processor to the implant. The internal implant magnet is retained by a single fixture and the sound processor snaps onto the external magnet placed on the skin. In addition to an intact skin flap, another advantage of this system is single-point transmission i.e. through the single implant, which enables increased sound transmission efficiency when compared to fixation with multiple screws [12].

Cochlear™ state that the average aided threshold over 0.5, 1, 2 and 4 kHz is 8.8 dB lower than with the percutaneous bone conduction aid with the greatest difference observed in the higher frequencies [12]. This is slightly better than the results obtained with the Sophono Alpha 1. With the use of a skull simulator, Hol et al. [13] demonstrated that the percutaneous bone conduction aid was 10 dB louder than the Sophono. The stated difference was equal to the benefit of percutaneous coupling compared with transcutaneous coupling as reported by Hakansson et al. [10].

In their study of 16 adult patients, comparing the BAHA Attract with a percutaneous bone conduction aid, Kurz et al. [14] demonstrated that there was a significant difference in the aided soundfield thresholds between the two devices with the percutaneous outperforming the transcutaneous device by approximately 10 dB at frequencies higher than 2 kHz and at 250 Hz. In aided speech understanding, they demonstrated no significant difference in speech in quiet and in noise between the BAHA Attract and the percutaneous device. They state that the additional attenuation of the BAHA Attract increases from approximately 5 dB at 1 kHz to 20–25 dB at 6 to 8 kHz when compared to the percutaneous device. Therefore, many of the speech frequencies remained unaffected.

Sophono Alpha 1

The Sophono Alpha 1 was introduced in 2006 in Europe and 2011 in USA. It comprises of a behind-the-ear external audio processor containing a bone conduction vibrator. The internal component consisted of two magnets attached to the skull with titanium screws to allow for osseointegration. However, there were several issues related to low gain. In their study of 23 patients implanted with the Sophono Alpha 1 for conductive hearing loss due to congenital canal atresia, Siegert et al. [15] demonstrated mean speech recognition scores of 77% in free-field speech testing at 65 dBHL. In two further studies of children implanted with the Sophono for bilateral canal atresia, Siegert et al. [16, 17] demonstrated sound-field speech recognition scores of 86% and 72%.

The reduced level of gain achieved by the Sophono significantly limits patient selection. In their comparative study of amplification options in patients with a mixed hearing loss, Zwartenkot et al. [18] demonstrated that the Sophono had the least gain when compared to the BAHA Divino, Cordelle and Vibrant Soundbridge. They stated that if an aided threshold of 35 dBHL was considered as acceptable, the Sophono could be used with bone conduction thresholds of 20 dBHL or better. In agreement with this, Sylvester et al. [19] in their study of patients with conductive or mixed hearing loss, demonstrated an average gain of 6.2 ± 5.3 dBHL for patients with bilateral mixed hearing loss and 21.9 ± 10.4 dBHL for those with bilateral conductive hearing loss. They concluded that the Sophono device could only be used in patients with normal or sub-normal cochlear function with bone conduction thresholds of 20 dBHL or better.

Expanding Indications

Both Cochlear and Oticon have developed a range of wireless products compatible with sound processors, allowing the user to speak on the phone or listen to a speaker or watch television with the devices streaming directly to the processor.

Bonebridge

The Med El Bonebridge (Fig. 10.2) is an active semi-implantable transcutaneous bone conduction device introduced in 2012. It consists of an external part, the audio processor and an internal part, the bone conduction implant (BCI), which consists of a receiver coil, a demodulator and a transducer. Sound information from the

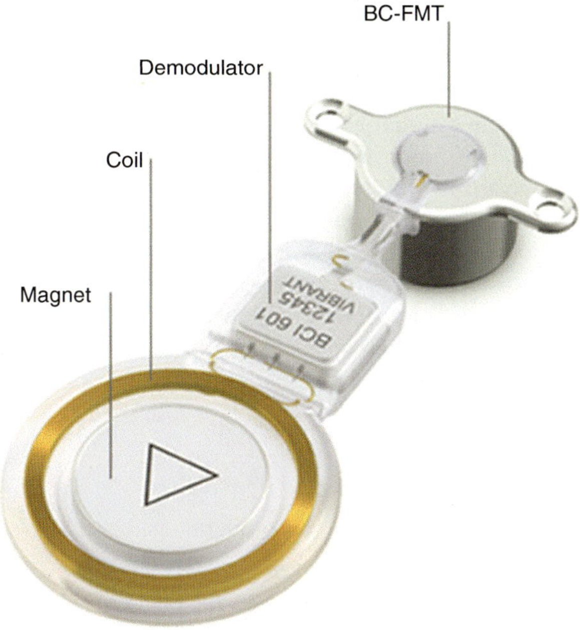

Fig. 10.2 MedEl Bonebridge device

audio processor is sent transcutaneously to the BCI, causing vibration of the transducer, the bone conduction floating mass transducer. Bone conduction thresholds must be no worse than 45 dB in the poorer hearing ear or at least 20 dB in the contralateral ear in SSD.

In their study of 24 patients, Riss et al. [20] demonstrated an overall functional hearing gain was 28.8 dB and a significant increase in monosyllabic word scores, concluding that the Bonebridge provided satisfactory improvements in functional gain and speech perception.

Surgery

Surgery for the percutaneous device has undergone several evolutionary steps.

The technique was initially described using a dermatome to create a skin flap followed by reduction of the subcutaneous soft tissue with hair follicle removal. There have been many variations of the procedure with many surgeons now performing a linear incision without soft tissue reduction and using a longer abutment which are associated with lower complication rates [21].

The transcutaneous device is positioned in the same manner as the percutaneous device. An inferiorly-based C-shaped incision is fashioned with the position of the implant at its centre and the implant magnet is anchored to the skull. All patients were loaded with a sound processor 6 to 8 weeks post-operatively

Middle Ear Implants

Middle ear implants are surgically implanted electronic devices, which are placed in the middle ear cleft and directly stimulate the ossicular chain or cochlea [22] leaving the EAC unobstructed. The basic components consist of a microphone, sound processor, battery, receptor and a vibration transducer, which is attached to the ossicular chain. The transducer can be either piezoelectric or electromagnetic and is capable of producing vibrational energy, which vibrates the ossicular chain, enabling the transfer of sound through the middle ear conduction mechanism [23]. Middle ear implants are indicated for patients who have failed to respond to other conservative therapies, including an optimally fitted hearing aid. They are of no benefit to the patient with profound hearing loss.

History

Fully implantable Middle Ear Implants have been the holy grail of hearing rehabilitation by amplification of sound for many years. Efforts can be traced back to the initial attempts by Wilska in 1935 [24] with iron particles placed directly on the tympanic membrane and activated by a magnetic field. Subsequent attempts in 1959 by Rutschmann in 1959 [25] and Fredrickson et al. in 1973 [26] were helped by advances in technology [26–30]. In 1995, Fredrickson et al. developed the Otologics MET, which was powered electromagnetically [29] and attached to the incus by a connecting rod. The transducer placed in the mastoid cavity was connected electrically to a receiving coil placed subcutaneously [31]. In 2005, a fully implantable version of the Otologics MET (now Cochlear CARINA™) was released.

A new device currently being developed by the Fraunhofer Institute for Manufacturing Engineering and Automation IPA in Stuttgart employs an electro-acoustic transducer with a piezoelectric micro-actuator, directly transmitting acoustic signals to the inner ear via the round window with a potential output of up to 120 dB [32].

Types of Implantable Middle Ear Devices

Implantable hearing devices can be either partially or totally implantable, the microphone and the power supply being incorporated into the fully implantable devices. The implanted microphone has the potential drawback of amplifying unwanted internal body sounds, therefore, many of the devices are partially implantable [32].

There are two types of transducer used by middle ear implants:

- Electromagnetic (Otologics, Vibrant Soundbridge)
- Piezoelectric (Envoy)

Electromagnetic devices consist of a magnet (made of rare earth metal either samarium cobalt or neodymium iron boron) and an energising coil. The magnet is attached to the ossicular chain, tympanic membrane or the round window of the cochlea. The external microphone of the device sends the signal through an inductive coil that creates a magnetic field. The implanted receiving coil detects the signal and connects to a transducer attached to an ossicle or the round window membrane and vibrates in synchrony with the magnetic field, transducing sound to the cochlea [32].

The piezoelectric devices pioneered by Yanagihara and Suzuki use a piezoelectric crystal, which can function as a microphone, generating electric charge in response to incoming sound energy which bend the crystal and act as a driver when attached to the ossicles, moving them in response to electric charge from the microphone [33].

Vibrant Soundbridge®

The Vibrant Soundbridge® (Fig. 10.3) is a middle ear hearing implant that was first implanted in 1996 for moderate to severe sensorineural hearing loss. Since 2007 it has been approved for conductive and mixed hearing loss and in 2009 was approved by EU authorities for implantation in children.

It consists of an implanted part, the vibrating ossicular prosthesis (VORP) and an external part, the audio processor (AP). This is worn behind the ear, attached by magnetic retention. The VORP consists of a receiver coil, a conductor link and the floating mass transducer (FMT) [34].

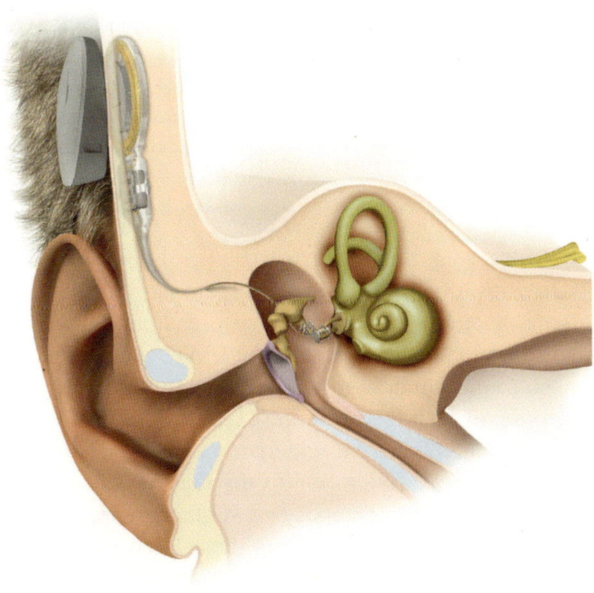

Fig. 10.3 MedEl Vibrant Soundbridge

Audiological Indications and Patient Selection

The Vibrant Soundbridge® or other middle ear implant is suitable mainly for two groups of patients. Firstly, patients with a stable, non-progressive sensorineural hearing loss with normal middle ear anatomy and function and no retrocochlear pathology [35].

Secondly, patients with a conductive or mixed hearing loss with stable bone conduction thresholds and healthy middle ear space [35].

The Vibrant Soundbridge® is indicated for all patients with a mild to severe hearing impairment with bone conduction thresholds of at least 45 dB HL in the low frequencies and 65 dB HL in the high frequencies.

Surgery

There are two main methods of implantation: incus coupling involves attachment of the FMT to the long process of the incus and round window vibroplasty, which involves placement of the FMT directly onto the round window.

The first patient with sensorineural hearing loss was implanted in 1996 by Ugo Fisch [36] using an incus coupling method. A partial mastoidectomy and posterior tympanotomy are performed, through which the FMT is passed into the middle ear space and attached to the incus using a titanium clip. In 2006, Colletti et al. [37, 38] proposed that the FMT could be placed in the round window to improve outcomes in patients with severe-profound conductive or mixed hearing loss. The round window vibroplasty technique is based upon the idea of sonoinversion as described by Garcia Ibanez [39] who stated that the cochlea can still hear sound if the sound is presented at the round window causing a reversal of the travelling wave.

Vibroplasty in Various Conditions

Published studies have demonstrated a mean functional gain of approximately 30 dB from vibroplasty in sensorineural loss [36, 40].

In atresia of the EAC, the middle ear can be approached directly through the atretic plate or via a cortical mastoidectomy and atticotomy. If there is associated malformation of the ossicles, the FMT can be attached to the stapes, oval window or the round window membrane. A more radical option, in patients with difficult anatomy, is via a fenestration [41].

In patients that have undergone canal wall down mastoidectomy with an open cavity, a staged obliteration of the mastoid cavity and placement of the FMT onto the round window or stapes or a subfacial approach can be used [42].

Complications are similar to those in cochlear implantation e.g. extrusions, partial or total flap necrosis and migration of the FMT.

The Envoy Esteem® Hearing Implant

This is a fully implantable hearing device developed by the Envoy Medical Corporation. The Esteem® consists of two separate piezoelectric transducers placed at different locations along the ossicular chain with one transducer coupled to the incus which communicates through a processor implanted under the postauricular scalp with a driver implanted coupled to the stapes. The design enables the user to have complete freedom compared to external hearing aids by allowing use while swimming, bathing and sleeping [43].

Indications

The Esteem® was approved for patients with stable moderate to severe hearing loss and speech discrimination scores greater than 60% along with normal Eustachian tube function and normal middle ear and tympanic membrane function and anatomy and radiographic evidence of an adequately sized mastoid to house the implant [44].

Surgery

A postauricular incision followed by a mastoidectomy with wide exposure of the body of the incus in the antrum and an enlarged posterior tympanotomy to expose the incudostapedial joint allow the transducers to be introduced into the middle ear space.

Complications

Due to the enlarged posterior tympanotomy for wide access to the facial recess, there is a risk of damage to the chorda tympani of between 30% [45] and 60% [46], temporary facial weakness can occur in up to 8% [45] and permanent in as many as 1% [46]. Kraus et al. quoted vertigo as high as 8% [46].

Ototronix MAXUM System

The Ototronix Maxum System (Ototronix LLC, Texas, USA) is a semi-implantable electromagnetic device that transfers energy from an external ear canal mould to an internally implanted magnet. A neodymium iron boron magnet mounted on the incudostapedial joint by collar prosthesis was powerful but small and lightweight [47]. The Maxum system is unique in that it has a combined digital sound processor and electromagnetic coil worn in the ear canal, known as the integrated processor and coil (IPC). The microphone, processor and transducer of the Maxum system are all housed within a single external ear canal mould. The charged coil produces an electromagnetic field, the magnet of which is synchronous to the original sound input, which is then transmitted to the stapes and cochlea. Feedback is overcome by not having an amplifying speaker. The implant magnet is composed of neodymium iron boron, housed in a titanium cylinder and attached to an open wireform ring. The open end of the attachment coil, which is composed of Nitinol, is placed around the ISJ and closes around the joint when exposed to heat [48].

Indications

The device is indicated in adult patients with moderate to moderately severe sensorineural hearing loss with normal middle ear anatomy and no previous middle ear surgery or active otitis media, retrocochlear lesions or central auditory system pathology. The canal must be 20 mm long, 4 mm wide at the canal aperture and 3 mm at the second bend of the canal to the tympanic membrane to accommodate the device [48]. It is recommended that patients should not undergo MRI, however, one study demonstrated that there were no problems at up to 0.3T [49].

Surgery

The electromagnetic coil of the MAXUM in the ear canal mold and the magnet should be aligned in parallel to maximise the magnet's vibratory capabilities and resulting functional gain of the device. Non-magnetic instruments are used to handle soft tissue.

Outcomes

Hough et al. [50] demonstrated that the SOUNDTEC system (now replaced by the MAXUM) device provided an average functional gain of 7.9 dB compared to conventional hearing aids while Roland et al. reported a mean 9.9 dB functional gain [51].

Cochlear Implantation

History

The history of cochlear implantation is one of the most interesting in electrically implanted devices to replace the function of a sense organ. In 1957, Andre Djourno, a professor of medical physics and C. Eyries, an otologist made a serendipitous discovery. Their original aim was to directly stimulate the facial nerve of a patient with bilateral facial palsy following cholesteatoma surgery by inserting a copper wire directly into the cochlea. Although unsuccessful in their original aim, they did manage to stimulate the cochlear nerve electrically using an alternating current, enabling the patient to perceive the rhythm of language [52]. In 1961, William House developed a single electrode implant. In conjunction with Doyle, he implanted three patients with a single gold electrode. This device stimulated the whole set of cochlear nerve fibres simultaneously. Although it was a major breakthrough, it only allowed patients to appreciate the timbre of speech.

In 1966, Blair Simmons [53], based at Stanford University developed a six-electrode system using a percutaneous plug, which he implanted in the trunk of the cochlear nerve. He demonstrated that stimulation of different groups of the cochlear nerve fibres generated sensations of different frequencies depending on the origin of the stimulated fibres on the cochlear.

In 1969, William House implanted the first hardwire five-electrode system into three patients. This was followed in 1973 by Michelson, based at UCSF who implanted an experimental multichannel implant [54]. These efforts would later lead to the formation of Advanced Bionics. In 1975 Claude Henri Chouard and P MacLeold demonstrated that electrical stimulation of 8 to 12 electrodes, isolated from one another and placed in different parts of the scala tympani enabled the recipients to appreciate different frequencies [55]. Following on from their initial success with patients with complete unilateral deafness, they proceeded to perform implantation in those with bilateral deafness.

In 1975, in Vienna, Kurt Burian launched the first Austrian implant, which eventually led to the formation of Med-El [56]. Ingeborg and Erwin Hochmair pursued Burian's work on single-channel intra- and extra-cochlear stimulation and then on multichannel stimulation. In 1977, the first microelectric multi-channel cochlear implant was implanted by Burian. The implant had eight channels, eight independent current sources and a flexible electrode, which Burian inserted through the round window. Later that year they implanted a multichannel system with sufficient flexibility to study the responses to various manipulations of the sound signal [57].

Simultaneously in 1978, in Melbourne, Graham Clark and colleagues developed a multi-channel prototype with an array of 20 electrodes, work that would eventually lead to the founding of Cochlear.

In 1984, the US Food and Drug Administration (FDA) approved the House/3M single-channel implant for adults. In the period 1987–2000, the FDA approved a multiple-channel implant for adults, multiple-channel cochlear implants for children 2 years and older, which was reduced to 18 months and older in 1998 and multiple channel for infants 1 year of age in 2000.

The main CI systems in current widespread use:

1. Cochlear system produced by Cochlear Ltd., Sydney Australia
2. Med-El system produced by Med-El of Innsbruck, Austria
3. Clarion system produced by Advanced Bionics of California, USA
4. Nuerelec system now produced by Oticon, Sweden.

CIs are licensed for patients with severe to profound hearing loss. There are approximately 800,000 people in the UK alone classified as severe to profoundly deaf. The British Cochlear Implant Group recently released figures demonstrating a steady increase in the number of CIs fitted with 1361 patients implanted between 2011 and 2012. According to the Food and Drug Administration (FDA), up until December 2012, approximately 324,000 people world-wide had received CIs. In 2008, a NICE appraisal document estimated the cost-effectiveness of single-sided CIs in post-lingually deaf adults at £14,200 per incremental QALY gained. For pre-lingually deaf children implanted at 1 year of age, this figure decreased to £13,400 [58].

Electrode Array

Once the auditory signal is processed, it is transduced by electrical pulses, which are fired from electrodes located along the array in close proximity to ganglion cells, which transmit the electrical impulses to the auditory cortex. The electrodes are composed of platinum-irridium alloy, which is both conductive and resistant to corrosion with each array containing between 4 and 22 electrodes. The electrodes are separated by poly(dimethylsiloxane) (PDMS) insulation, which is flexible enough to enable the array to be either straight or curved.

The organisation of the electrodes in the array is in accordance with the tonotopic arrangement of the cochlea i.e. each area of the cochlea detects a different frequency with high frequency sound being detected at the basal turn progressing to low frequency sounds at the apex.

The functionality of the CI depends on several array-related factors. The shape of the array may be straight or contoured. The advantage of a contoured electrode (the first prototype introduced by Cochlear in 1989) is that it enables closer apposition with a greater proportion of the nerves positioned on the inner aspect of the cochlea. The disadvantage of the straight electrode is that it has a tendency to be pushed along the outer aspect of the cochlea, which reduced the contact between the array and the nerves they are aiming to stimulate. It has also been associated with a greater risk of damage to the cochlea, either at spiral ligament, osseous spiral lamina, basilar membrane and Reissner's membrane [59].

The depth of insertion and number of electrodes influence the functionality of the CI.

As the implant is advanced along the cochlea, more neurons are activated, which leads to an increase in the range of frequencies that can be stimulated. It is well recognised that multichannel implants are superior to single-channel due to the place coding of frequency. However, the optimum number of channels has not yet been determined. Throughout the development of the CI, numerous arrangements have been trialled with 4 in the Ineraid [60], to 7 or 8 with the Clarion S and Chorimac 8 to 12 with the Chorimac 12 and Combi-40 [61] to 22 with the Nucleus 22 and 24 systems [62]. Blamey et al. [63] demonstrated a correlation between increasing number of electrodes and speech perception whilst Holmes et al. [64] found that open-set word recognition and continuous discourse tracking results for the Nucleus F0/F1/F2 speech processor improved for the use of up to 15 electrodes.

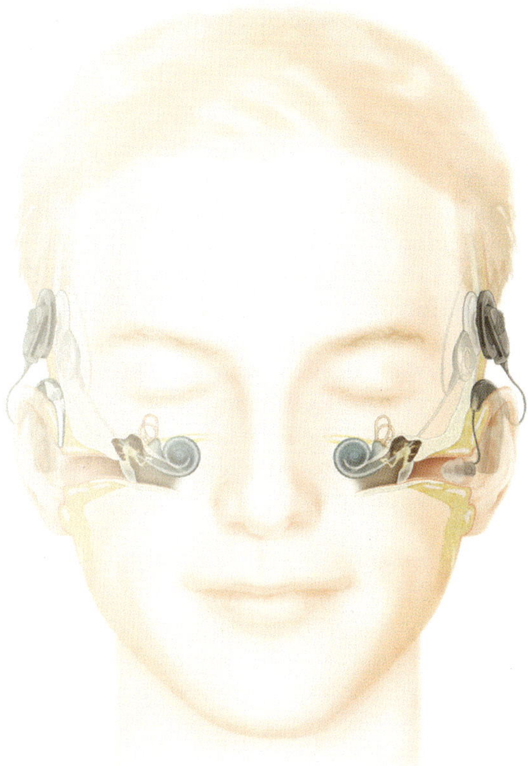

Fig. 10.4 Cochlear Nucleus 6 cochlear implant in right ear and electroacoustic implant in left ear

The density of auditory neurons can vary throughout the cochlea, especially in the presence of pathology; the greater number of electrodes in the Nucleus conveys an advantage in that there are more electrodes available in areas of the cochlea where stimulation is more effective (Fig. 10.4).

To distinguish the most complicated of sentences composed of the full array of vowel sounds at least eight channels are necessary. Many commercially available electrode arrays have far in excess of eight channels [59].

Indications

In the UK, cochlear implantation is governed by NICE [65]. Their guidelines state that patients should have thresholds of 90 dBHL or greater at 2 and 4 kHz. In addition, they should have word discrimination scores of 50% or less at 70 dB in optimal aided conditions using Bamford-Kuwal-Bench (BKB) open sentences. Prior to consideration of implantation, all adults are given a three-month trial of hearing aids. In post-lingual adults, there is only funding currently for a unilateral implant in adults, unless they are deaf-blind, in which they are increasingly reliant on their hearing.

In children, the same audiological criteria exist, but it is not possible to assess their speech using BKB scores, especially in the congenitally deaf child. These children are fitted with hearing aids and assessed as to whether they are achieving their speech milestones. Bilateral simultaneous implantation (or sequential implantation for children who had unilateral implantation prior to NICE guidelines) is funded and most children undergo this. This is due to the recognition that pre-lingual children who have binaural hearing have greater access to language.

Pre-lingually deaf children should be implanted before the age of 4. This is due to the development of the auditory pathway and language centres. Prior to this, neural plasticity is such that these pathways will develop once stimulated. However, if these children are implanted after this age, the necessary pathways will not develop and that patients are unlikely to understand speech or develop language. The cortical areas destined for hearing are taken over by other sensory modalities resulting in failure of auditory perception even when subsequently stimulated by implants. These patients fail to develop spoken language and have a high possibility of becoming non-users of cochlear implants.

The ultimate goal of hearing rehabilitation is to be able to understand open-set speech in everyday environments. Predicting individual outcomes from CI is difficult due to the heterogeneity of implant candidates. It is now widely accepted that in pre-lingual children, earlier implantation results in better outcomes. Implanting pre-lingual children before the age of two will result in almost normal language development with approximately 90% able to be in mainstream education [66]. A number of factors influence outcomes including aetiology of hearing loss, level of residual hearing, mode of communication, rehabilitation (speech therapy, education) and device type [67].

Surgery

Incisions and Flaps

The initial incision used, for the 3M single-electrode implant was C-shaped [68] changed to an inverted J-shape [69] for larger multichannel devices with a receiver-stimulator unit. A modification of this incision by Lehnhardt [70] replaced the upward postauricular limb of the inverted J with an incision in the external auditory canal (extended endaural). This progressed to the S-shaped incision with a postauricular incision extended onto the scalp [59]. More recently, minimal access techniques have led to smaller incisions and minimal hair shaving [71].

Although a variety of designs can be used, a separate anteriorly-based flap of deep fascia and periosteum should be raised to stabilise the implant and protect it from a breakdown of the anterior limb of the incision.

Pockets

Minimal access approaches make it more difficult to achieve bony fixation but this has been made possible by fashioning a pocket in the temporalis fascia [72, 73] or a subperiosteal pocket [74].

Wells and Anchorage

A well in the squamous temporal bone is fashioned to house the receiver-stimulator to prevent it from migration and protrusion. Due to slimmer receiver-stimulators, a well can be drilled down to dura in an infant's skull with a thickness of 1–2 mm [75, 76].

Insertion

Round Window Versus Cochleostomy

In both techniques, a limited cortical mastoidectomy is performed in order to expose the mastoid antrum, short process of incus and the lateral semi-circular canal. A posterior tympanotomy, bounded by the facial nerve posteriorly, chorda tympani anteriorly and fossa incudis superiorly, is performed to access the facial recess of the middle ear and to visualise the round window niche.

In 1975, Clark et al. [77] demonstrated that it was possible to pass an electrode array around the turns of the cochlea to the region of the speech frequencies by drilling into the upper and middle turns directly below the facial nerve and passing the array in a retrograde fashion back toward the round window. The initial issue with a round window insertion was that the array was prevented from lying near the speech frequencies due to the sharp basal turn and friction at the insertion site, which was overcome by developing an array with graded stiffness and a soft flexible tip [78].

The electrode array is inserted into the scala tympani to stimulate the peripheral processes of the auditory nerve if present, in addition to residual spiral ganglion cells. It is important to avoid damage to the spiral lamina and basilar membrane during insertion as this can lead to the loss of ganglion cells [79].

The advantage of performing a cochleostomy over round window insertion is that there is improved access to the scala tympani and the array can pass more easily into it with minimal trauma. Secondly, animal studies have demonstrated that the middle ear infection is more likely to pass between the array and the round window membrane than along the protective fibrous tissue sheath formed around the array at a cochleostomy [59]. However, the vogue has moved towards round window insertion than cochleostomy for improved hearing preservation surgery.

Device Failures

Failure of the implant may be due to malfunction of the electronics, lack of cochlear nerve, damage to the electrodes or extracochlear insertion in a hypotympanic cell.

It is, therefore, imperative for the patient to undergo preoperative CT and MRI scans in order to check for the presence of a cochlear nerve and appreciate the anatomy of the cochlea.

Complications

Cochlear implantation is a very safe procedure with overall major complication rates being extremely low. Suppurative labyrinthitis and meningitis are rare but serious complications. Meningitis following middle ear infection can occur in the early post-operative period prior to the round window seal forming or at a later stage from a superimposed infection. In the 20-year period from 1982–2002, 18 patients were reported as having suffered from meningitis in the USA. In order to prevent this, all patients undergoing cochlear implantation receive the pneumococcal and meningococcal vaccines pre-op.

Facial nerve stimulation occurs in 3.1% of adults and 1.2% of children and is more common in patients with cochlear otosclerosis. If it does occur, the offending electrodes can be turned off [59].

Special Cases

Ossified Cochlea

This can occur following meningitis or as a result of cochlear otosclerosis. In this scenario, a bifid array consisting of two short arrays with dual insertion in order to maximise stimulation of the remaining neurons. One array is inserted along the basal turn and the other into the apical or middle turns through a cochleostomy drilled into the overlying bone [80]. In the case of obliteration of all the cochlear turns, an initial approach involved drilling out the entire basal turn to enable insertion of the multiple-electrode array. Gantz et al. [81] created a channel in the basal turn around the modiolus. Cohen and Waltzman [82] described an alternative approach of inserting a short 8 mm array into a tunnel created along the scala tympani.

Congenital or Genetic Malformation of the Cochlea

Mondini dysplasia of the cochlea results in a reduced number of turns, of which there are usually 2.5. The principal defect is the absence of the interscalar septum between the two upper turns, which leads to a scala communis. It can also be associated with enlarged vestibular aqueduct syndrome. Implantation in this scenario can result in damage to the membranous structures due to the absence of the interscalar septum. The internal auditory meatus may be entered through a dehiscence or a perilymph gusher may be encountered. The risk of meningitis is greater. If the modiolus is well formed, a perimodiolar array can be inserted to stimulate the spiral ganglion cells lying centrally. If absent, a straight array should be inserted to stimulate the nerves as they lie peripherally [59].

Vestibular Schwannoma

If the cochlea nerve remains intact following extirpation of a vestibular schwannoma, (VS) a cochlear implant can be inserted to help restore useful hearing [83].

High-Tone Sensorineural Hearing Loss

In certain patients, their hearing thresholds at 2 and 4 kHz are 90 dB or greater i.e. they have a severe-profound high frequency hearing loss with preservation of the lower frequencies, a so called 'ski-slope' hearing loss. In these patients, a short array can be inserted so that just the high frequencies are stimulated by the CI. This can be used in conjunction with an acoustic hearing aid which aids the low and mid frequencies, a process known as electro-acoustic stimulation (Fig. 10.5).

Results

In 1999, Summerfield and Marshall [84] published the initial large UK multicentre study of patients implanted between 1990 and 1994. Ninety-five percent of patients identified more words correctly when using their implants in conjunction with lipreading. Fifty percent of patients managed to correctly identify some words cor rectly without lipreading. Thirty-five percent of patients demonstrated some level of understanding of questions posed over the telephone. Seventy percent demonstrated improvements in the quality and intelligibility of their speech. These outcomes were sustained 18 months after implantation. The patients most likely to benefit from implantation were those that had recent onset of deafness and lipreading.

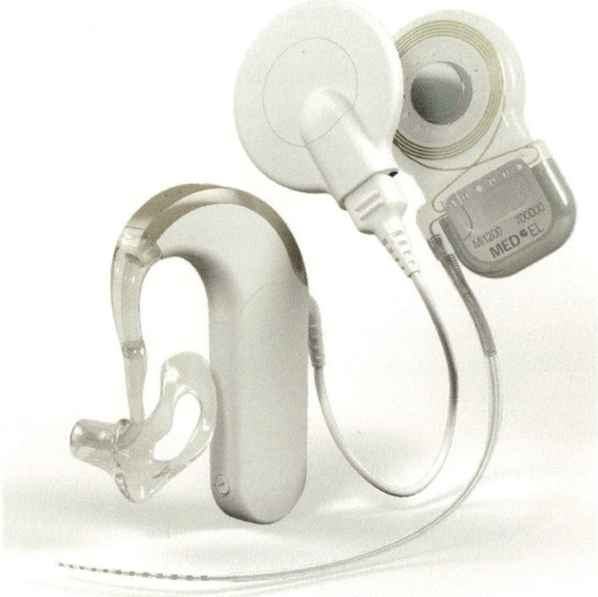

Fig. 10.5 Med El Synchrony electroacoustic stimulation

Future Developments

Total Implantability

The concept of the implant being invisible is attractive to many and would also reduce the energy consumption used to transmit signals through the skin. However, it has not been fully achieved to date, possibly as it will bring with it its own issues. The surgery may become more technically difficult and any technical failures will require further surgery and replacement of the entire device or of certain failed modules. Also, there is ongoing work on robotic assisted electrode insertions for increased accuracy and reduced insertion trauma.

Auditory Brainstem Implants

The insertion of an auditory brainstem implant (ABI) is primarily for Neurofibromatosis 2 (NF2), the main feature of which is bilateral VS. They can also be used for cochlear or cochlear nerve agenesis or hypoplasia.

Damage to the cochlea nerve as a result of VS excision would render a CI useless and, therefore, an ABI can be used to stimulate the cochlea nerve in the brainstem.

House and Hitsleberger first used the ABI in 1979 [85–87]. The electrode of the ABI is introduced into the lateral recess of the fourth ventricle and placed over the area of the ventral and dorsal cochlear nuclei after tumour removal. The ABI is similar in design and function to multichannel cochlear implants except for differences in the design of the stimulating electrode arrays [88–90]. The programming also differs in several important aspects from cochlear implant programming.

In NF2, the ABI is placed during removal of the first tumour even if they have hearing on the contralateral side. This allows the patient to become more familiar with the use of the device and prepares them for the loss of hearing on the other side.

In addition to NF2, ABIs have been implanted for cochlear nerve aplasia and severe cochlear malformations in children, as well as complete cochlea ossification or cochlear nerve disruption die to cochlear trauma in adults [91–94, 95].

Surgical Technique and the Anatomy of the Cochlear Nucleus

The cochlear nucleus complex (dorsal and ventral cochlear nuclei) is part of the floor of the lateral recess of the fourth ventricle [94, 96]. The target for the placement of the electrode array is partially obscured by the cerebellar peduncles. A surface electrode introduced in the lateral recess crossing the tinea choroidea will stimulate viable cells in the cochlear nuclei.

The ABI can be inserted in a translabyrinthine approach, which provides direct access to the cochlear nuclei. The jugular bulb is skeletonized to provide greater access. Anatomical landmarks for placement of the implant are glossopharyngeal nerve, facial nerve and the tinea choroidea as well as the foramen of Luschka where all these structures converge [95].

Device

The ABI electrode is composed of 21 electrodes embedded in a silicone carrier fixed to a fabric mesh and connected to an implantable internal receiver/stimulator. The external component consists of a transmitter coil held in place by magnetic tape placed on the scalp over the receiver/stimulator coil and connected to a sound processor. In patients with NF2 who are likely to need serial MRI scans, the internal magnet is removed. Scans can proceed as long as the magnetic tape and external magnet is removed [97].

ABIs differ from CIs in that CIs usually employ a relatively standard pattern of neural stimulation due to the homogenous arrangement of neurons in the cochlea. ABIs are more varied due to variations in brainstem anatomy, electrode array placement and tumour effects that require the use of more individualised stimulus patterns to code frequency cues and manage nonauditory sensations.

The hearing results of the ABI are poorer compared to a CI. Approximately, 16% of patients achieve open-set discrimination speech [88, 90]. The majority of patients recognise some environmental sounds; speech understanding ability is enhanced by an average of 30% when ABI sounds is added to lip-reading cues.

Colletti et al. [92] described the outcomes for ABI in NF2 patients compared to non-tumour patients. Some of the non-tumour patients achieved good speech discrimination without lipreading and they compared well with the best cochlear implant results. The tumour of NF2 was believed to have damaged specialized cells in the cochlear nucleus, which are important for speech perception. The improved outcomes for non-tumour patients led to the ABI being used for children with congenital cochlear nerve aplasia or hypoplasia [98].

References

1. Branemark PI, Hansson BO, Adell R. Osseointegrated implants in the treatment of the edentulous jaw. Experience from a 10-year period. Scand J Plast Reconstr Surg Suppl. 1977;16:1–132.
2. Tjellstrom A, Lindstrom J, Hallen O, Albrektsson T, Branemark PI. Osseointegrated titanium implants in the temporal bone. A clinical study on bone-anchored hearing aids. Am J Otol. 1981;2:304–10.
3. de Wolf MJ, Hendrix S, Cremers CW, Snik AF. Better performance with bone-anchored hearing aid than acoustic devices in patients with severe air-bone gap. Laryngoscope. 2011;121(3): 613–6.
4. Wazen JJ, Spitzer JB, Ghossaini SN, Fayad JN, Niparko JK, Cox K, et al. Transcranial contralateral cochlear stimulation in unilateral deafness. Otolaryngol Head Neck Surg. 2003;129(3): 248–54.
5. Stelmachowicz PG, Pittman AL, Hoover BM, Lewis DE. Effect of stimulus bandwidth on the perception of/s/in normal- and hearing-impaired children and adults. J Acoust Soc Am. 2001;110(4):2183–90.
6. Calvo Bodnia N, Foghsgaard S, Nue Moller M, Caye-Thomasen P. Long-term results of 185 consecutive osseointegrated hearing device implantations: a comparison among children, adults, and elderly. Otol Neurotol. 2014;35(10):e301–6.
7. de Wolf MJ, Hol MK, Mylanus EA, Cremers CW. Bone-anchored hearing aid surgery in older adults: implant loss and skin reactions. Ann Otol Rhinol Laryngol. 2009;118(7):525–31.
8. Dun CA, de Wolf MJ, Mylanus EA, Snik AF, Hol MK, Cremers CW. Bilateral bone-anchored hearing aid application in children: the Nijmegen experience from 1996 to 2008. Otol Neurotol. 2010;31(4):615–23.
9. Gates GA, Hough JV, Gatti WM, Bradley WH. The safety and effectiveness of an implanted electromagnetic hearing device. Arch Otolaryngol Head Neck Surg. 1989;115(8):924–30.
10. Hakansson B, Tjellstrom A, Carlsson P. Percutaneous vs. transcutaneous transducers for hearing by direct bone conduction. Otolaryngol Head Neck Surg. 1990;102(4):339–44.
11. Gatehouse S, Browning GG. The output characteristics of an implanted bone conduction prosthesis. Clin Otolaryngol Allied Sci. 1990;15(6):503–13.
12. Flynn MC. Design concept and technological considerations for the Cochlear Baha 4 Attract System. Cochlear Bone Anchored Solutions AB. 2013: E82744.
13. Hol MK, Nelissen RC, Agterberg MJ, Cremers CW, Snik AF. Comparison between a new implantable transcutaneous bone conductor and percutaneous bone-conduction hearing implant. Otol Neurotol. 2013;34(6):1071–5.
14. Kurz A, Flynn M, Caversaccio M, Kompis M. Speech understanding with a new implant technology: a comparitive study with a new nonskin penetrating Baha system. Biomed Res Int. 2014:1–9.
15. Siegert R, Kanderske J. A new semi-implantable transcutaneous bone conduction device: clinical, surgical, and audiologic outcomes in patients with congenital ear canal atresia. Otol Neurotol. 2013;34(5):927–34.

16. Siegert R. Magnetic coupling of partially implantable bone conduction hearing aids without open implants. Laryngorhinootologie. 2010;89(6):346–51.
17. Siegert R. Partially implantable bone conduction hearing aids without a percutaneous abutment (Otomag): technique and preliminary clinical results. Adv Otorhinolaryngol. 2011;71:41–6.
18. Zwartenkot JW, Snik AFM, Mylanus EAM, Mulder JJS. Amplification options for patients with mixed hearing loss. Otol Neurotol. 2014;35:221–6.
19. Sylvester DC, Gardner R, Reilly PG, et al. Audiologic and surgical outcomes of a novel, non-percutaneous, bone conducting hearing implant. Otol Neurotol. 2013;34:922–6.
20. Riss D, Arnoldner C, Baumgartner WD, Blineder M, Flak S, Bachner A, et al. Indication criteria and outcomes with the Bonebridge transcutaneous bone-conduction implant. Laryngoscope. 2014;124(12):2802–6.
21. Carr SD, Moraleda J, Baldwin A, Ray J. Bone-conduction hearing aids in an elderly population: complications and quality of life assessment. Eur Arch Otorhinolaryngol. 2015. 273(3):567–571.
22. Manrique M, Valdivieso A, Ruba D, Gimeno-Vilar C, Montes-Jovellar L, Manrique R. Review of audiometric criteria in treatment of neurosensorial deafness with hearing aids and implantable hearing devices. Acta Otorrinolaringol Esp. 2008;59(1):30–8.
23. Kulkarni K, Hartley DE. Recent advances in hearing restoration. J R Soc Med. 2008;101(3): 116–24.
24. Wilska A. Einmethode zur bestimmung der horsch wellanamplituden des trommelfells bei verscheiden frequenzen. Skand Arch Physiol. 1935;72:161–5.
25. Rutschmann J. Magnetic audition: auditory stimulation by means of alternating magnetic fields acting on a permanent magnet fixed to the eardrum. IRE Trans Med Electron. 1959;6: 22–3.
26. Fredrickson J, Tomlinson D, David E, Odvist M. Evaluation of an electromagnetic implantable hearing aid. Can J Otolaryngol. 1973;2:53–62.
27. Goode RL. An implantable hearing aid. State of the art. Trans Am Acad Ophthalmol Otolaryngol. 1970;74(1):128–39.
28. Goode RL. Electromagnetic implantable hearing aids. In: Suzuki J-I, editor. Advances in otology. Basel: Karger; 1988. p. 44–31.
29. Fredrickson JM, Coticchia JM, Khosla S. Ongoing investigations into an implantable electromagnetic hearing aid for moderate to severe sensorineural hearing loss. Otolaryngol Clin N Am. 1995;28(1):107–20.
30. Fredrickson J, Coticchia JM, Khosla S. Current status in the develpment of implantable middle ear hearing aids. In: Advances in Otolaryngology. St. Louis: Mosby; 1996. p. 189–204.
31. Snik A. Implantable hearing devices for conductive and sensorineural hearing impairment. In: Zeng FG, Popper AN, Fay RR, editors. Auditory prostheses new horizons. New York: Springer Science + Business Media LLC; 2011.
32. Mankekar G. Implantable hearing devices besides cochlear and brain stem implants. In: Mankekar G, editor. Implantable hearing devices other than cochlear implants. New Delhi: Springer; 2014. p. 25–41.
33. Snik AF, Mylanus EA, Cremers CW. Implantable hearing devices for sensorineural hearing loss: a review of the audiometric data. Clin Otolaryngol Allied Sci. 1998;23(5):414–9.
34. Mankekar G. Bone conduction implant devices. In: Mankekar G, editor. Implantable hearing devices other than cochlear implants. New Delhi: Springer; 2014. p. 41–71.
35. Green K. The role of active middle-ear implants in the rehabilitation of hearing loss. Expert Rev Med Devices. 2011;8(4):441–7.
36. Fisch U, Cremers CW, Lenarz T, Weber B, Babighian G, Uziel AS, et al. Clinical experience with the Vibrant Soundbridge implant device. Otol Neurotol. 2001;22(6):962–72.
37. Colletti V, Soli SD, Carner M, Colletti L. Treatment of mixed hearing losses via implantation of a vibratory transducer on the round window. Int J Audiol. 2006;45(10):600–8.
38. Colletti L, Mandala M, Colletti V. Long-term outcome of round window Vibrant SoundBridge implantation in extensive ossicular chain defects. Otolaryngol Head Neck Surg. 2013;149(1): 134–41.

39. Garcia-Ibanez L. Sonoinversion: a new audiosurgical system. Arch Otolaryngol. 1961;73: 268–72.
40. Snik AF, Mylanus EA, Cremers CW, Dillier N, Fisch U, Gnadeberg D, et al. Multicenter audiometric results with the Vibrant Soundbridge, a semi-implantable hearing device for sensorineural hearing impairment. Otolaryngol Clin N Am. 2001;34(2):373–88.
41. Pau HW, Just T. Third window vibroplasty: an alternative in surgical treatment of tympanosclerotic obliteration of the oval and round window niche. Otol Neurotol. 2010;31:225–7.
42. Zernotti ME, Grasso P. Middle ear implants: vibrant Soundbridge. In: Mankekar G, editor. Implantable hearing devices othe than cochlear implants. New Delhi: Springer; 2014.
43. Sweeney AD, Carlson ML, Glasscock ME. The envoy esteem hearing implant. In: Mankekar G, editor. Implantable hearing devices other than cochlear implants. New Delhi: Springer; 2014. p. 85–97.
44. FDA. FDA – esteem implantable hearing system – P090018. 2014. Available from: http://www.fda.gov/MedicalDevices/ProductsandMedicalProcedures/DeviceApprovalsandClearances/Recently-ApprovedDevices. Cited 29 Jan 2015.
45. Klein K, Nardelli A, Stafinski T. A systematic review of the safety and effectiveness of fully implantable middle ear hearing devices: the carina and esteem systems. Otol Neurotol. 2012;33(6):916–21.
46. Kraus EM, Shohet JA, Catalano PJ. Envoy Esteem totally implantable hearing system: phase 2 trial, 1-year hearing results. Otolaryngol Head Neck Surg. 2011;145(1):100–9.
47. Baker RS, Wood MW, Hough JV. The implantable hearing device for sensorineural hearing impairment. The hough ear institute experience. Otolaryngol Clin N Am. 1995;28:147–53.
48. Pelosi S, Carlson ML, Glasscock ME. The ototronix MAXUM system. In: Mankekar G, editor. Implantable hearing devices other than cochlear implants. New Delhi: Springer; 2014. p. 97–109.
49. Dyer Jr RK, Nakmali D, Dormer KJ. Magnetic resonance imaging compatibility and safety of the SOUNDTEC Direct System. Laryngoscope. 2006;116(8):1321–33.
50. Hough JV, Matthews P, Wood MW, Dyer Jr RK. Middle ear electromagnetic semi-implantable hearing device: results of the phase II SOUNDTEC direct system clinical trial. Otol Neurotol. 2002;23(6):895–903.
51. Roland PS, Shoup AG, Shea MC, Richey HS, Jones DB. Verification of improved patient outcomes with a partially implantable hearing aid, The SOUNDTEC direct hearing system. Laryngoscope. 2001;111(10):1682–6.
52. Djourno A, Eyries C. Auditory prosthesis by means of a distant electrical stimulation of the sensory nerve with the use of an indwelt coiling. Presse Med. 1957;65(63):141.
53. Simmons FB. Electrical stimulation of the auditory nerve in man. Arch Otolaryngol. 1966;84(1):2–54.
54. Michelson RP, Merzenich MM, Pettit CR, Schindler RA. A cochlear prosthesis: further clinical observations; preliminary results of physiological studies. Laryngoscope. 1973;83(7): 1116–22.
55. Mac Leold P, Pialoux P, Chouard CH, Meyer B. Physiological assessment of the rehabilitation of total deafness by the implantation of multiple intracochlear electrodes. Ann Otolaryngol Chir Cervicofac. 1975;92(1–2):17–23.
56. Burian K. Letter: significance of cochlear nerve electric stimulation in totally deaf patients. Laryngol Rhinol Otol. 1975;54(6):530–1.
57. Hochmair ES, Hochmair-Desoyer IJ, Burian K. Investigations towards an artificial cochlea. Int J Artif Organs. 1979;2(5):255–61.
58. Actiononhearingloss. Facts and figures on deafness and tinnitus. 2012. Available from: http://www.actionhearingloss.org.uk/your-hearing/aboyt-deafness-and-hearing-loss/statistics.
59. Clark GM. In Cochlear implants: fundamentals and application. Beyer RT, editor. New York: Springer; 2003.
60. Eddington DK. Speech recognition in deaf subjects with multichannel intracochlear electrodes. Ann N Y Acad Sci. 1983;405:241–58.

61. Fugain C, Meyer B, Chabolle F, Chouard CH. Clinical results of the French multichannel cochlear implant. Acta Otolaryngol Suppl. 1984;411:237–46.
62. Clark GM, Black R, Forster IC, Patrick JF, Tong YC. Design criteria of a multiple-electrode cochlear implant hearing prosthesis [43.66.Ts, 43.66.Sr]. J Acoust Soc Am. 1978;63(2): 631–3.
63. Blamey PJ, Pyman BC, Gordon M, Clark GM, Brown AM, Dowell RC, et al. Factors predicting postoperative sentence scores in postlinguistically deaf adult cochlear implant patients. Ann Otol Rhinol Laryngol. 1992;101(4):342–8.
64. Holmes AE, Kemker FJ, Merwin GE. The effects of varying the number of cochlear implant electrodes on speech perception. Am J Otol. 1987;8(3):240–6.
65. Cochlear implants for children and adults with severe to profound hearing loss. NICE. 2009.
66. Holt RF, Svirsky MA. An exploratory look at pediatric cochlear implantation: is earliest always best? Ear Hear. 2008;29(4):492–511.
67. Osberger MJ, Fisher L. Preoperative predictors of postoperative implant performance in children. Ann Otol Rhinol Laryngol Suppl. 2000;185:44–6.
68. House WF. Surgical considerations in cochlear implantation. Ann Otol Rhinol Laryngol Suppl. 1982;91(2 Pt 3):15–20.
69. Clark GM, Pyman BC, Bailey QR. The surgery for multiple-electrode cochlear implantations. J Laryngol Otol. 1979;93(3):215–23.
70. Lehnhardt E, Hirshorn MS. Cochlear implants. Cochlear implants. Berline: Springer; 1986. p. 128–32.
71. Prager JD, Neidich MJ, Perkins JN, Meinzen-Derr J, Greinwald Jr JH. Minimal access and standard cochlear implantation: a comparative study. Int J Pediatr Otorhinolaryngol. 2012;76(8):1102–6.
72. Balkany TJ, Whitley M, Shapira Y, Angeli SI, Brown K, Eter E, et al. The temporalis pocket technique for cochlear implantation: an anatomic and clinical study. Otol Neurotol. 2009;30(7): 903–7.
73. Shelton C, Warren FM. Minimal access cochlear implant fixation: temporalis pocket with a plate. Otol Neurotol. 2012;33(9):1530–4.
74. Jethanamest D, Channer GA, Moss WJ, Lustig LR, Telischi FF. Cochlear implant fixation using a subperiosteal tight pocket without either suture or bone-recess technique. Laryngoscope. 2014;124(7):1674–7.
75. Burton MJ, Cohen LT, Rickards FW, McNally KI, Clark GM. Steady-state evoked potentials to amplitude modulated tones in the monkey. Acta Otolaryngol. 1992;112(5):745–51.
76. Burton MJ, Shepherd RK, Xu SA, Xu J, Franz BK, Clark GM. Cochlear implantation in young children: histological studies on head growth, leadwire design, and electrode fixation in the monkey model. Laryngoscope. 1994;104(2):167–75.
77. Clark GM. A surgical approach for a cochlear implant: an anatomical study. J Laryngol Otol 1975;89(1):9–15. Epub 1975/01/01.
78. Clark GM, Patrick JF, Bailey Q. A cochlear implant round window electrode array. J Laryngol Otol. 1979;93(2):107–9.
79. Franz BK, Clark GM, Bloom DM. Surgical anatomy of the round window with special reference to cochlear implantation. J Laryngol Otol. 1987;101(2):97–102.
80. Chouard CH, Meyer B, Fugain C, Koca O. Clinical results for the DIGISONIC multichannel cochlear implant. Laryngoscope. 1995;105(5 Pt 1):505–9.
81. Gantz BJ, McCabe BF, Tyler RS. Use of a multichannel cochlear implants in obstructed and obliterated cochleas. Otolaryngol Head Neck Surg. 1989;98:72–81.
82. Cohen NL, Waltzman SB. Partial insertion of the nucleus multichannel cochlear implant: technique and results. Am J Otol. 1993;14(4):357–61.
83. Hulka GF, Bernard EJ, Pillsbury HC. Cochlear implantation in a patient after removal of an acoustic neuroma. The implications of magnetic resonance imaging with gadolinium on patient management. Arch Otolaryngol Head Neck Surg. 1995;121(4):465–8.

84. Summerfield AQ, Marshall DH. Cochlear implantation in the UK 1990–1994. Report by the Medical Research Council Institute of Hearing Research: HMSO Books; 1999.
85. Edgerton BJ, House WF, Hitselberger W. Hearing by cochlear nucleus stimulation in humans. Ann Otol Rhinol Laryngol Suppl. 1982;91(2 Pt 3):117–24.
86. Eisenberg LS, Maltan AA, Portillo F, Mobley JP, House WF. Electrical stimulation of the auditory brain stem structure in deafened adults. J Rehabil Rses Dev. 1987;24(3):9–22.
87. Portillo F, Nelson RA, Brackmann DE, Hitselberger WE, Shannon RV, Waring MD, et al. Auditory brain stem implant: electrical stimulation of the human cochlear nucleus. Adv Otorhinolaryngol. 1993;48:248–52.
88. Brackmann DE, Hitselberger WE, Nelson RA, Moore J, Waring MD, Portillo F, et al. Auditory brainstem implant: I. Issues in surgical implantation. Otolaryngol Head Neck Surg. 1993;108(6):624–33.
89. Schwartz MS, Otto SR, Brackmann DE, Hitselberger WE, Shannon RV. Use of a multichannel auditory brainstem implant for neurofibromatosis type 2. Stereotact Funct Neurosurg. 2003;81(1–4):110–4.
90. Shannon RV, Fayad J, Moore J, Lo WW, Otto S, Nelson RA, et al. Auditory brainstem implant: II. Postsurgical issues and performance. Otolaryngol Head Neck Surg. 1993;108(6):634–42.
91. Colletti V, Carner M, Miorelli V, Guida M, Colletti L, Fiorino F. Auditory brainstem implant (ABI): new frontiers in adults and children. Otolaryngol Head Neck Surg. 2005;133(1): 126–38.
92. Colletti V, Shannon RV. Open set speech perception with auditory brainstem implant? Laryngoscope. 2005;115(11):1974–8.
93. Colletti V, Fiorino FG, Carner M, Giarbini N, Sacchetto L, Cumer G. The retrosigmoid approach for auditory brainstem implantation. Am J Otol. 2000;21(6):826–36.
94. Terr LI, Edgerton BJ. Surface topography of the cochlear nuclei in humans: two- and three-dimensional analysis. Hear Res 1985;17(1):51–59. Epub 1985/01/01.
95. Fayad JN, Otto SR, Brackmann DE. Auditory brainstem implants: surgical aspects. In: Møller AR, editor. Cochlear and brainstem implants. Munich: Karger; 2006. p. 144–54.
96. Kuroki A, Moller AR. Microsurgical anatomy around the foramen of Luschka in relation to intraoperative recording of auditory evoked potentials from the cochlear nuclei. J Neurosurg. 1995;82(6):933–9.
97. Heller JW, Brackmann DE, Tucci DL, Nyenhuis JA, Chou CK. Evaluation of MRI compatibility of the modified nucleus multichannel auditory brainstem and cochlear implants. Am J Otol. 1996;17(5):724–9.
98. Colletti V, Carner M, Fiorino F, Sacchetto L, Miorelli V, Orsi A, et al. Hearing restoration with auditory brainstem implant in three children with cochlear nerve aplasia. Otol Neurotol. 2002;23(5):682–93.

Chapter 11
Functional Electrical Stimulation to Treat Foot Drop as a Result of an Upper Motor Neuron Lesion

Marietta L. van der Linden and Thomas H. Mercer

Abstract Foot drop or dropped foot is a common gait problem in many people with an upper motor neuron lesion such as people after a stroke, people with Multiple Sclerosis and children and adults with Cerebral Palsy. This chapter explains the action of Functional Electrical Stimulation (FES) to the pre-tibial muscles in order to treat foot drop and how it can be adapted to the walking pattern of the individual patients by altering the stimulation patterns. The potential benefits of using FES to treat foot drop, the outcome measures used to assess these benefits and evidence for these benefits for three different clinical populations form the main part of this chapter. Finally, future directions of research into FES are summarised.

Keywords Functional Electrical Stimulation • Peroneal nerve stimulation • Foot drop • Dropped foot • Stroke • CVA • Multiple Sclerosis • Cerebral Palsy • Upper Motor Neuron lesion

Introduction

Functional electrical stimulation is increasingly used in people with an upper motor neuron lesion to aid their mobility and upper limb function. This chapter will examine the application of electrical stimulation (ES) of the peroneal nerve in order to achieve dorsiflexion of the ankle during the swing phase of gait to treat people who present with foot drop during gait as a result of an upper motor neuron pathology. This application of ES is therefore called 'functional', as it directly provides a function in gait, i.e. lifting the foot, as opposed to modes of ES such as TENS (Transcutaneous Electrical Nerve stimulation) where the muscle is stimulated below

M.L. van der Linden, PhD, MSc (✉) • T.H. Mercer, PhD, FBASES
Department of Rehabilitation Sciences, Queen Margaret University,
Centre for Health Activity and Rehabilitation Research,
Queen Margaret University Dr, Musselburgh EH21 6UU, UK
e-mail: mvanderlinden@qmu.ac.uk; tmercer@qmu.ac.uk

A. Majid (ed.), *Electroceuticals*, DOI 10.1007/978-3-319-28612-9_11

the threshold where a contraction takes place. It can be argued that all applications of electrical stimulation which lead to a clear contraction of the muscle (often called neuromuscular electrical stimulation or NMES) are 'functional' as its aim is to enhance muscle function, for example through strengthening. However, this chapter will only focus on Functional Electrical Stimulation (FES) with the primary aim to enhance dorsiflexion of the ankle during the swing phase gait, e.g. a 'neuroprosthetic' or orthotic function to treat foot drop.

Foot drop is the result of insufficient ankle dorsiflexion during the swing phase of gait. The lack of dorsiflexion is typically caused by caused by weakness, lack of selective voluntary motor control, increased spasticity of the plantar flexors or a combination of these. Foot drop can lead to foot dragging, toe scuffing, tripping and falls. People experiencing foot drop may have increased fear of falling [1] that can lead to a reduction of their habitual physical activity and/or an increase in the time spent sedentary, both of which have negative implications for health. Further, it is believed that the gait compensation "strategies" of people with foot drop, to ensure foot clearance such as hip hitching and circumduction, can also result in an increased effort of walking [2] and in some people back pain.

The conventional treatment approach for foot drop is the provision of an ankle foot orthosis (AFO), which encompasses the lower leg and foot, or a simple brace such as the 'foot up'. However, because of issues with comfort, appropriate fitting and the fact that AFOs often do not allow active ankle control, there has been increased consideration and implementation of FES for the treatment of foot drop.

Foot drop can be caused by peripheral nerve damage, but FES to treat foot drop is mainly prescribed for people with and upper motor lesion but intact peripheral nerve system, such as people after a stroke, Cerebral Palsy, multiple sclerosis, Traumatic Brain Injury, familial/hereditary spastic paraparesis, Parkinson's disease, and incomplete spinal cord injuries. The majority of the patients who use FES to treat foot drop in the UK are stroke survivors and people with Multiple Sclerosis [3]. Interestingly, there is also a considerable body of evidence regarding the effect of FES on the gait of children with Cerebral Palsy. The cause of foot drop and the immediate and long-term effects of FES to treat foot drop will differ in these clinical populations. To illustrate this, we describe in detail the evidence for the efficacy of FES to treat foot drop for three clinical populations: people after a CVA or stroke survivors, people with Multiple Sclerosis and children with Cerebral Palsy.

Normal Gait

Figure 11.1 shows the ankle kinematics in normal and foot drop gait. At heel strike, the ankle briefly plantar flexes until the whole foot contacts the ground and the shank starts to move over the foot, hence dorsiflexion of the ankle. Toward the end of the stance phase, the heel starts to rise from the ground, and the ankle starts to plantar flex again just before the toe-off, which is the start of the swing phase. During the second phase of the swing phase, the ankle dorsiflexes again to ensure adequate foot clearance. Peak dorsiflexion in swing occurs just before ipsi-lateral

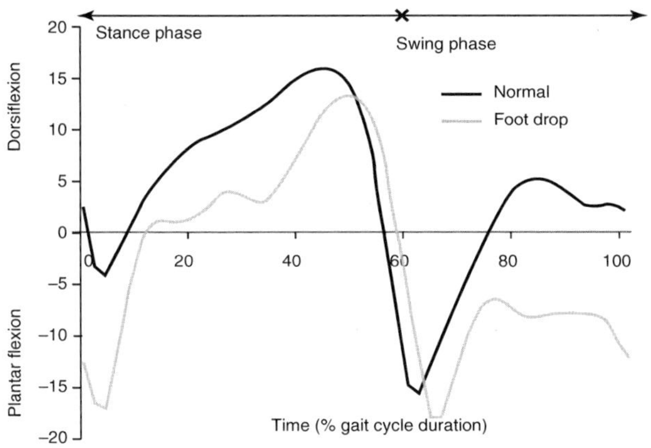

Fig. 11.1 Illustration of the ankle angle (foot-shank) movement (kinematics) of a person with foot drop (*grey line*) and a healthy control (*black line*). The horizontal x axis represents the duration of one gait cycle, i.e. from initial contact of the foot with the ground (0%) through the stance phase until approximately 60% when the toe leaves the ground, and to 100% when the same foot makes contact with the ground again. The person with foot drop has an ankle joint which is plantar flexed (i.e. foot is dropped) at initial contact (time 0%), then dorsiflexes during the stance phase when the shank moves over the foot. The ankle then plantar flexes during the last part of the stance phase and the start of the swing phase similar to the ankle of a healthy control. However, during the swing phase, the ankle of the person with foot drop shows increased plantar flexion just before initial contact

heel strike. In normal gait the Tibialis Anterior (TA) is active during the first part of the stance phase to prevent foot slap and throughout the swing phase to ensure foot clearance. In people with foot drop, the dorsiflexion in swing is reduced, often leading to initial contact by the forefoot or the whole foot instead of the heel.

How Does FES Work?

Although a range of commercially available stimulators are currently available (Fig. 11.2), they all work on the principle that the dorsiflexors need to be activated during the swing phase of gait and sometimes during the first part of stance to prevent foot slap. The instant of heel rise and the end of swing phase ('initial contact') are detected using either a foot switch, which is inserted into the shoe, or a tilt sensor attached to the shank.

On detection of heel rise or the appropriate shank ankle, the common peroneal nerve is stimulated via two electrodes either attached to the skin or incorporated into a cuff, activating the TA which dorsiflexes and inverts the foot and the peroneal muscles, which evert the foot. By slightly changing the positions of the electrodes the result of the stimulation can be adjusted to achieve the desired motion in both the sagittal (i.e. more or less dorsiflexion) and frontal plane (i.e. more inversion or eversion).

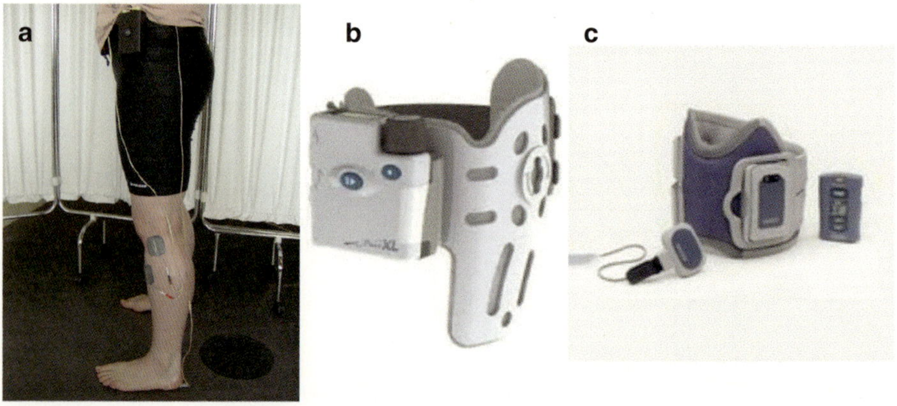

Fig. 11.2 Examples of commercially available FES systems to treat foot drop. (**a**) Odstock ODFS III, now upgraded to ODFS Pace (own picture); (**b**) ODFS Leg Cuff (http://odstockmedical.com/products/odfs-leg-cuff) surface-stimulator) (With permission © Odstock Medical); (**c**) Bioness L300 (http://www.bioness.com/Products/L300_for_Foot_Drop.php) (With permission © Bioness)

In some FES systems wires connect the footswitch and the electrodes with the stimulator itself (ODFS III and ODFS Pace), while other designs only use a wire connecting electrodes with the stimulator (ODFS Pace XL) or do not use any external wires at all (WalkAide, Bioness L300, Ottobock MyGait, ODFS Leg Cuff) Stimulators using implanted electrodes, until recently only for research purposes are now commercially available (StimuStep®, ActiGait®). This option could be attractive for a selection of patients including those who experience difficulties placing the electrodes correctly or those with skin irritation. People who have reduced hand function may also benefit from using a system with implantable electrodes. For this type of stimulators electrodes are implanted in the peroneal nerve just under the skin. This procedure can be done in day surgery under a general anaesthetic.

Not all patients with foot drop are suitable candidates for FES. Patients need some level of mobility in order to benefit from FES to assist with their walking, i.e. they need to be able to stand up from sitting without assistance and be able to walk a short distance (about 10 m) either with or without walking aids. If the patient does not live with a carer, he or she needs be able to correctly fit and place the electrodes or cuff and operate the equipment independently. Other medical exclusion criteria are poor skin condition, poorly controlled epilepsy, and a cancerous tumour in the area of the electrical stimulation as well as the presence of some medical implanted devices such as pace makers.

Stimulation Parameters

There are no optimum stimulation parameters for FES to treat foot drop as the parameters resulting in the best movement pattern and with the highest degree of comfort varies between patients and sometimes will change in a patient over time.

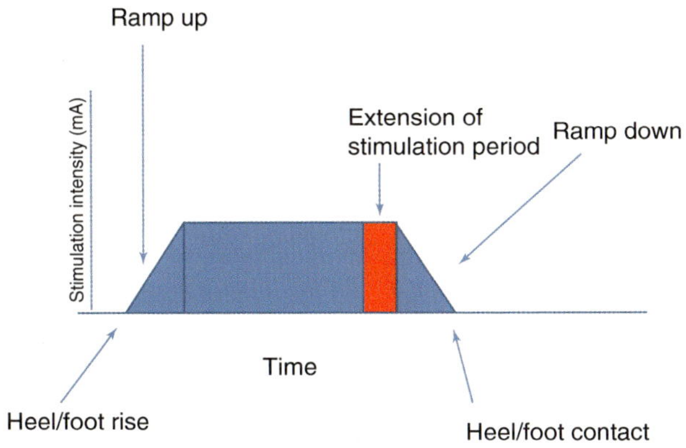

Fig. 11.3 Illustration of the sections of the stimulation period, which can be adjusted on most stimulators using a foot switch to detect the gait events. In patients who lack heel contact, the foot switch, which is usually placed under the heel, can be moved further forward. Van der Linden et al. [5] used a pressure sensitive strip placed along part of the foot to account for a variable foot contact pattern

However, most manufacturers recommend stimulation frequencies between 25 and 40 Hz as this frequency provides a smooth contraction without tiring the muscle too quickly. Increasing the stimulation frequency produces a stronger contraction but will also fatigue the muscle more quickly. Reducing the frequency can increase comfort and reduce spasticity, which may explain why some studies with children with CP have used a lower frequency of 25 Hz [4].

Most types of commercially available stimulators also allow the setting of other simulator parameters such as the waveform (asymmetrical or symmetrical) the rising and falling ramp, extension (Fig. 11.3), pulse duration (pulse width) and current amplitude (in mA). These can be adjusted for each individual patient to optimise the amount and timing of the dorsiflexion and the comfort of the stimulation. In the set-up phase of some stimulators, walking data is collected that is used by the stimulator software to optimise the stimulation parameters, which can then be further adjusted by a trained clinician if necessary.

Adjusting the rising and falling ramp can influence the strength and comfort of the stimulation. By adjusting the extension time, the stimulation time can be extended after contact with the floor in order to prevent sudden plantar flexion ('foot slap').

Pulse width (pulse duration) can also be set in most types of stimulators mostly ranging from 25 to 300 μs. Interestingly, both in relation to FES for children with CP, Prosser et al. [4], stated that the pulse width was set to 25 or 30 μs in order increase comfort while Carmick [6] argued that longer pulse widths are more comfortable. It is possible that the optimum pulse width depends on the individual child as was shown in the table by Pool et al. [7] which showed pulse durations of 12 children ranging from 25 to 300 μs.

Optimal electrode placement (both of surface electrodes and those incorporated in a cuff) is also essential. By altering the positions of the electrodes the amount of inversion (Tibialis Anterior) and eversion (Peroneus Longus and Peroneus Brevis)

can be adjusted as well as the magnitude of the dorsiflexion. By placing one electrode in the popliteal fossa a stronger flexion withdrawal reflex can be achieved, i.e. dorsiflexion of the ankle will be accompanied by knee flexion and hip flexion.

Is FES an Efficacious Treatment for Foot Drop?

Since Liberson et al. [8] first reported the results of using FES for people with a hemiplegia in 1961, evidence has accumulated regarding the efficacy of FES to treat foot drop in neurological populations. The published evidence on safety and efficacy of FES resulted in the publication of the 2009 National Institute for Health and Clinical Excellence (NICE) guideline 'Functional electrical stimulation for drop foot of central neurological origin' [9]. This report supported the use of FES for foot drop of central neurological origin. However, it was also suggested that further investigations addressing the efficacy of FES on patient-reported outcomes, such as quality of life and activities of daily living would usefully complement the existing evidence. These evidence-based guidelines were primarily based on studies with stroke survivors. However, since their publication, evidence has also accumulated with regard to the use of FES both for stroke survivors and in a range of other patient populations, which has been summarised in several recent systematic reviews into the evidence for stroke survivors [10–12] and children with Cerebral Palsy [13–15]. The following sections will: (i) detail the potential benefits of FES treatment of foot drop, (ii) summarise the most common outcome measures used to assess the efficacy of FES and (iii) consider the evidence for its efficacy and effectiveness in three different patient populations, stroke survivors, people with MS and children with CP.

Benefits of FES

FES to treat foot drop has the potential to improve the walking function of a patient both with immediately use (when it is switched on) and after a longer period of use (Fig. 11.4). In this chapter we adopt the terminology where the 'orthotic' effect is the

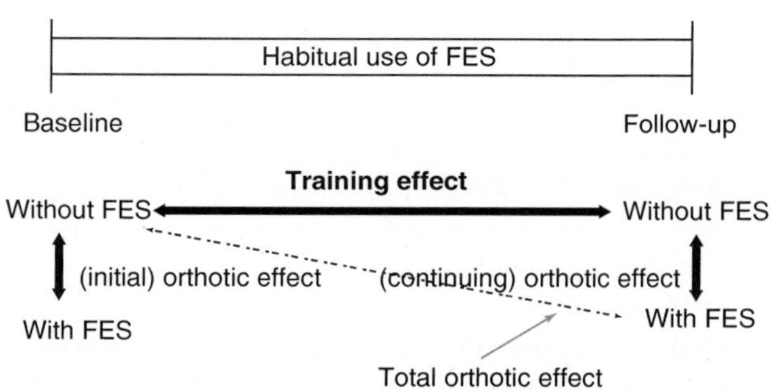

Fig. 11.4 Illustration of the types of potential benefits of FES to treat foot drop

difference between, for example, a person's walking speed with the stimulator switched on compared to the walking speed without the stimulation at the same assessment point. The orthotic effect can thus be evaluated in a single assessment. Taylor et al. [16] also define an 'initial orthotic effect,' when the stimulator is used first, from the 'continuing' orthotic effect which is measured after the person has regularly used the stimulator for a certain amount of time.

There is also a possibility of eliciting a positive "carryover" effect on the person's function, in the absence of stimulation, as a result of the prolonged/habitual use of the stimulator. To use the example of walking speed again, this so-called training effect is defined as the difference between a person's walking speed without stimulation after a period of FES use and the person's walking speed without stimulation at the baseline assessment. This change is also referred to as a 'carry over', 'treatment' or 'therapeutic' effect.

There are several possible mechanisms which could result in a training effect on walking performance or function including (i) increased strength of the Tibialis Anterior (as a result of hypertrophic adaptation) due to its repeated stimulation and possibly increased blood flow to the muscle; (ii) a strengthening of the neural pathways, possibly through synaptic plasticity; or (iii) the result of a general improvement in physical fitness (i.e. aerobic fitness, increased strength of other muscles involved in walking) as the patient increases his or her physical activity. Only a few authors have looked into the mechanisms behind a possible training effect as a result of FES. Everaert et al. [17] measured the Motor Evoked Potential (MEP) in the Tibialis Anterior from transcranial magnetic stimulation over the motor cortex, the Maximum motor wave (Mmax) by stimulating the common peroneal nerve, and the maximum voluntary contraction (MVC) in a group of non-progressive (mainly stroke) and progressive (mainly MS) patients before and after 3–12 months use of a foot drop stimulator. In both groups, both the MVC and MEP increased significantly but the increases in Mmax due to hypertrophy were small and did not correlate with the changes in MEP. The authors concluded that repeated use of the stimulator may strengthen the activation of motor cortical areas and their residual descending connections and that this increased activation of the motor cortical areas may have contributed to the training effect on walking speed. Unfortunately, the possible mechanisms of how exactly this may have produced an increase in walking speed were not discussed. Damiano et al. [18] measured the Tibialis Anterior muscle thickness using ultrasound after 1 month of FES device accommodation during which the child was getting used to FES and again after 3 months of habitual use. Although muscle size was increased after the intervention no permanent improvements in dorsiflexion during gait were found.

Finally, a total orthotic effect is the difference in performance between the person's walking performance with FES after a period of FES use compared to the performance without FES at the initial (baseline) assessment. Although of course of clinical importance, this effect is the sum of the (continuing) orthotic effect and the training effect, and therefore the specific evidence for this effect will not be discussed below as this effect can be inferred from the orthotic and training effects.

The next section will describe the most common outcome measures used in investigations into the efficacy of FES to the pretibial muscles to treat foot drop.

Outcomes

When describing the outcome measures used to evaluate the effects of FES to treat foot drop, the ICF (International **Classification** of Functioning, Disability and Health) [19] provides an appropriate framework. The ICF classifies outcomes in three domains: 'Body structures and Function', 'Activity' and 'Participation'. Examples of the outcomes used to evaluate the effect of FES for each domain are shown in Table 11.1.

Body Structures and Function

Outcomes of the first domain, which are relevant to FES to treat foot drop are passive and active range of motion, muscle strength, muscle spasticity, selective voluntary motor control and neurophysiological variables such as those recorded in the study by Everaert et al. [17]. Gait kinematics such as the ankle and knee angles are classified under 'Body Function'. Joint angles can be estimated from visual observation or recorded using electrogoniometry or computerised three-dimension gait analysis (3DGA).

Interestingly, although the primary aim of FES to treat foot drop is to dorsiflex the ankle, not many studies, except those involving children with CP, have used gait analysis to assess the effect of FES on the gait pattern. As well as the quantification of improvement in dorsiflexion on foot clearance, three dimensional gait analysis also permits the assessment of the effects of FES on the kinematics of the more proximal joints and the contra-lateral leg. Knee, hip and pelvic kinematics can be

Table 11.1 Example of outcome measures used in studies assessing the benefits of FES, using the ICF classification

Body structures and function	Activity	Participation
Muscle strength	Timed walking performance tests short (10mWT, 25FWT):	Daily physical activity (step count) through activity monitoring
Muscle neuro-physiology	Timed walking performance tests long (2, 3, 4, 5 and 6 min walk tests)	Quality of life (sf36, sf12, EQ-5D)
Selective motor control	PCI, VO_2	Impact disease on daily living (MSIS29, SIS)
Fugl-Meier assessment	MSWS12	Falls diary
Gait kinematics and kinetics	COPM	
	Berg Balance Scale	
	mEFAP	

mEFAP modified emory functional ambulation profile, *PCI* physiological cost index, *MSWS12* multiple sclerosis impact scale 12, *COPM* Canadian occupational performance measure, *sf12/sf36* short form 12, short form 36, *MSIS29* multiple sclerosis impact scale 29, *SIS* stroke impact scale, *FES* functional electrical stimulation, *ICF* the international **classification** of functioning, disability and health relevant as some patients who suffer from foot drop alter their gait pattern to ensure foot clearance via compensatory mechanisms such as hip hitching, circumduction or increased ankle plantar flexion of the contra-lateral ankle.

As applying FES to treat foot drop is thought to decrease the effort of walking, studies have also assessed the energy costs of walking with and without FES (e.g. [2]). Energy cost can be estimated by measuring the heart rate or by measuring oxygen uptake. The Physiological Cost Index (PCI) is defined as the number of heart beats per meter walked. Oxygen uptake can either be expressed as millilitres per minute or per meter with the latter being a measure of efficiency (most often during walking measured as ml/kg/min).

Activity

The most commonly used outcome in FES studies is walking speed over a relatively short distance such as 10 m or 25 ft. This distance is, however, shorter than the usual distance walked with FES during daily life which is why several studies also have included walking tests over a longer duration, mostly ranging from 2 (2minWT) to 6 (6minWT) min. It must be noted however, that the length of these tests needs to be carefully selected depending on the physical fitness of the patient. Distances that are too long will result in some patients not being able to complete the test while a short test for some patients will not appropriately assess their endurance.

To attach a clinical meaning to changes in walking speed of patients as result of using FES, studies have referred to work by Perry et al. [20] and Perrara et al. [21]. Perry et al. [20] reported the average walking speed of 147 stroke survivors in six functional categories; (1) physiological walker (0.1 m/s), (2) most limited household walkers (0.23 m/s), (3) least limited house hold walker (0.27 m/s), (4) most limited community walker (0.40 m/s), (5) least limited community walker (0.58 m/s) and (6) community walker (>0.8 m/s). Walking speed differentiated the three community walking categories. Perera et al. [21] compared changes in walking speed with changes in the self-reported Short Form 36 mobility items and a global mobility change scale in a group of elderly people with a variety of health conditions. They calculated that the minimum meaningful change in walking speed was 0.05 m/s while a change of 0.1 m/s or more was considered a substantial meaningful change. It should be noted however, that the functional walker categories by Perry et al. [20] and clinical change values [21] were derived from elderly populations and thus may not apply to children with Cerebral Palsy or younger and higher functioning adults with neurological conditions.

Walking performance and balance in activities of daily living has been assessed using the Timed Up and Go (TUG) test [22], the stroke specific Modified Emory Functional Ambulation Profile (mEFAP [23] and the Berg Balance Scale (BBS) which assesses the person's balance performance on a series of static and dynamic balance tasks [24]. As opposed to the aforementioned measures, which are recorded by a clinician, the Multiple Sclerosis Walking Scale (MSWS-12) is a self-report measure of the patient's walking performance [25]. Finally, the Canadian Occupational Performance Measure is an individualized outcome measure designed to detect change in a person's self-perception of their performance and satisfaction with one or more identified activities of daily living over time [26].

Participation and Quality of Life

The aims of using FES to treat foot drop may also include increasing the user's confidence in their walking ability, increasing walking performance and decrease the effort of walking. It has therefore been hypothesised that as a result, people will increase their level of habitual physical activity [27, 28]. Objective habitual physical activity can be measured by a simple pedometer or more accurately using an accelerometer (activity monitor), which records the number of steps (i.e. ActivPal and ActiGraph). Accelerometers to assess physical activity behaviour are increasingly used in studies assessing the effect of variety of interventions in neurological populations [29].

The number of falls is another important outcome when evaluating the effect of FES to treat foot drop. Surprisingly, only a few studies have recorded the number of falls and near falls before and after prolonged use of FES either using falls diaries [30, 31] or self-reported number of falls over the intervention period [7]. Finally, researchers have tested the hypotheses that an improved walking ability and function in activities of daily living, as a result of using FES, leads to improved health related quality of life. Quality of life is frequently reported using general health outcomes questionnaires such as the Short Form 36 [32] or Short Form 12, EQ -5D [33] or outcomes specific to a clinical population, such as Multiple Sclerosis Impact Scale 29 [34] and the stroke specific Stroke Impact Scale [35].

Evidence for the Efficacy in Different Clinical Population

The next sections will summarise the evidence for the clinical effectiveness of FES to treat foot drop for those three patient populations for which FES is most often prescribed and/or for which considerable evidence for its efficacy is available. These three patient groups selected for this review are: those after Cerebral Vascular Accident, in this chapter referred to as 'stroke survivors', people with Multiple Sclerosis (pwMS) and children with Cerebral Palsy (CP).

Stroke Survivors

It is estimated that every year 15 million people worldwide experience a new stroke [36]. Although the majority of stroke survivors regain the ability to walk, many will experience the continuing and/or residual effects of spasticity, muscle weakness and poor balance. It is estimated that foot drop resulting from dorsiflexor weakness and/or increased spasticity in the gastrocnemius affects approximately 20% of the stroke survivors [37]. Three phases of recovery are commonly described; acute (up to 2 weeks), sub-acute (2 weeks to 6 months) and chronic (more than 6 months after a stroke). Most of the natural recovery is thought to occur within the first 6 months, although this may depend on the individual and complexity of the task assessed [38].

Orthotic Effect

Body Structures and Function

Relatively few studies have looked at the effect of FES to treat foot drop on outcomes in this domain. Kesar et al. [39] and Lee et al. [40] confirmed the orthotic action of FES showing a decrease in plantar flexion/increase in dorsiflexion during swing with FES compared to without. Kesar et al. [39] also compared the orthotic effect of stimulation both the dorsiflexors (during swing) and plantar flexors (during stance) to that of the stimulation of the dorsifexors alone. The orthotic effect on peak dorsiflexion in swing was similar in the single and dual stimulation groups, but the dual stimulation resulted in an avoidance of the reduction in the plantar flexion at toe-off, which was observed when only the dorsiflexors were stimulated.

FES to treat foot drop has been shown to significantly reduce physical effort, as measured by the PCI by between 0.16 to 0.2 beats/m [41, 42], in contrast no orthotic effect on PCI was reported by Everaert et al. [43].

Activity

Walking speed over a relatively short distance (5–10 m/25 ft) has been the most common outcome measure used to assess the initial and continuing orthotic effect of FES to treat foot drop in studies with stroke survivors. Nearly all reported a statistically significant improvement of walking speed with FES compared to without FES [3, 16, 41–44]. Improvements ranged from 0.07 m/s (from 0.42 to 0.49 m/s, for an initial orthotic effect reported Kluding et al. [44] to 0.23 m/s (from 0.83 to 1.06 m/s for a continuing orthotic effect at 3 months) as reported by Laufer et al. [42].

Using the clinically meaningful change values proposed by Perera et al. [21], Taylor et al. [3] reported that 14 of 56 stroke survivors increased their walking speed by more than 0.1 m/s and 17 of 56 between 0.05 and 0.1 m/s in the first 16.5 months (continuing orthotic effect).

In walking performance tests over a longer distance (4 min or more), statistically significant initial and/or continuing effects were reported by Everaert et al. [43] (improvement of 5.7 m, in 4minWT), and in the 6minWT by Kluding et al. [44] and Laufer et al. [42]; who reported improvements of 19.3 m and 43 m respectively.

FES to treat foot drop also has shown to result in direct orthotic effect by improving functional walking and balance tests. Kluding et al. [44] reported improvements on the Timed Up and Go test (3.3 s) and Berg Balance Scale test (0.9 points) when the device was used. However, it should be noted that similar improvements were noticed in the control group when using an Ankle Foot Orthosis compared to no device.

Training Effects

Body Structures and Function

Only a few studies have looked at the training effects of FES to treat foot drop on outcomes in the 'Body structures and Function' domain. Both Sheffler et al. [45] and Kluding et al. [44] failed to detect an improvement over time in the Lower limb section of the Fugl-Meyer assessment (FMA), which is a measure of stroke motor impairment. Only one study, with an intensive programme combining 5 sessions of FES a week with a conventional rehabilitation for a period of 12 weeks, reported greater improvements in plantar flexor spasticity, dorsiflexor strength and voluntary ankle dorsiflexion than the control group who only received conventional rehabilitation [46]. As described earlier, Everaert et al. [17] reported that a strengthening of cortical spinal pathways after a period of using FES to treat foot drop, but whether this improved active dorsiflexion of the ankle is not known.

The 110 participants in the study by Sheffler et al. [45] underwent 3D gait analysis but no statistically significant training effects in the sagittal ankle angle were observed, i.e. the ankle kinematics during unassisted walking were not improved after 12 weeks of habitual FES use.

Activity

The majority of the studies on FES to treat foot drop in stroke survivors have reported on findings of the training effect of medium to long-term use of FES on the walking performance over short distances of mostly 10 m. Follow-up ranged from 6 weeks [43], 12 weeks [41, 45], 18 weeks [16], 30 weeks [44] and 1 year [42]. In the audit by Taylor et al. [3], the medium time of FES use was 3.6 years. Many studies reported statistically significant training effects on walking speed over 10 m [41–45]. Average improvements from baseline ranged from 0.045 m/s after 12 weeks of use [45] to 0.16 m/s after a year [42]. Putting these results in a more clinically relevant perspective, Taylor et al. [3] reported that 27 of the 56 (34%) stroke survivors increased their unassisted walking speed by 0.05 m/s or more, with the majority showing an increase of more than 0.1 m/s after using FES for a median of 3.6 years.

Prolonged use of FES also resulted in a training effect on walking speed over a longer distance in studies by Laufer et al. [42]; 61 m (6 minWT), Everaert et al. [43];

24 m (4 minWT) and Kluding et al. [44]; 15.6 m, 6minWT) and into a reduction in the effort of walking as measured by the PCI [3, 43].

Other statistically significant training effects after FES use for 30 weeks have been reported on the Timed Up and Go tests of 2.52 s [44] and 1.65 points on the Berg Balance score [44]. Sheffler et al. [45] reported an improvement of 10.2 s on total mEFAP score after 12 weeks of FES use.

Participation

Although FES to treat foot drop has been shown to result in improved outcomes of 'activity' after prolonged use, such improvements have not always translated into statistically significant improvements in objective habitual physical activity as measured by step count [28, 44]. This lack of a statistically significant effect on habitual physical activity could be explained by the fact that an increase in physical activity requires a behavioural change, which may be harder to elicit or simply because of a lack of statistical power because of the often considerable variation in physical activity pattern between patients. However, quality of life reported using a variety of measures (SF36, Stroke Impact Scale, Stroke Specific Quality of Life Scale) after prolonged use of FES has been shown to improve [44, 45, 47–49].

AFO Versus FES

Several recent RCTs [43–45, 48, 49] have compared the effects of FES and AFO on orthotic and training effects in stroke survivors. In a multi centre RCT (30 centres, 384 participants at follow-up), Berthoux et al. [49] followed up their participants for up to a year but the performance was only measured with the assistance of the device, hence unfortunately, a 'training' effect ('off vs 'off') using the terminology defined in this chapter was not reported. The long-term effects on the outcomes (as assessed with the device) showed an improvement in both FES (10 mWT, 6 minWT, mEFAP) and AFO groups (10mWT only) but no statistically significant (level of significance was set at $p < 0.002$ after Bonferroni correction) differences were found between the changes in the two groups in any of the outcome measures. However, although there was no statistically significant ($p = 0.008$) difference between the groups, after 12 months the obstacle course component of the mEFAP improved in the FES group but deteriorated in the AFO group. Better obstacle avoidance performance using FES compared to AFO was also reported by van Swighem et al. [50].

Sheffler et al. [28] reported a small but statistically significant *decrease* in peak dorsiflexion in swing without the assistance of FES after the 12-week intervention period over the whole sample. i.e. both hinged AFO and FES groups ('time effect') and hypothesized that peroneal nerve stimulation during walking may decrease the concurrent motor cortical drive which may a have detrimental effect on DF in swing when the device is switched off. A closer inspection of the data, however, shows that the average peak DF in swing only decreased by 1° in the FES group after 12 week intervention). In the hinged AFO group, however, peak dorsiflexion in swing was decreased by 2.9° and the ankle at initial contact was 2.3° more plantar flexed when walking without the AFO. However, no statistically significant group by time interaction was found. Although one could question the clinical significance of an average of 1° change in the FES group and 2.3° in the AFO group, Winter [51] showed that individual changes in foot angles as small as 2° can impact foot clearance during gait.

In summary, none of the studies comparing the orthotic or training effects of FES with those of AFOs reported a clear difference between the two devices. The only statistically significant differences were found in obstacle performance [47, 49], user preference [43] and satisfaction [43] in favour of the FES group.

Concluding Remarks

The mechanisms behind the training effect reported in outcomes in the ICF 'activity' domain are still not clear. Increased training effects are suggested to occur over longer time intervals (>42 weeks) in younger patients with greater mobility levels [51, 52] as well as those receiving FES in the sub-acute compared to the 'chronic' phase stage of recovery. Another issue, potentially confounding the results when interpreting the training effect of FES, is what constitutes 'usual care'. For example, in the systematic review of Dunning et al. [10], in 3 of 6 studies, both FES and control group participants received additional physiotherapy [41, 44, 45].

People with Multiple Sclerosis

Recent research indicates a growing number of studies exploring the efficacy of FES for the treatment of foot drop for people with Multiple Sclerosis (pwMS).

Multiple Sclerosis is a complex neurological disorder, which is characterised by demyelination within the central nervous system [53]. Progressive destruction of the myelin layer, which insulates the axons within the CNS, causes disturbed neural transmission along the spinal cord. Consequently, a reduced volume of electrical activity is delivered to the intended destination which can result in marked physical disability in people with MS. Motor deficits most commonly affect the lower extremities, with about 80% of people with MS reporting gait disturbance as their main complaint [54].

Orthotic Effect

The majority of the research studies into FES to treat foot drop in pwMS have assessed the orthotic effect of FES, i.e. the performance with the assistance of FES compared to that without.

Body Structures and Function

Studies using three dimensional gait analysis have demonstrated that both peak dorsiflexion in swing and knee flexion in swing, which further improved foot clearance, improved with the assistance of FES in both new users [55] and after 6 and 12 weeks of use of FES [27].

Energy cost during walking was shown to be statistically significantly improved with the assistance of FES in studies, which measured PCI over 10 m [16] and 4 min [56] and in the study by Paul et al. [2], which measured oxygen cost per meter walked. Interestingly, Miller et al. [57] noticed that people who walked faster than 0.8 m/s did not improve their walking speed and had an increased instead of decreased oxygen uptake per m distance walked, while those walking slower than 0.8 m/s showed clear reductions in their oxygen uptake per m walked (i.e. increased efficiency). However, all participants in the faster walking group were established users of FES who subjectively reported benefits of FES use. This finding may illustrate that the measurement of walking speed and oxygen cost, over a duration of 5 min, may not be entirely appropriate and/or sensitive enough outcomes to assess the benefits of FES in a group of people with a milder disability. Benefits of FES in this group of people may be only apparent over longer distances, or more 'ecologically valid (real world) environments as opposed to laboratory settings. Alternatively, benefits seen in this group may be possibly related to an increased confidence when walking and a reduction in number of trips and falls.

Activity

As in the stroke population, statistically significant improvements in the performance in the 10 m and 25 foot walking tests have been reported both at base line (first time of FES use) and after a period of use (continuing orthotic effect [3, 16, 27, 56, 58, 59]. Observed improvements in walking speed varied from 0.07 m/s to 0.11 m/s. In their audit report Taylor et al. [3] reported that at their first follow-up assessment at 20 weeks, of the 35 people with MS, 10 increased their speed by more than 0.1 m/s and 6 between 0.05 and 0.1 m/s, while after the using FES for16.5 months (continuing orthotic effect), 10 increased their walking speed by more than 0.1 m/s and 10 between 0.05 and 0.1 m/s.

An alternative analysis of this audit data was performed by Street et al. [58] who reported the number of people 'moving up and down' the functional walking categories described by Perry et al. [20]. The analysis of their audit data showed that after 20 weeks of using FES, 49 of the 153 pwMS moved up a functional walking category when using FES. Eleven of the 153 moved down a functional walking category.

Orthotic effects on the longer walking performance tests (2–5 min duration) have been reported in most studies [27, 31, 56, 60]. Average improvements in walking speed in these tests ranged from 0.03 to 0.05 m/s. Although an initial orthotic effect on the 10 m test was found, Scott et al. [55] did not find an improvement in the 6 min walk tests, in the 8 participants who had not used FES before ('initial orthotic effect'). This may possibly have been because the stimulated muscles were not conditioned to prolonged stimulation over a longer walking test.

Sample sizes of the studies evaluating the orthotic effect of FES to treat foot drop ranged from 9 [27] to 153 [58] the latter being derived from audit data. In the majority of the studies participants used either the ODFS III or ODFS pace. Participants in the studies by Stein et al. [56] and Downing et al. [59] used the Walkaide. Miller et al. [61] compared the orthotic effect between the ODFS and the WalkAide in 20 pwMS but did not find any statistically significant differences between the two devices.

Training Effect

Body Structures and Function

Only a few studies looked at the training effect of FES to treat foot drop on outcomes in the 'Body structures and function' domain. In a small scale study, after 12 weeks of FES use, the average dorsiflexion angle in swing of 9 participants improved by 3° compared to baseline [27] which however failed to reach statistical significance. A lack of training effect on PCI in people with MS was reported by Stein et al. [56] and Taylor et al. [16] following interventions of 3 months and 18 weeks, respectively.

Activity

Several studies have investigated the effects of long-term use of FES on the walking performance of pwMS when walking without the assistance of FES. The time span across these studies, between the initial (baseline) assessment of the patient's function and the follow-up, ranged from 2 weeks to more than 12 months. This time span is of importance when interpreting the results of the studies especially in a progressive disease such as MS. With increasing length of the time interval between the baseline and follow-up assessments there is likely to be a higher proportion of participants experiencing a disease progression-related deterioration in their gait pattern. This is clearly shown when evaluating the results of those studies assessing the training effect. Only one study [56] reported a statistically significant training effect on the 10-m walk test, i.e. after both 3 months and 11 months of use with increases of 0.08 m/s and 0.04 m/s respectively. Participants in a small scale study with 9 participants [27] showed an average increase in speed of 0.04 m/s over both 10 m and 2 min after 12 weeks of FES use but this improvement was not statistically significant. A study using audit data of 187 people also failed to find a training effect on walking speed after 20 weeks [58] with no change in the average walking speed over 10 m.

A lack of improvement in walking performance and walking effort, or even a slight deterioration, which becomes more pronounced with longer time intervals, is perhaps not surprising in a population with a progressive disease. However, this does not mean individuals with MS cannot experience a training effect after long-term use. The aforementioned studies reported the mean values of the whole sample. In such cases, if half of the participants improved and the other half deteriorated, the net effect is described as no overall change. However, this nomothetic approach may be "masking" the potential therapeutic benefit to some patients. This was illustrated by Street et al. [58] who showed that 31% of the pwMS increased their (unassisted) walking speed by 0.1 m/s compared to 39% who showed a decrease in their walking speed when walking without FES.

Participation

Patient Reported Outcome Measures (PROMS) have only recently been used in a few studies on FES to treat foot drop. The nine participants in the study by Taylor et al. [31] reported a reduction of both the psychological (16.5 points) and physical impact (18 points) of their MS on daily life after 6 weeks of FES use, but only the improvement in the psychological component was statistically significant. Downing et al. [59] however, showed a statistically significant improvement of both physical and psychological components of the MSIS29 after as early as 2 weeks of FES use.

Esnouf et al. [30] used the COPM as an outcome measure and showed that the most commonly reported problematic activities of daily living, 'not tripping' and 'walking a certain distance', were given an improved (higher average) performance rating after 18 weeks of FES use. Self-reported falls have also been reported to decrease significantly over the period when participants started to use FES, with the majority of the falls in this period occurring when the FES was not used [31].

AFO Versus FES in MS?

To date, only one small scale study comparing the benefits of FES compared that of AFOs has been published. Sheffler et al. [62] reported on a study with only four participants. Although the dorsiflexion angle at initial contact was increased with FES compared to AFO and no device in 3 of the 4 participants, other outcomes such as walking speed and other gait kinematics were more variable.

A qualitative study with separate focus groups for FES (n = 6) and AFO users (n = 4) reported that similar numbers of positive and negative aspects were described for the use of AFO and FES. Both interventions were reported to reduce fatigue, improve gait, reduce trips and falls, increase participation, and increase confidence. Interestingly, increased walking distance, fitness and physical activity was only reported by FES users and greater balance/stability only by those using an AFO.

Cerebral Palsy

Cerebral Palsy (CP) is an umbrella term used to describe children with a group of disorders associated with injury to the developing brain. In Europe the incidence of CP ranges from 1.5 to 3 per 1000 live births [63, 64]. Over 66% of the children is able to walk but may need walking aids [65].

Children with CP demonstrate muscle weakness and diminished selective voluntary motor control with the ankle joint most often affected [66, 67]. Ambulatory children with CP are often prescribed AFOs to provide support and prevent deformities due to high tone in the plantar flexors. However, the use of the often rigid AFOs has also been criticised as they prevent active dorsiflexion in swing and plantar flexion during push-off.

FES to the dorsiflexors may for some children be an appropriate alternative to an AFO and it was first proposed in the1980s as a treatment option for children with Cerebral Palsy (CP). In the 1990s Carmick published several case studies showing the beneficial effects of FES to a variety of muscles to improve gait [68, 69].

As in the case of some stroke survivors, the origin of foot drop is often increased spasticity of the gastrocnemius in addition to dorsiflexor weakness. Several authors have therefore proposed that stimulating the medial gastrocnemius during stance can also alleviate foot drop, stating that the spastic muscle is often the weakest [70] and hypothesising that appropriate stimulation in time with the gait cycle may interrupt the pattern of spasticity and contraction [71].

Orthotic Effects

Body Structures and Function

Gait analysis has historically been used much more often in children with Cerebral Palsy compared to adults with stroke and MS, probably driven by the need to evaluate the need for and outcome of various surgical procedures. This probably explains why many studies investigating the effects of FES to treat foot drop in children with CP have been evaluated using gait analysis. All studies in which the data was analysed using inferential statistics reported an statistically significant increase in dorsiflexion angle (or decreased plantar flexion) both at initial contact and in swing as a result of stimulating the Tibialis Anterior using surface electrodes [4, 5, 72], percutaneous stimulation [73] or stimulation of the Gastrocnemius with and without Tibialis Anterior [71].

Activity

None of the aforementioned studies showed a statistically significant improvement in walking speed or in any other spatio-temporal stride parameters. This is in contrary to the findings in the MS and Stroke population where an improvement in walking speed was the most often reported benefit. A possible reason for this is that children with CP who are candidates for FES may walk faster than adults with MS or stroke. Also, many children with CP who walk with 'toe gait' have difficulty controlling forward progression because of problems with balance due to the lack of heel contact. Indeed van der Linden et al. [5] reported a significant decrease in walking speed with FES possibly indicating a more controlled gait pattern because of an improvement in foot contact, which was also noted.

Training Effect

All Domains

Although an increased orthotic effect was found after 8 weeks [5] and 3 months [4] of using FES to the Tibialis Anterior, a statistically significant training effect on ankle kinematics as a result of long-term use of FES has not been demonstrated in children with CP.

Damiano et al. [18] reported on the training effects for the same sample for which Prosser et al. [4] described the orthotic effects. Tibialis Anterior muscle size (thickness and cross sectional area) showed significant increases after the primary three-month intervention phase. However, this increase in muscle size did not translate into an improved dorsiflexion in barefoot walking over the same period and in some children the muscle size decreased over the intervention period.

Using somewhat different outcome measures, a recent study with a with 12 children [7] showed that dorsiflexor strength, Range of Motion, spasticity in the gastrocnemius and Selective Motor Control significantly improved after a period of 6 weeks of FES, as well as the number of reported falls. It must be noted however, that although to be included in the study, the children had to be at least 3 month after their Botox injections, 9 of the 12 children received 6 monthly Botox injections, which may partly explain the more positive outcomes of this study.

Clinical Acceptability, Patient Perception of FES (All Populations)

The perception of the patient both with regard to the benefits of FES and the difficulties and drawbacks relating to FES are important issues for the clinician to consider. If the patient perceives that the barriers of using FES outweigh the benefits or if no benefits are perceived, the device will not be used which is a clear waste of resources. Selecting appropriate candidates for FES and educating the patient both require an understanding of the benefits and barriers perceived by both current and past FES users.

Taylor et al. [74] reported on the results of a user's survey (78 out of 107 were stroke survivors) and found that the most reported benefits were 'increased confidence', 'less effort', 'less likely to trip' and 'faster walking speed'. Current users of the ODFS III encountered difficulties with the positioning of electrodes (43.9%), unreliable equipment (39.3%) and skin irritation (22.4%). Reasons for stopping for past users were problems with electrode positioning, 'equipment too much bother', and deterioration or improvement of mobility. An audit into skin problems more than 10 years later showed this problem to be drastically reduced to only 2.4% of users after introduction of different electrodes in 2005 [75].

A more recent small scale survey [76] of user experiences of the ODFS III and ODFS Pace in people with MS only (n = 30), showed similar findings with the benefits most often reported to be reductions in both physical (70%) and mental (47%)

effort when walking', 'reduced risk of tripping', 'increased confidence' (both 65%) and 'reduced fatigue' (41%). Main disadvantages were the appearance of the wires (59%), cost of the device (47%), problems with electrode positioning (41%) and bulkiness of device at waistline (47%). The most important reason for stopping/not continuing reported by past users were painful stimulation sensation (36%) and time taken to set up equipment (18%). Interestingly, past users noted similar benefits to current users with 'reduced physical (64%) and mental (46%) effort when walking', 'reduced risk of tripping' (64%), 'increased confidence' (63%) and 'reduced fatigue' (46%) being the most commonly identified. However, it seems that for the past users the disadvantages outweighed the benefits.

Information regarding FES user experiences derived from surveys has also been augmented by participants in focus groups reported by Bulley et al. with stroke survivors [77] and people with MS [63]. In the study with 9 stroke survivors who had used both FES and AFOs, all but one preferred FES and cited a more normal walking pattern, movement of the ankle, and greater independence as the main reasons. However, some preferred an AFO for occasional use, for example when travelling or walking near water.

Clinical acceptability and practicality is probably an even more important issue for children with CP. The presence of wires of some devices can be a problem especially for younger children [5]. The device used in the studies by Prosser et al. [4] and by Poon et al. [7] were wireless and this may have contributed to the high acceptability reported in these studies. Other important strategies to increase acceptability of the device include support such as follow-on phone calls and visits to the child's house and a period of neuromuscular electrical stimulation (used passively) prior to FES to improve the responsiveness of the muscle and to get the child used to the sensation [4, 5]. Results from the parental questionnaire [5] showed that reasons for not using the stimulator were embarrassment, skin problems (unrelated to the use of the stimulator) and unpracticality for 'non-standard activities' such as playing out of doors or participating in organised sports. It proved less of a burden when used by older children, who could take responsibility for the units themselves. Older children are often reluctant to continue to use their ankle foot orthoses, and FES may be a practical alternative for these children.

Conclusion

There is mounting evidence of the benefits of FES to treat drop foot in all three clinical populations discussed above. However, appropriate selection of outcomes to capture these benefits is of critical importance. This is illustrated for example by the findings in children with Cerebral Palsy and people with MS with near normal walking speeds, that FES use does not increase walking speed. Outcomes such as the frequency of toe dragging' or tripping or altered confidence levels when walking may be more appropriate outcome measures in studies on the application of FES for these individuals.

Furthermore, little is known about the effects of long-term FES use on outcomes on the 'body structures' domain, which may (or may not) explain the training effects on walking speed as noted in stroke survivors and in some people with MS.

Another important area of investigation is the cost-effectiveness of FES to treat foot drop. Taylor et al. [3] used the estimated QALY gain of 0.041 associated with FES use, published in an economic report by the NHS Centre for Evidence Purchasing [78] and the estimated mean costs of FES of £3.096, to calculate the mean cost per QALY, which was £15,406. The authors concluded that with the willingness to pay threshold of the National Institute for Health and Clinical Excellent (NICE) of £20,000 per QALY, FES is a cost-effective treatment for the correction of foot drop. Further studies, using an alternative estimation of QALY gain associated with the use of FES and from other research groups should be conducted to confirm this conclusion.

Future Directions: Advantages in Technology

Commercial stimulators are continuing to develop in order to optimise the effect of the stimulation and to improve the acceptability/user friendliness of the device. Odstock Medical Limited which supplies FES devices to the majority of NHS patients in the UK, recently developed a simulator in which the wires from the footswitch to the simulator were removed (Pace XL) and also produced a device which uses a leg cuff. Other companies (WalkAide®, Bioness) provide smaller cuffs for paediatric patients. Stimulators using implanted electrodes, until recently only for research purposes are now commercially available (StimuStep®, ActiGait®) and have shown to be feasible and effective [47, 79–81].

Identifying the correct sites to place the electrodes is a problem for some users and in particular those for whom the optimal position may change over time. Some recent studies have looked at the possibility of using 'virtual electrodes', which involves the process of stimulating a subset of electrodes chosen from an array, which allows the site of stimulation to be moved electronically rather than physically [82, 83].

Others have looked into the type of stimulation pattern (variable-frequency vs constant frequency trains) or into the stimulation profile (intensity depending on the phase in the gait cycle as opposed to a constant intensity) to achieve a more physiological stimulation resulting in a more pronounced action of the muscle and reduced fatigue [39, 79]. In a review of technological developments of functional electrical stimulation to correct foot drop, Melo et al. [84] recommends further development of the current commercially available systems to focus on incorporating closed-loop control strategies and the stimulation of more than one muscle. These developments should lead to stimulation patterns which are closer to those present in healthy individuals and thus result in more normal movement patterns and reduced muscle fatigue. Moreover, although not discussed in this chapter, consideration needs to be given to any potential additive or interactive benefits of FES to treat foot drop when combined with other therapeutic interventions such as Botox [85], compression (lycra-type) garments, treadmill training [86] or orthopaedic surgery [87].

References

1. Peterson EW, Cho CC, Finlayson ML. Fear of falling and associated activity curtailment among middle aged and older adults with multiple sclerosis. Mult Scler. 2007;13(9):1168–75.
2. Paul L, Rafferty D, Young S, Miller L, Mattison P, McFadyen A. The effect of functional electrical stimulation on the physiological cost of gait in people with multiple sclerosis. Mult Scler. 2008;14(7):954–61.
3. Taylor P, Humphreys L, Swain I. The long-term cost-effectiveness of the use of functional electrical stimulation for the correction of dropped foot due to upper motor neuron lesion. J Rehabil Med. 2013;45(2):154–60.
4. Prosser LA, Curatalo LA, Alter KE, Damiano DL. Acceptability and potential effectiveness of a foot drop stimulator in children and adolescents with cerebral palsy. Dev Med Child Neurol. 2012;54(11):1044–9.
5. van der Linden ML, Hazlewood ME, Hillman SJ, Robb JE. Functional electrical stimulation to the dorsiflexors and quadriceps in children with cerebral palsy. Pediatr Phys Ther. 2008; 20(1):23–9.
6. Carmick J. Letters to the editor. Effect of functional electrical stimulation on activity in children with cerebral palsy: a systematic review. Pediatr Phys Ther. 2014;26(4):487–8.
7. Pool D, Blackmore AM, Bear N, Valentine J. Effects of short-term daily community walk aide use on children with unilateral spastic cerebral palsy. Pediatr Phys Ther. 2014;26(3):308–17.
8. Liberson WT, Holmquest HJ, Scott HJ, Dow M. Functional electrotherapy stimulation of the common peroneal nerve synchronised with the swing phase of gait of hemiplegic subjects. Arch Phys Med Rehabil. 1961;42:101–5.
9. National Institute for Health and Clinical Excellence (NICE) Guideline. Functional electrical stimulation for drop foot of central neurological origin. Available at: https://www.nice.org.uk/guidance/ipg278/chapter/1-guidance. Accessed 12 Oct 2015.
10. Dunning K, O'Dell MW, Kluding P, McBride K. Peroneal stimulation for foot drop after stroke: a systematic review. Am J Phys Med Rehabil. 2015;94(8):649–64.
11. Kottink AI, Oostendorp LJ, Buurke JH, Nene AV, Hermens HJ, IJzerman MJ. The orthotic effect of functional electrical stimulation on the improvement of walking in stroke patients with a dropped foot: a systematic review. Artif Organs. 2004;28(6):577–86.
12. Robbins SM, Houghton PE, Woodbury MG, Brown JL. The therapeutic effect of functional and transcutaneous electric stimulation on improving gait speed in stroke patients: a meta-analysis. Arch Phys Med Rehabil. 2006;87(6):853–9.
13. Wright PA, Durham S, Ewins DJ, Swain ID. Neuromuscular electrical stimulation for children with cerebral palsy: a review. Arch Dis Child. 2012;97(4):364–71.
14. Chiu HC, Ada L. Effect of functional electrical stimulation on activity in children with cerebral palsy: a systematic review. Pediatr Phys Ther. 2014;26(3):283–8.
15. Cauraugh JH, Naik SK, Hsu WH, Coombes SA, Holt KG. Children with cerebral palsy: a systematic review and meta-analysis on gait and electrical stimulation. Clin Rehabil. 2010;24(11):963–78.
16. Taylor PN, Burridge JH, Dunkerley AL, Wood DE, Norton JA, Singleton C, Swain ID. Clinical use of the Odstock dropped foot stimulator: its effect on the speed and effort of walking. Arch Phys Med Rehabil. 1999;80(12):1577–83.
17. Everaert DG, Thompson AK, Chong SL, Stein RB. Does functional electrical stimulation for foot drop strengthen corticospinal connections? Neurorehabil Neural Repair. 2010;24(2):168–77.

18. Damiano DL, Prosser LA, Curatalo LA, Alter KE. Muscle plasticity and ankle control after repetitive use of a functional electrical stimulation device for foot drop in cerebral palsy. Neurorehabil Neural Repair. 2013;27(3):200–7.
19. World Health Organization. International classification of functioning, disability and health (ICF). Geneva: WHO; 2001.
20. Perry J, Garrett M, Gronley JK, Mulroy SJ. Classification of walking handicap in the stroke population. Stroke. 1995;26(6):982–9.
21. Perera S, Mody SH, Woodman RC, Studenski SA. Meaningful change and responsiveness in common physical performance measures in older adults: meaningful change and performance. J Am Geriatr Soc. 2006;54:743–9.
22. Podsiadlo D, Richardson S. The timed "Up & Go": a test of basic functional mobility for frail elderly persons. J Am Geriatr Soc. 1991;39(2):142–8.
23. Wolf SL, Catlin PA, Gage K, Gurucharri K, Robertson R, Stephen K. Establishing the reliability and validity of measurements of walking time using the Emory Functional Ambulation Profile. Phys Ther. 1999;79(12):1122–33.
24. Berg K, Wood-Dauphinee S, Williams JI. The Balance Scale: reliability assessment with elderly residents and patients with an acute stroke. Scand J Rehabil Med. 1995;27(1):27–36.
25. Hobart JC, Riazi A, Lamping DL, Fitzpatrick R, Thompson AJ. Measuring the impact of MS on walking ability: the 12-Item MS Walking Scale (MSWS-12). Neurology. 2003;60(1):31–6.
26. Law M, Polatajko H, Pollock N, McColl MA, Carswell A, Baptiste S. Pilot testing of the Canadian Occupational Performance Measure: clinical and measurement issues. Can J Occup Ther. 1994;61:191–7.
27. van der Linden ML, Hooper JE, Cowan P, Weller BB, Mercer TH. Habitual functional electrical stimulation therapy improves gait kinematics and walking performance, but not patient-reported functional outcomes, of people with multiple sclerosis who present with foot-drop. PLoS One. 2014;9(8):e103368.
28. Sheffler LR, Taylor PN, Bailey SN, Gunzler DD, Buurke JH, IJzerman MJ, Chae J. Surface peroneal nerve stimulation in lower limb hemiparesis: effect on quantitative gait parameters. Am J Phys Med Rehabil. 2015;94(5):341–57.
29. Motl RW, McAuley E, Snook EM, Scott JA. Validity of physical activity measures in ambulatory individuals with multiple sclerosis. Disabil Rehabil. 2006;28(18):1151–6.
30. Esnouf JE, Taylor PN, Mann GE, Barrett CL. Impact on activities of daily living using a functional electrical stimulation device to improve dropped foot in people with multiple sclerosis, measured by the Canadian Occupational Performance Measure. Mult Scler. 2010;16(9):1141–7.
31. Taylor P, Barrett C, Mann G, Wareham W, Swain I. A feasibility study to investigate the effect of functional electrical stimulation and physiotherapy exercise on the quality of gait of people with multiple sclerosis. Neuromodulation. 2014;17(1):75–84.
32. Ware JE, Kosinski M, Dewey JE. How to score Version 2 of the SF-36® Health Survey Lincoln: Quality Metric Incorporated; 2001.
33. Brazier J, Jones N, Kind P. Testing the validity of the Euroqol and comparing it with the SF-36 health survey questionnaire. Qual Life Res. 1993;2(3):169–80.
34. Hobart J, Lamping D, Fitzpatrick R, Riazi A, Thompson A. The Multiple Sclerosis Impact Scale (MSIS-29): a new patient-based outcome measure. Brain. 2000;124:962–73.
35. Lin KC, Fu T, Wu CY, Hdieh YW, Chen CL, Lee PC. Psychometric comparisons of the Stroke Impact Scale 3.0 and Stroke-Specific Quality of Life Scale. Qual Life Res. 2010;19(3): 435–43.
36. Go AS, Mozaffarian D, Roger VL, et al. Heart disease and stroke statistics—2013 update: a report from the American Heart Association. Circulation. 2013;127:e6–e245.
37. Wade DT, Wood VA, Heller A, Maggs J, Langton HR. Walking after stroke: measurement and recovery over the first 3 months. Scand J Rehabil Med. 1987;19:25–30.
38. Skilbeck CE, Wade DT, Langton HR, Wood VA. Recovery after stroke. J Neurol Neurosurg Psychiatry. 1983;46:5–8.
39. Kesar TM, Perumal R, Jancosko A, Reisman DS, Rudolph KS, Higginson JS, Binder-Macleod SA. Novel patterns of functional electrical stimulation have an immediate effect on dorsiflexor muscle function during gait for people poststroke. Phys Ther. 2010;1:55–66.

40. Lee YH, Yong SY, Kim SH, Kim JH, Shinn JM, Kim Y, Kim S, Hwang S. Functional electrical stimulation to ankle dorsiflexor and plantarflexor using single foot switch in patients with hemiplegia from hemorrhagic stroke. Ann Rehabil Med. 2014;38(3):310–6.
41. Burridge JH, Taylor PN, Hagan SA, Wood DE, Swain ID. The effects of common peroneal stimulation on the effort and speed of walking: a randomized controlled trial with chronic hemiplegic patients. Clin Rehabil. 1997;11(3):201–10.
42. Laufer Y, Hausdorff JM, Ring H. Effects of a foot drop neuroprosthesis on functional abilities, social participation, and gait velocity. Am J Phys Med Rehabil. 2009;88(1):14–20.
43. Everaert DG, Stein RB, Abrams GM, Dromerick AW, Francisco GE, Hafner BJ, Huskey TN, Munin MC, Nolan KJ, Kufta CV. Effect of a foot-drop stimulator and ankle-foot orthosis on walking performance after stroke: a multicenter randomized controlled trial. Neurorehabil Neural Repair. 2013;27(7):579–91.
44. Kluding PM, Dunning K, O'Dell MW, Wu SS, Ginosian J, Feld J, McBride K. Foot drop stimulation versus ankle foot orthosis after stroke: 30-week outcomes. Stroke. 2013;44(6):1660–9.
45. Sheffler LR, Taylor PN, Gunzler DD, Buurke JH, Ijzerman MJ, Chae J. Randomized controlled trial of surface peroneal nerve stimulation for motor relearning in lower limb hemiparesis. Arch Phys Med Rehabil. 2013;94(6):1007–14.
46. Sabut SK, Sikdar C, Kumar R, Mahadevappa M. Functional electrical stimulation of dorsiflexor muscle: effects on dorsiflexor strength, plantarflexor spasticity, and motor recovery in stroke patients. NeuroRehabilitation. 2011;29(4):393–400.
47. Kottink AI, Ijzerman MJ, Groothuis-Oudshoorn CG, Hermens HJ. Measuring quality of life in stroke subjects receiving an implanted neural prosthesis for drop foot. Artif Organs. 2010;34(5):366–76.
48. Bethoux F, Rogers HL, Nolan KJ, et al. The effects of peroneal nerve functional electrical stimulation versus ankle-foot orthosis in patients with chronic stroke: a randomized controlled trial. Neurorehabil Neural Repair. 2014;28(7):688–97.
49. Bethoux F, Rogers HL, Nolan KJ, et al. Long-term follow-up to a randomized controlled trial comparing peroneal nerve functional electrical stimulation to an ankle foot orthosis for patients with chronic stroke. Neurorehabil Neural Repair. 2015;29:911–922. pii: 1545968315570325.
50. van Swigchem R, van Duijnhoven HJ, den Boer J, Geurts AC, Weerdesteyn V. Effect of peroneal electrical stimulation versus an ankle-foot orthosis on obstacle avoidance ability in people with stroke-related foot drop. Phys Ther. 2012;92(3):398–406.
51. Winter DA. Foot trajectory in human gait: a precise and multifactorial motor control task. Phys Ther. 1992;72:45–66.
52. O'Dell MW, Dunning K, Kluding P, Wu SS, Feld J, Ginosian J, McBride K. Response and prediction of improvement in gait speed from functional electrical stimulation in persons with poststroke drop foot. PM R. 2014;6(7):587–601.
53. Smith KJ, McDonald WI. The pathophysiology of multiple sclerosis: the mechanisms underlying the production of symptoms and the natural history of the disease. Philos Trans R Soc Lond B Biol Sci. 1999;354(1390):1649–73.
54. Larocca NG. Impact of walking impairment in multiple sclerosis: perspectives of patients and care partners. Patient. 2011;4:189–201.
55. Scott SM, van der Linden ML, Hooper JE, Cowan P, Mercer TH. Quantification of gait kinematics and walking ability of people with multiple sclerosis who are new users of functional electrical stimulation. J Rehabil Med. 2013;45(4):364–9.
56. Stein RB, Everaert DG, Thompson AK, Su LC, Whittaker M, Robertson J, et al. Long-term therapeutic and orthotic effects of a foot drop stimulator on walking performance in progressive and nonprogressive neurological disorders. Neurorehabil Neural Repair. 2010;24:152–67.
57. Miller L, Rafferty D, Paul L, Mattison P. The impact of walking speed on the effects of functional electrical stimulation for foot drop in people with multiple sclerosis. Disabil Rehabil Assist Technol. 2015;31:1–6.
58. Street T, Taylor P, Swain I. Effectiveness of functional electrical stimulation on walking speed, functional walking category, and clinically meaningful changes for people with multiple sclerosis. Arch Phys Med Rehabil. 2015;96(4):667–72.

59. Downing A, Van Ryn D, Fecko A, Aiken C, McGowan S, Sawers S, McInerny T, Moore K, Passariello L, Rogers H. Effect of a 2-week trial of functional electrical stimulation on gait function and quality of life in people with multiple sclerosis. Int J MS Care. 2014;16(3): 146–52.
60. Barrett CL, Mann GE, Taylor PN, Strike P. A randomized trial to investigate the effects of functional electrical stimulation and therapeutic exercise on walking performance for people with multiple sclerosis. Mult Scler. 2009;15(4):493–504.
61. Miller L, Rafferty D, Paul L, Mattison P. A comparison of the orthotic effect of the Odstock Dropped Foot Stimulator and the Walkaide functional electrical stimulation systems on energy cost and speed of walking in Multiple Sclerosis. Disabil Rehabil Assist Technol. 2014;10(6): 482–5.
62. Sheffler LR, Bailey SN, Chae J. Spatiotemporal and kinematic effect of peroneal nerve stimulation versus an ankle-foot orthosis in patients with multiple sclerosis: a case series. PM R. 2009;1(7):604–11.
63. Bulley C, Mercer TH, Hooper JE, Cowan P, Scott S, van der Linden ML. Experiences of functional electrical stimulation (FES) and ankle foot orthoses (AFOs) for foot-drop in people with multiple sclerosis. Disabil Rehabil Assist Technol. 2015;10(6):458–67.
64. Surveillance of Cerebral Palsy in Europe (SCPE). Prevalence and characteristics of children with cerebral palsy in Europe. Dev Med Child Neurol. 2002;44:633–40.
65. Surman G, Bonellie S, Chalmers I, Colver A, Dolk H, Hemming K, King A, Kurinczuk I, Parkes I, Platt MJ. UKCP: a collaborative network of cerebral palsy registers in the United Kingdom. J Public Health (Oxf). 2006;28(2):148–56.
66. Wiley ME, Damiano DL. Lower-extremity strength profiles in spastic cerebral palsy. Dev Med Child Neurol. 1998;40:100–7.
67. Fowler EG, Staudt LA, Greenberg MB. Lower-extremity selective voluntary motor control in patients with spastic cerebral palsy: increased distal motor impairment. Dev Med Child Neurol. 2010;52:264–9.
68. Carmick J. Managing equinus in children with cerebral palsy: electrical stimulation to strengthen the triceps surae muscle. Dev Med Child Neurol. 1995;37(11):965–75.
69. Carmick J. Clinical use of neuromuscular electrical stimulation for children with cerebral palsy, part 1: lower extremity. Phys Ther. 1993;73(8):505–13.
70. Brown JK, Rodda J, Walsh EG, Wright GW. Neurophysiology of lower-limb function in hemiplegic children. Dev Med Child Neurol. 1991;33(12):1037.
71. Comeaux P, Patterson N, Rubin M, Meiner R. Effect of neuromuscular electrical stimulation during gait in children with cerebral palsy. Pediatr Phys Ther. 1997;9:103–9.
72. Postans NJ, Granat MH. Effect of functional electrical stimulation, applied during walking, on gait in spastic cerebral palsy. Dev Med Child Neurol. 2005;47:46–52.
73. Orlin MN, Pierce SR, Stackhouse CL, Smith BT, Johnston T, Shewokis PA, McCarthy JJ. Immediate effect of percutaneous intramuscular stimulation during gait in children with cerebral palsy: a feasibility study. Dev Med Child Neurol. 2005;47(10):684–90.
74. Taylor PN, Burridge JH, Dunkerley AL, Lamb A, Wood DE, Norton JA, Swain ID. Patients' perceptions of the Odstock Dropped Foot Stimulator (ODFS). Clin Rehabil. 1999;13(5):439–46.
75. Dalton H, Taylor P, New letter Winter 2011 http://www.odstockmedical.com/sites/default/files/skin_irritation_audit.pdf. Accessed 17 Oct 2015.
76. Van der Linden ML, Hooper JE, Mercer TM. Functional electrical stimulation to treat foot drop for people with MS; user perceptions of benefits, disadvantages and service provision in Edinburgh. In: Proceedings of rehabilitation in MS (RIMS) meeting, 6–7 June 2014; Brighton.
77. Bulley C, Shiels J, Wilkie K, Salisbury L. User experiences, preferences and choices relating to functional electrical stimulation and ankle foot orthoses for foot-drop after stroke. Physiotherapy. 2011;97(3):226–33.
78. Economic Report. Functional electrical stimulation for dropped foot of central neurological origin [Internet]. NHS Purchasing and Supply Agency. 2010. CEP10012. Available from: http://www.cedar.wales.nhs.uk/sitesplus/documents/1091/CEP10012%20FES%20econ%20report.pdf. Accessed 19 July 2016.

79. Ernst J, Grundey J, Hewitt M, von Lewinski F, Kaus J, Schmalz T, Rohde V, Liebetanz D. Towards physiological ankle movements with the ActiGait implantable drop foot stimulator in chronic stroke. Restor Neurol Neurosci. 2013;31(5):557–69.
80. Kottink A, Hermens HJ, Nene AV, Tenniglo MJ, van der Aa HE, Buschman HP, Ijzerman MJ. A randomized controlled trial of an implantable 2-channel peroneal nerve stimulator on walking speed and activity in poststroke hemiplegia. Arch Phys Med Rehabil. 2007;88(8):971–8.
81. Schiemanck S, Berenpas F, van Swigchem R, van den Munckhof P, de Vries J, Beelen A, Nollet F, Geurts AC. Effects of implantable peroneal nerve stimulation on gait quality, energy expenditure, participation and user satisfaction in patients with post-stroke drop foot using an ankle-foot orthosis. Restor Neurol Neurosci. 2015;33(6):795–807.
82. Heller BW, Clarke AJ, Good TR, Healey TJ, Nair S, Pratt EJ, Reeves ML, van der Meulen JM, Barker AT. Automated setup of functional electrical stimulation for drop foot using a novel 64 channel prototype stimulator and electrode array: results from a gait-lab based study. Med Eng Phys. 2013;35(1):74–81.
83. O'Halloran T, Haugland M, Lyons GM, Sinkjaer T. An investigation of the effect of modifying stimulation profile shape on the loading response phase of gait, during FES-corrected drop foot: stimulation profile and loading response. Neuromodulation. 2004;7(2):113–25.
84. Melo PL, Silva MT, Martins JM, Newman DJ. Technical developments of functional electrical stimulation to correct drop foot: sensing, actuation and control strategies. Clin Biomech. 2015;30(2):101–13.
85. Johnson CA, Burridge JH, Strike PW, Wood DE, Swain ID. The effect of combined use of botulinum toxin type A and functional electric stimulation in the treatment of spastic drop foot after stroke: a preliminary investigation. Arch Phys Med Rehabil. 2004;85(6):902–9.
86. Ng MF, Tong RK, Li LS. A pilot study of randomized clinical controlled trial of gait training in subacute stroke patients with partial body-weight support electromechanical gait trainer and functional electrical stimulation: six-month follow-up. Stroke. 2008;39(1):154–60.
87. Johnston TE, Finson RL, McCarthy JJ, Smith BT, Betz RR, Mucahey MJ. The use functional electrical stimulation to augment traditional orthopaedic surgery in children with cerebral palsy. J Pediatr Orthop. 2004;24:283–91.

Chapter 12
Electrical Stimulation for Modification of Memory and Cognition

Ioan Opris

Abstract A major challenge in neuroscience research is to develop stimulation systems (both minimally invasive and noninvasive) that can safely, flexibly and efficiently tap into the human brain, to coordinate complex cognitive and behavioral tasks. In this regard, neural technology is targeting new therapeutic approaches to improve mental performance for patients with cognitive disorders. Herein, we discuss recent developments in electro-stimulation therapies that have been instrumental in improving memory and cognition, including working memory, decision making and executive control, by enhancing cognitive performance. The use of various stimulation devices and technologies developed recently is examined in terms of preclinical (nonhuman primate experiments) and clinical applications to human brain disorders.

Keywords Cognition • Memory • Decision • Electrical Stimulation • Therapy • Nanitechnology • TMS • tDCS

Introduction

The use of electrical stimulation to uncover the functional links between neural activity and mental phenomena spans over more than 200 years. Luigi Galvani and Alessandro Volta were the first to test the 'electricity' of animal cells (nerve and muscle) in the 1790s [1]. By 1801, Galvani's nephew, Giovanni Aldini, used electrical stimulation in human patients to improve melancholy [2]. In 1870, Fritsch and Hitzig applied electrical stimulation to locate the primary motor cortex [3]. David Ferrier identified the frontal eye field in monkeys by stimulating in prefrontal cortex and describing a visual orienting response – the eyes opened wide (the pupils dilated), and the eyes and head turned toward the opposite side of stimulation [4]. Then,

I. Opris, PhD
Miller School of Medicine, Department of Neurological Surgery,
Lois Pope Life Center 4th floor, 1095 NW 14th Ter, Miami, FL 33136, USA
e-mail: ixo82@med.miami.edu

A. Majid (ed.), *Electroceuticals*, DOI 10.1007/978-3-319-28612-9_12

Penfield's findings in human patients beautifully demonstrated that applying an artificial signal to the conscious brain could induce complex psychic processes, including percepts and memories so "vivid" that patients felt as if they were "reliving" events from their past [5]. In nonhuman primates (NHPs), Stamm and Rosen tested the effect of electrical stimulation on delayed response tasks, providing evidence that prefrontal and inferotemporal cortices are crucial for short-term memory [6].

The principle of inductive brain stimulation with eddy currents has been known since the late 19th century. Using noninvasive approaches, early attempts to stimulate the brain using magnetic fields occurred in 1896 by d'Arsonval [7]. Jaques-Arsène d'Arsonval has reported his experience with noninvasive brain magnetic stimulation to the scientific French community. However, the first successful transcranial magnetic stimulation (TMS) study was performed only in 1985 by Anthony Barker in Sheffield [8]. As compared to the transcranial stimulation method, that applies direct electric current to the scalp [9, 10], the use of electromagnets greatly reduced the discomfort of the electrical procedure (sometimes painful because the skull has a high electrical resistance) and allowed the mapping of the cerebral cortex and its connections. The goal of the chapter is, therefore, to uncover the functional links between neural activity and cognitive phenomena by both invasive and noninvasive stimulation approaches.

Rationale for Using Electrical Stimulation

The major reasons for using electrical stimulation in cognitive neuroscience are: (i) to map the microanatomy of the frontal lobe to specific cognitive functions, (ii) to demonstrate links between cognitive function and behavior, and, (iii) to manipulate neural activity in neural prosthetics. Electrical stimulation approaches have been employed to modify memory and/or cognition mainly because the applied electrical micro-current interacts directly with the neural signals of the cognitive circuit and have the ability to bias, repair or enhance cognitive performance. This ability of neuromodulation is ideally suited for implementation in cognitive neural prosthetics in various human brain dysfunctions/disorders. There are two major categories of electrical stimulation in cognitive prosthetics for human brain deficits: one uses minimally invasive approaches while the other is based on noninvasive tools.

Electrical stimulation has been used in both humans (to map cognitive functions) and NHPs (to test hypotheses about cognitive function). NHPs are the best animal models for human cognition because they allow for: (i) minimally invasive microstimulation procedures in behavioral tasks (involving memory and cognition), in a manner that has not yet been shown in rodents or other species that allow for similar manipulations; (ii) electrical microstimulation is particularly useful for precisely timed manipulation of neural activity, that may normally fire in a relatively synchronous manner, like with microstimulation [11, 12] and is causally related to working memory [13, 14] and motor planning updating [13], antisaccade [15] perceptual decision [16], target selection [14], executive control [17], arousal [18]; (iii) electrical

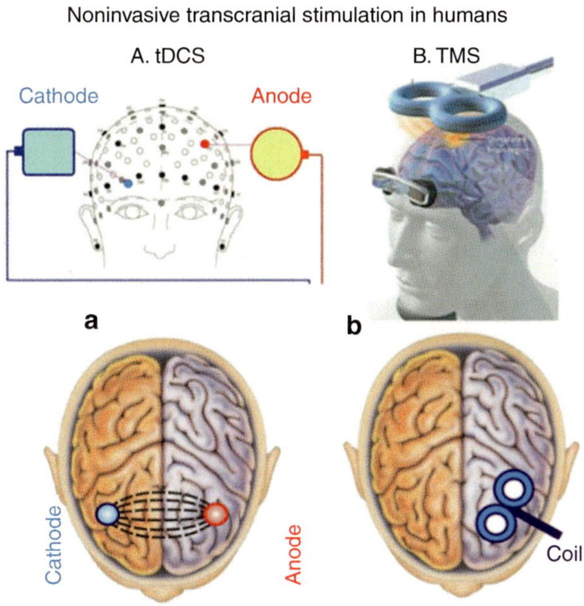

Fig. 12.1 Human brain stimulation. (**a**) Transcranial direct current stimulation (*tDCS*), and (**b**) Transcranial magnetic stimulation (*TMS*). Illustration on the human brain of the flow of direct current between anode and cathode in the tDCS and of the placement of the magnetic coil over prefrontal cortex in TMS

microstimulation is currently more reliable in NHPs than any other manipulation tool, under most conditions [19–25]. A new optogenetic stimulation approach is gaining momentum in rodent neuroscience research, mainly because of its ability to dissect the functions of neural circuits [26]. However, in NHPs a down fall of optogenetics is that only about 40–50% of cells are expressed by viral vectors [25]. Moreover, this technique comes with some complex requirements that, for the moment, hinder its application to humans.

Manipulation of neural activity in the human brain: (i) provides direct observation about the localizations of perceptual and behavioral functions that are reported during focal electrical stimulation [27]; (ii) links specific brain regions to specific cognitive tasks (processes) through tDCS (Fig. 12.1a), that can generate cortical changes (neuroplasticity) even after stimulation has ended [28], (iii) TMS has been effective in reversing symptoms (Fig. 12.1b) in various psychiatric disorders, such as depression and schizophrenia [29, 30]. (iv) TMS and tDCS have limited spatial and/or temporal specificity for targeting subcortical regions [31–33].

Memory and Cognition

The seat of higher brain functions, including memory and cognition, has been identified in the prefrontal cortex (PFC). Indeed, the cognitive role of PFC was demonstrated by lesion studies that have shown impaired performance on delayed response tasks in monkeys with selective lesions on the lateral PFC [34, 35]. Additional insight came from single unit recordings [36, 37], in prefrontal cortical

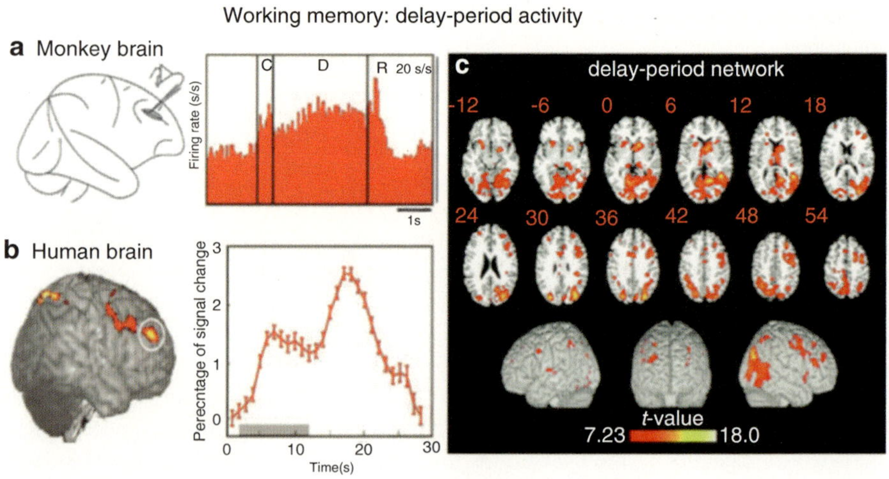

Fig. 12.2 Comparison of prefrontal cortical activity in a spatial occulomotor delayed response (ODR) task in monkey (**a**) and human (**b**). (**a**) Monkey: average of single-unit recordings from 46 neurons with delay-period activity from the monkey lateral PFC (brain area (*BA*) area 46; adapted from Ref. [14]). (*C*) cue, (*D*) delay, (*R*) response. (**b**) Human: significant delay-period activity (*left*) and average fMRI signal (*right*) from right lateral PFC (BA area 46; *circled*) in a human performing an ODR task (D'Esposito 2007). The *grey bar* represents the length of the delay interval. Note that in both cases the level of PFC activity persists throughout the delay, seconds after the stimulus cue has disappeared. (**c**) Delay-period correlation map with right FFA seed (Ref. [20]). Activations are thresholded at $p < 0.05$ (corrected) and shown overlaid on both axial slices and a three-dimensionally rendered MNI template brain. The color scale indicates the magnitude of the t-values (With permission © the Society for Neuroscience [19])

cells (Fig. 12.2a), displaying persistent, sustained levels of neuronal firing during the retention delay period, in tasks that required the NHP to retain information over a short period of time e.g. [36–39]. Such "sustained activity" is thought to provide a "bridge across time" between the stimulus cue (e.g. the location of a flash of light) and its contingent response (e.g. a later delayed saccade to the remembered location). These results have been supported by functional neuroimaging studies in humans that have shown activity in lateral PFC during performance on delay response tasks [40]. For example, in a functional magnetic resonance imaging (fMRI) study using an oculomotor delay task similar to that used in NHP studies, it was observed not only the frontal cortical activity during the retention period (Fig. 12.2b), but also the magnitude of the activity correlated positively with the accuracy of memory-guided saccade that followed later.

This relationship suggests that the neural correlate of the actively maintained location is reflected in the delay-period activity [41, 42]. Therefore, the persistent neural activity during memory delay tasks is a powerful empirical finding, which lends strong support for the hypothesis that such activity represents a neural mechanism for the active maintenance or storage of task-relevant representations. Moreover, a network of brain regions (including the prefrontal, parietal and temporal cortices) consistently correlated with the Fusiform Face Area (FFA) "seed" during the delay period and hence associated with the active maintenance of the represented stimulus [42] was identified (Fig. 12.2c). The neural mechanisms of memory and cognitive processes within functionally specialized brain regions support the concept of "persistent functional connectivity" between brain regions [43].

The Use of Electrical Stimulation in Cognition

A growing interest for therapeutic neural technologies emerged recently, mainly because novel technologies have the potential to improve mental performance of patients with various cognitive disorders [44–47]. To address these therapeutic needs, both pre-clinical approaches, such as focal intra-cortical [48–51] and patterned microstimulation [52], as well as clinical brain stimulation approaches are discussed [53]. The latter includes the transcranial current stimulation (tCS), which has been shown to improve cognitive performance [54, 55]. tCS distinguishes between transcranial direct current stimulation (tDCS; [56]), transcranial alternating current stimulation (tACS) and transcranial random noise stimulation (tRNS).

Pre-clinical Stimulation

This section includes recent experimental results in nonhuman primates that demonstrated relationships between perception, memory (short and long term) and cognitive function. One widely used modality to depict causal relations in processes of biological/neural, physical/engineering or economic systems is the "S" shape representation with sigmoid functions (Fig. 12.2). For example, the life cycle for manufacturing a product (including phases of predevelopment, take off, acceleration, stabilization) fits nicely with the lower, central and upper parts of the sigmoid curve. Similarly, during electric stimulation brain microcircuits slowly adapt to the new stimuli (pre-development), then take off, accelerate processing (on the sigmoid curve's slope), and then stabilize (depending on the intensity of the micro-current). The speed and acceleration of neural processing is quantified by the slope of the sigmoid curve (that can be more or less steeper).

Intra-cortical Stimulation

To describe causal relationships in extra-striate cortex during perceptual decisions, Newsome and collaborators [51, 59] employed a random dot kinetogram for examining correct perceptual discrimination in NHPs, as a function of sensory input (moving dots to the right; Fig. 12.3a). Such sigmoid-shaped input-output functions

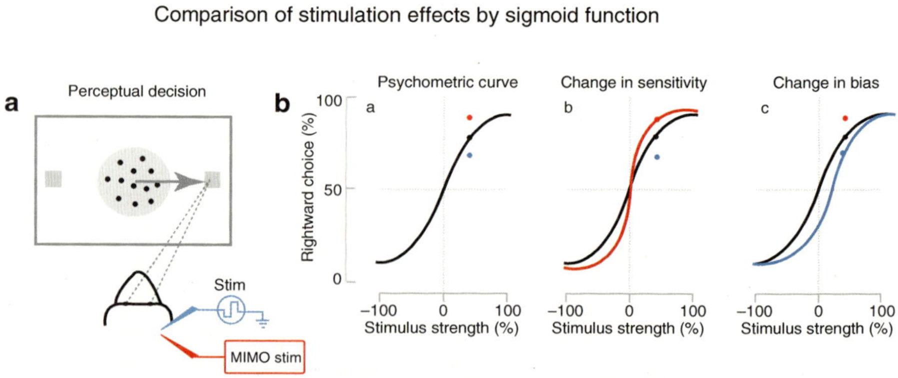

Fig. 12.3 Characterization of electrical stimulation by psychometric curves. (**a**) Monkey makes a perceptual decision, by evaluating the direction of the moving dots (in this case a rightward saccade to the target). (**b**) (*a*) Interpretation of the psychometric functions for an electrical stimulation experiment relating the rate of one of the responses (ordinate) to the relative strength of the corresponding stimulus (abscissa). *Black dot* is one of the underlying measurements. *Blue dot* is a measurement made in a different experimental condition, where performance is reduced. Two interpretations of a new measurement (*blue dot*): that may reflect a change in sensitivity (*b*), or a change in bias (*c*). In all plots, the *blue curves* represent the psychometric function in the control condition and the *black curve* is the same for the stimulation condition while the two data points have similar interpretations (Adapted with permission © Nature Publishing. [57])

can be mathematically described as: **output** = tanh (b.**input**), where b is the gain/slope [57]. An example of sigmoid curve, known as psychometric function (Fig. 12.3ba), depicts the perceptual choice (selection of the right target, output) as a function of the percentage of dots motion strength (sensory input), expressed as the percent coherence of random dots [58, 59]. Sigmoid (psychometric) curves may be regarded as transitions between different psychological states corresponding to different percepts/directions. The effect of stimulation on choice performance may be represented as a change in slope/sensitivity (faster or slower processing; Fig. 12.3bb), or as a shift in behavior, in which the probability (Fig. 12.3bc) of a certain behavioral state is biased over the others.

Patterned Stimulation

The multi-input multi-output (MIMO) model provides a novel type of microstimulation approach, based on selecting the configuration/pattern of stimulating current [52]. This approach allows task-related firing patterns in infra-granular layer to be substituted with electrical stimulation pulses in the same microcircuits, during columnar transmission from supra-granular to infra-granular layers at the time of target selection. Such patterned stimulation ensures a change in selectivity (i.e. an increase in the slope of psychometric curve; Fig. 12.3bb). More importantly, patterned stimulation improved cognitive performance [14, 60, 61].

Clinical Stimulation

Electrical Stimulation of Human Brain

Electrical stimulation is a routine clinical practice consisting of electrical discharges delivered intra-cortically to the brain region of interest in awake human patients, to map their functional involvement in cognitive functions such as language [62, 63], decision-making and memory [53, 64–66]. This method has brought unique insights into the modulation of neuronal activity within a localized, but distributed, micro-anatomical network that might explain the perceptual and behavioral phenomenology, reported during focal stimulation [53]. Actually, this was the only tool (prior to the neuroimaging era) that allowed neurologists to examine the human mind in conscious patients [67]. The classical studies provided the most direct evidence about the localization of functions in the human brain. A prime example is the map of somatosensory homunculus in the primary sensory cortex [67–70].

Transcranial Stimulation with Electrical Current

This form of stimulation is a group of neural technologies that use electrical current for therapy purpose. If the stimulation approach uses constant, low current, delivered to the brain region of interest through the electrodes on the scalp, the method is known as transcranial direct current stimulation (tDCS) [56]. This stimulation method was developed with the goal of helping patients with brain injuries (strokes). tDCS is capable of improving cognitive performance in healthy subjects in a variety of tasks, depending on the region of the brain being stimulated [45]. tDCS was employed to enhance attention span [71], memory [72–74], problem solving ability [75], language [76, 77] and math ability [78, 79]. Three different types of stimulation are in use: anodal, cathodal, and sham [80]. The *anodal* stimulation increases neuronal excitability [75, 81], while the *cathodal* stimulation decreases the neuronal excitability of stimulated area (treating hyper-activity, [82]). *Sham* stimulation emits a brief current and remains off for the rest of stimulation period, thus serving as a control for experiments [83]. By comparing the stimulation outcomes in subjects undergoing sham stimulation with those exposed to anodal or cathodal stimulation, one can dissociate the effect caused by current stimulation from the placebo effect [82]. One recurring question asks why is this technique not accepted and used widely? One group (Buzsáki, [84]) found that only 10 % of the applied current reached the brain, the rest is not entering the brain, likely being redirected by the skin. In fact, it is well known that tDCS doesn't cause neurons to fire (Biksom, [84]), but tDCS may affect brain plasticity (i.e. the degree to which the brain changes with experience). It is believed that even though tDCS may be over-hyped, it is still possible that it could be a very useful technique to find out more about how brain functions, or even to help those distressed by unusual experiences (hearing voices or seeing phosphenes).

Transcranial Magnetic Stimulation

The TMS technique of brain stimulation utilizes a magnetic coil held above the region of interest on the scalp [44]. It uses a rapidly changing magnetic field to induce a small electrical current in the brain (according to the Faraday's law of electromagnetism). TMS causes neural cell to actually fire action potentials [85]. There are two types of magnetic stimulation techniques used in research therapy: (i) a repetitive TMS and (ii) a single pulse TMS. The repetitive TMS is using higher frequency to induce excitatory neuronal activity and lower frequency to generate neural inhibition. The repetitive version of TMS provides longer lasting effects than the stimulation period [86]. Also, TMS can be used superficially [44, 47] and deep [86–88]. TMS was shown to improve cognitive performance by targeting the specific microcircuits involved in the deficits [47, 89–91]. TMS is FDA approved for use in depression, autism spectrum disorder, anxiety, post-traumatic stress and other disorders. A recurring question is why is this technique accepted and used widely? One of the reasons is that TMS causes neurons to fire and tDCS does not. Then, TMS has minimal side effects while treating patients within a broad spectrum of symptoms.

Overview of Preclinical Data

Causal Role of Prefrontal Cortex in Executive Function

Intracortical Microstimulation of Cognitive Circuits

To manipulate the cognitive functions of perception, attention, working memory, decision making and executive control, one needs to tap into the cognitive neural circuit [92]. In this regard, intra-cortical microstimulation with low microcurrents has been instrumental in modifying these cognitive states. Opris and Ferrera (2014) reviewed recent preclinical data showing primate neurophysiological evidence from prefrontal, parietal or infero-temporal cortices, as well as the subcortical structures of basal ganglia and thalamus, in a multitude of cognitive processes that are outlined below [92]. To demonstrate causal links to cognition, focal intra-cortical stimulation with microcurrents below the behavioral threshold has been successfully used. This allowed the experimenter to manipulate neural activity of memory fields with spatial and temporal precision [13–16, 59, 93]. A sub-threshold electrical micro-current applied during the delay period helps to localize the processing site of memory (maintenance or updating) or the selection of behavioral target. Recent primate literature [13–16, 92] provides clear causal links to working memory (saccade target selection, decision making, behavioral inhibition, saccade motor planning and updating), as revealed by delay period microstimulation in prefrontal cortex. There are also potential applications of microstimulation to higher cognitive functions and their 'read-out' mechanisms for interpreting memory fields in executive control.

Motor Plan Updating in Working Memory

An intriguing aspect of visual working memory deals with the updating of an oculomotor plan [73, 92]. Microstimulation applied to nonhuman primate brain during the remembering period (delay) of a memory guided saccade (MGS) task, provided insights into how prefrontal cortical neuron firing and the mechanism of spatial updating work together during saccadic eye movement plans [13, 94–98]. Stimulation caused a reduction in saccade amplitude, as the electrically elicited saccade was shorter than the desired voluntary saccade [13]. The change in saccade amplitude at the preferred location was greater than that at opposite location, and the directional shift of saccades was away from the preferred location. Both saccade direction and amplitude changes obeyed a vector subtraction scheme (analogous to a difference of casted "votes" in political elections or preferences of two populations of neurons). This suggests that FEF microstimulation may, in fact, induce a re-mapping of visual space that may result in an update (change) of a saccade plan [13, 99]. This finding seems consistent with the view that FEF is involved in maintaining and updating a spatially accurate representation of target location that compensates for eye movements, intervened between target disappearance and movement onset [13, 94, 100–104].

Causal Role of Prefrontal Cortex in Target Selection

Spatial working memory is considered a part of an executive mechanism involved in the association (including selection) and transformation of visual signals in voluntary behavior. Memory delay period stimulation experiments in nonhuman primates, performing the selection of spatial target in the match-to-sample (MTS) task, shed light on the mechanism used in saccade target selection (an example is shown in Fig. 12.4) [14]. Applying sub-threshold microcurrents has induced a selection bias that deflected the saccades towards the receptive/memory field. This is a neat causal effect since the memory field shown by the tuning plot in Fig. 12.4a and the direction of deflected saccades in Fig. 12.4b coincide to each other. In the absence of stimulation, monkey was choosing correctly the matching target, while the microcurrent introduced a consistent bias away from the matching target, but towards the memory field. Overall, the stimulation of prefrontal cortex taps into the selection/decision mechanism signals responsible for target selection, biasing saccade choices towards or away from memory. These and other results open the door for cognitive therapies to enhance memory and decision processes.

Patterned Microstimulation

A novel paradigm in the microstimulation approach occurred when the pattern of stimuli (a sequence of microcurrent pulses derived in real time from the input neurons recorded simultaneously) was fed into the output neurons. This stimulation

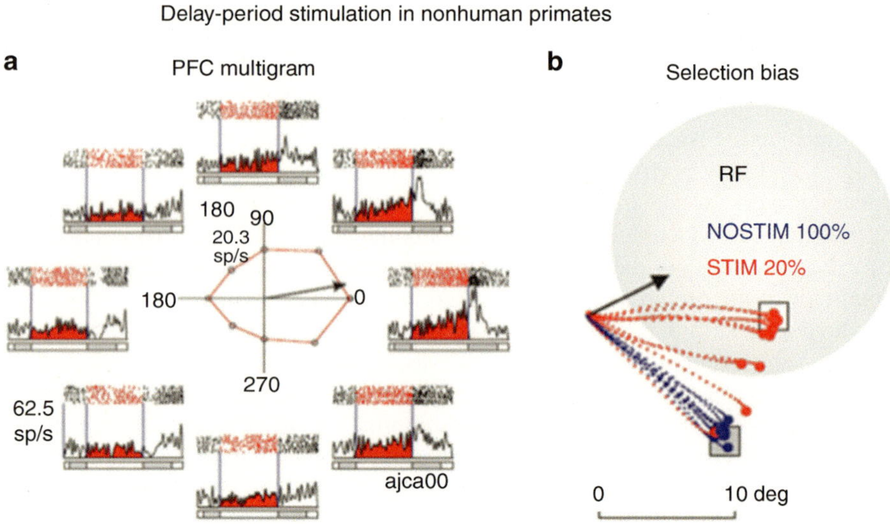

Fig. 12.4 Illustration of the functional role of prefrontal cortical activity to target selection. (a) Prefrontal cortical cell showing delay period activity and spatial preference (neural tuning). (b) Electrical stimulation induced bias towards the receptive field (Adapted from [92])

approach employing multiple inputs and multiple outputs (MIMO), known as the MIMO model (see Fig. 12.5), is based on the principle of multiplexing. Basically, this principle allows a high rate signal to be split into several lower rate signals, which are then sent to multiple recipients, via multiple channels. With multiple channels of information transfer, the MIMO model provides a more reliable communication alternative [52]. A key difference between focal stimulation and MIMO model is reflected in the sigmoid curves of the psychometric plots (Fig. 12.3bb, bc). While focal microstimulation mainly induces a shift/bias, the MIMO microstimulation increases the curve's slope that depicts processing rate/sensitivity [59]. This implies an increase in correct performance that represents the cognitive enhancement substrate.

Inter-laminar Prefrontal Cortical Microcircuit Stimulation

As it was initially proposed by Vernon Mountcastle, the primate neocortical circuitry has a modular architecture with a multitude of sensory (visual, auditory, touch), motor, cognitive (attention, memory, decision) and emotional functions [105–108]. These modules are composed of elementary building blocks formed by vertical arrangements of cortical neurons, called minicolumns [106, 109]. Within minicolumns, cortical neurons are aggregated into six horizontal layers (or laminae): supra-granular (L1-L3), granular (L4) infra-granular layers (L5/L6) (Fig. 12.5a). The granular layer receives sensory input from thalamus [110], and the infra-granular layers execute the associative computations elaborated in supra-granular layers [111, 112].

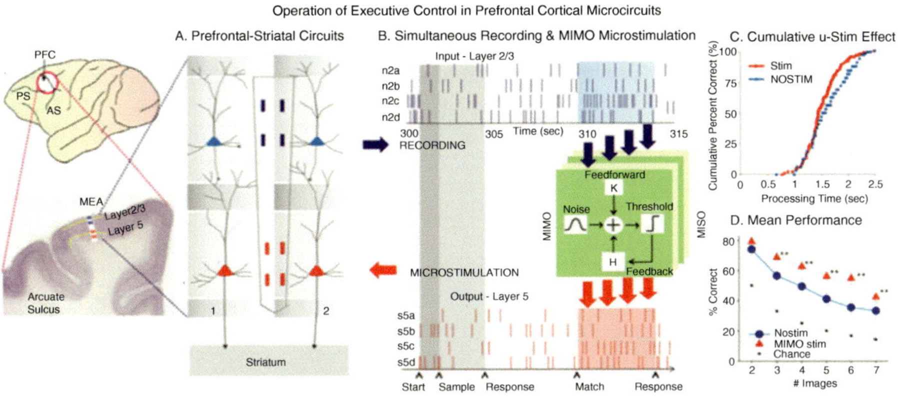

Fig. 12.5 Illustration of the executive control operation in prefrontal cortical microcircuits. *Left*: Monkey brain with a coronal section through the prefrontal cortex showing the display of multi-electrode array (*MEA*) across the cortical layers. *Right*: (**a**) Diagram of two adjacent cortical mini-columns with the recording multielectrode array in place. (**b**) The type of input and output firing patterns recorded and analyzed by the MIMO model. (**c**) Cumulative effect of microstimulation depicted in percent correct performance as a function of processing time (reaction time + movement time). (**d**) Comparison of mean performance with and without MIMO stimulation (Adapted from [92])

The neuromorphic MEAs provided a basis for applying the columnar specific MIMO model to control firing of cells via of electrical stimulation [61, 113–117]. Figure 12.5 depicts the operation of a multi-input multi-output nonlinear model, applied to the prefrontal cortical cells in layer L2/3 and L5 [61, 116–118]. Figure 12.5b shows the input and output firing patterns, recorded and analyzed by the MIMO model and illustrates how the output pattern of L5 cell firing is duplicated via a multichannel stimulator that is capable of delivering predetermined patterns (that mimic firing on correct trials) of pulses to the same L5 pads. The advantage of the MIMO model stimulation is that it: (i) detects when an inappropriate L2/3 firing pattern occurs, (ii) triggers the delivery of the appropriate L5 stimulation pattern, (iii) provides the means to override errors, and (iv) enhances performance (Fig. 12.5c, d). [116, 117]. Stimulation consisted of 1.0 ms bipolar pulses (50–70 uA) delivered to L5 recording locations following presentation of the Match phase screen and prior to the completion of the Match Response. This nicely illustrated that MIMO derived stimulation induces an enhanced cognitive processing (Fig. 12.5d) [116, 117].

Enhancement of Cognitive Performance

Cognitive enhancement may be explained by an increase in the columnar processing of cortical circuit seen in Fig. 12.2bb and by the increased percentage of trials performed correctly (Fig. 12.5d). These enhancement methods employed the multi-input/multi-output (MIMO) model, which converted the firing of neurons in layer

2/3 into microstimulation patterns applied to layer 5 [28, 117]. Such stimulation improved normal task performance, but more importantly, recovered performance after being impaired by a pharmacological disruption of the decision process [117]. These findings provided the first successful demonstration of a microcircuit-based neuroprosthesis designed specifically to restore or repair the disrupted cognitive function.

Transformation of Spatial Perception into Action

PFC microcircuits play a key role in the transformation of sensation/perception into action, known as the perception to action cycle (Fig. 12.6). Multi-neuron firing from synaptically interconnected PFC cells was recorded in supra-granular layer L2/3, infra-granular layer L5 and the caudate nucleus CN. The results [61] nicely show that during the perception and selection phases of the task, cell firing in the localized prefrontal layers L2/3, L5 and caudate-putamen region (Fig. 12.6a) exhibited a similar location preference on spatial-trials (single session, in Fig. 12.6b, and all sessions in Fig. 12.6c), but not on object- trials. The same MIMO model was capable of extracting relevant L2/3-to-L5 spatiotemporal firing patterns during task performance (Fig. 12.6d). These findings suggest that inter-laminar PFC microcircuits play key roles in bridging perception and action to coordinate the executive control of behavior across the entire spectrum of sensory and motor functions [61, 117–121].

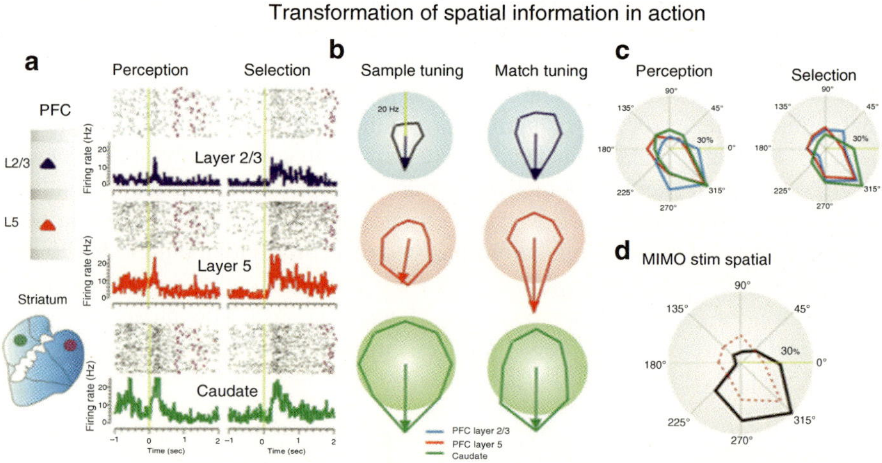

Fig. 12.6 Transformation of spatial information in action. (**a**) Neural activity in prefrontal cortical layers L2/3, L5 and caudate during perception and selection. (**b**) Spatial tuning during the perception and selection phases of the task. (**c**) Distribution of neural tuning in prefrontal cortical layers L2/3, L5 and caudate nucleus during perception and selection functions. (**d**) Distribution of MIMO stimulation induced tuning during correct performance (Adapted from [38])

Enhancement of Memory Performance by Hippocampal Stimulation

The primary factor that defines Alzheimer's disease, ageing and dementia is the deterioration of memory accuracy [118]. Memory deterioration is coming from the impaired function of the hippocampal microcircuits in the medial temporal lobe. Therefore, the development of a hippocampal memory neuroprosthesis that can improve natural memory encoding in nonhuman primates (NHPs), could provide memory improving in human memory disorders. To demonstrate enhancement of memory performance, NHPs were trained to perform the same standard memory task [118], i.e. the delay match to sample task (DMS). Multi-neuron recordings from synaptically interconnected hippocampal cell fields, CA1 and CA3, show neural firing associated to encoding of spatial target (in Fig. 12.7aa, b). The application of patterned stimulation derived from the MIMO model to the hippocampal CA3 and CA1 subfields in NHPs, enhances spatial preference (tuning) in correct performance across spatial types of memory variables (for single session in Fig. 12.7ba, and for all sessions in Fig. 12.7bb). The MIMO model demonstrated that specific CA3-to-CA1 firing patterns were crucial for the successful encoding of spatial features in memory. This was validated by the successful delivery of memory encoding patterns via electrical stimulation of the same CA1 recording sites during the encoding phase, which improved task performance in the subsequent retrieval phase. A potential clinic interest is likely to emerge along the memory prosthesis concept, developed by Berger's team that may allow patients with memory deficits to improve

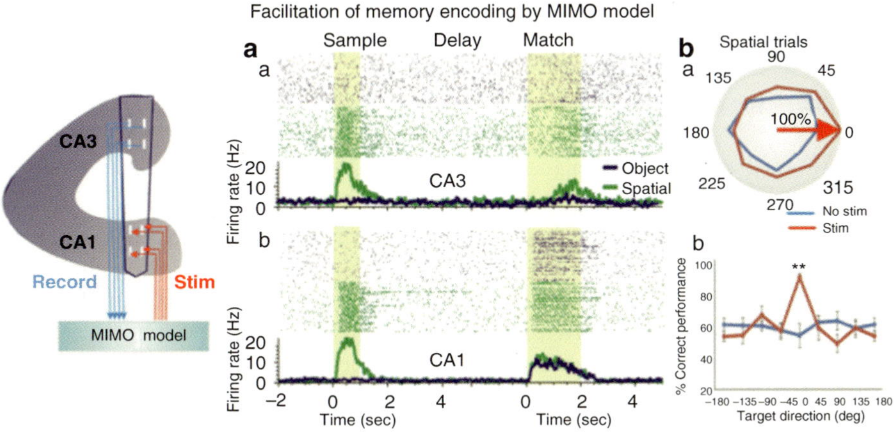

Fig. 12.7 Microstimulation induced memory performance enhancement. (**a**) Encoding of the spatial location of target images by hippocampal subfields CA1-CA3. Two hippocampal cells from CA3 (*a*) and CA1 (*b*) respond to the presentation of the sample target location when the spatial rule is in effect, but did not increase firing on object trials. (**b***a*). Facilitated spatial tuning by the delivery of MIMO stimulation. The facilitative effect of MIMO stimulation (Stim) vs. control (no-stim) trials shows both tuning and enhancement. (**b***b*). Overall facilitation effect (n = 20 sessions) on correct performance between MIMO stimulation and control (no-stim) conditions for "Spatial" tuning (Adapted from [118])

their cognitive performance. Overall, these unique results [36] provided the first evidence for a memory neuroprosthesis in the primate brain, and indicate the potential use for recovering hippocampal dysfunction, related to Alzheimer's disease and ageing in humans [122].

Overview of Clinical Data

Minimally Invasive Electrical Brain Stimulation

In humans, electrical stimulation of the frontal lobe was reported in the dorsolateral prefrontal cortex [123], ventromedial, orbitofrontal, and anterior cingulate locations (for review see ref. 29). Depending on the stimulation site, the following responses were reported: oculomotor response i.e., smooth pursuit and saccadic eye movements (frontal eye fields, [124] adjustment of posture (supplementary motor area, SMA), [125, 126] reaching and grasping (anterior cingulate and pre-SMA), [127, 128] and non-conscious movements (premotor and primary motor area); [129] emotional facial expression and smile/laughter (anterior cingulate and SMA), [130–132] feelings of pain and discomfort (dorsal, ventromedial and orbital), [133, 134] disequilibrium sensations (anterior cingulate and SMA), [128] somatic sensations (primary motor area); [44] speech arrest, reading and singing problems, autonomic reactions such as blushing, mydriasis, and increase in heart or respiration rate (anterior cingulated) [128].

Use of Noninvasive tDCS in Prefrontal Cortex

A number of tDCS studies have shown improved cognitive performance during attention, working memory, (motor) learning, and even complex problem solving [135–139]. For example, application of tDCS over frontal brain regions, show an increase on working memory performance. When anodal tDCS was applied over left prefrontal dorsolateral cortex (DLPFC) to study its effects on working memory performance, the number of errors people make on a 3-back working memory task, increased accuracy of performance [140]. Another finding demonstrates the effect of cognitive state when subjects are not involved in a cognitive task, by modulating activity in task-positive vs. task-negative networks (as measured with fMRI [141] and EEG [142]. Thus, this stimulation effects provide evidence for the relevance of tDCS as a tool for the implementation of noninvasive neuroprosthetics.

Use of Noninvasive TMS on Cognitive Disorders

Transcranial magnetic stimulation (TMS) is a powerful technique for non-invasive brain stimulation in awake alert humans [143] and nonhuman primates [144]. The use of TMS is focused to understand the interplay between induced firing and the neural activity in neural systems that control cognition and behavior, under various behavioral contexts. In humans, repetitive TMS is increasingly used to perturb non-invasively specific brain sites, to test for causal effects on cognitive performance [145, 146]. Additionally, many researchers are investigating the therapeutic effects of repetitive TMS in depression [147, 148], schizophrenia [148], autism [24, 69, 149–151] and other brain disorders. A large amount of work has been done to demonstrate that daily use of prefrontal TMS can improve symptoms in major depression [21, 152–154].

There are two versions of TMS types in use currently: superficial and deep stimulation that have been approved for treating depressions. The superficial TMS using the butterfly coil over the prefrontal cortex can treat depression by causing a change in the brain state [153]. A routine clinical treatment for acute episodes of depression is using rTMS. Deep TMS is used for the treatment of drug-resistant major depressive disorder. The deep TMS [67, 154] can induce increases or decreases in the excitability of large assemblies of neurons in the deep areas of the brain by using cone coils (or H-coil). Moreover, for major depressive disorders resistant to treatment, the use of high frequency rTMS for the left dorsolateral PFC (dlPFC) proved effective, while low-frequency rTMS on the right dlPFC has shown "probable" efficacy [155–157]. High frequency rTMS applied to the left dlPFC also has promising efficacy in treating the negative symptoms of schizophrenia, by improving excitatory firing in pyramidal cells [155].

To further characterize the relevance of rTMS effect on memory delay-period activity the modulation of alpha-band power by rTMS [158] is presented. Figure 12.8a shows a sustained increase in alpha-band power under both conditions: with and without rTMS [158]. The effect was more enhanced for object than for location memory ($p < 10^{-5}$). Overall, there were no significant changes in power with rTMS (Fig. 12.8b, c). At the individual level, rTMS produced large, sustained changes in delay-period alpha-band power, with some subjects showing an increase, and others a decrease in power. These differences in the TMS effect on alpha-band power predicted its effect on behavior and thus illustrate its therapeutic role.

Error Correction in Autism

Low frequency rTMS stimulation in autistic children has been shown to improve the inhibitory mechanism (Fig. 12.9) of the frontal cortex [148, 159]. Similar treatment was used for the loss of brain function caused by stroke, i.e. applying low frequency rTMS on the corresponding brain region has shown a "probable" efficacy [155]. One important executive function, which is known to be compromised in autism relates to response error monitoring and post-error response correction [24]. Several reports indicate that children with autism have reduced error processing and deficient behavioral correction, after an error is committed [160–162]. Sokhadze and colleagues (2012) has shown that prefrontal neuromodulation using rTMS improves error monitoring and correction in autism. These cognitive deficits (depression, dementia, autism and others) may be repairable by means of noninvasive brain machine interfaces [163–165] that can restore neural communications, memory and cognition [28, 166].

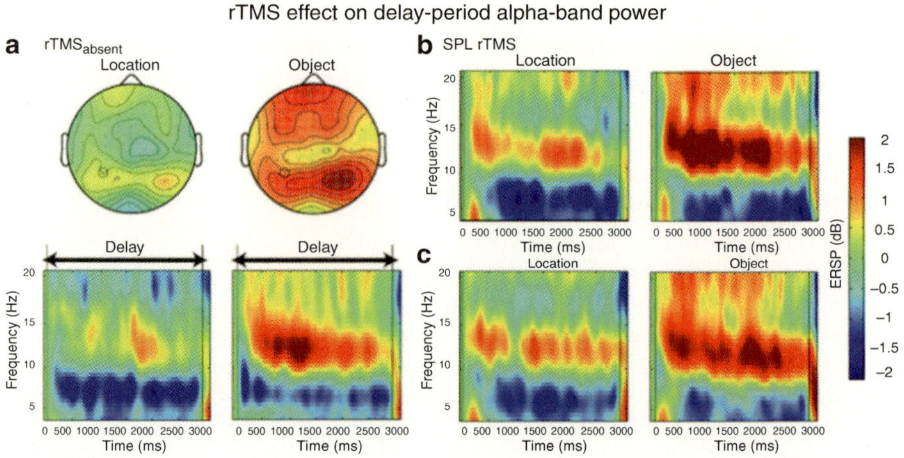

Fig. 12.8 Effect of rTMS on delay-period alpha-band power. (**a**) During the delay-period there was an increase in power between 10 and 15 Hz for both memory tasks, predominantly over posterior scalp regions. The magnitude of power change between the two memory conditions differed significantly mean difference across all channels: $t(14) = 7.58$; $p < 10^{-5}$, with delay period alpha band power being significantly greater during object memory trials compared to location memory trials. (**b**, **c**) During rTMS trials, there was a brief increase in power at 4–8 Hz associated with the onset of the stimulation train. However, compared to the rTMS absent trials, there was no significant change in power within the alpha-band range in rTMS present trials. Topographic plots in (**a**) represent the mean alpha-band power over the 3-s delay period during rTMS absent trials (© Frontiers Media S.A. [158])

Neural Technologies

The use of various stimulation devices and technologies, developed recently, are further examined and the potential clinical application to human brain disorders is discussed.

Neural Devices

Neural devices including brain machine interfaces (BMIs, [167]) and cognitive neural prosthetics [163] have been recently developed to repair a damaged brain or its disrupted function. Electrical stimulation, whether in its invasive [168] or noninvasive [47, 89], can be implemented in cognitive neuroprosthetics. Recent research sheds light on the difficult task of restoring memory or executive abilities [52, 60]. Such cognitive devices might be able to read out neural representations, percepts or thoughts for the selection of a certain behavioral goal [169, 170]. Nicolelis (2001) suggested that "hybrid brain–machine interfaces" have the potential to enhance our perceptual, motor and cognitive capabilities". Nevertheless, other questions remain

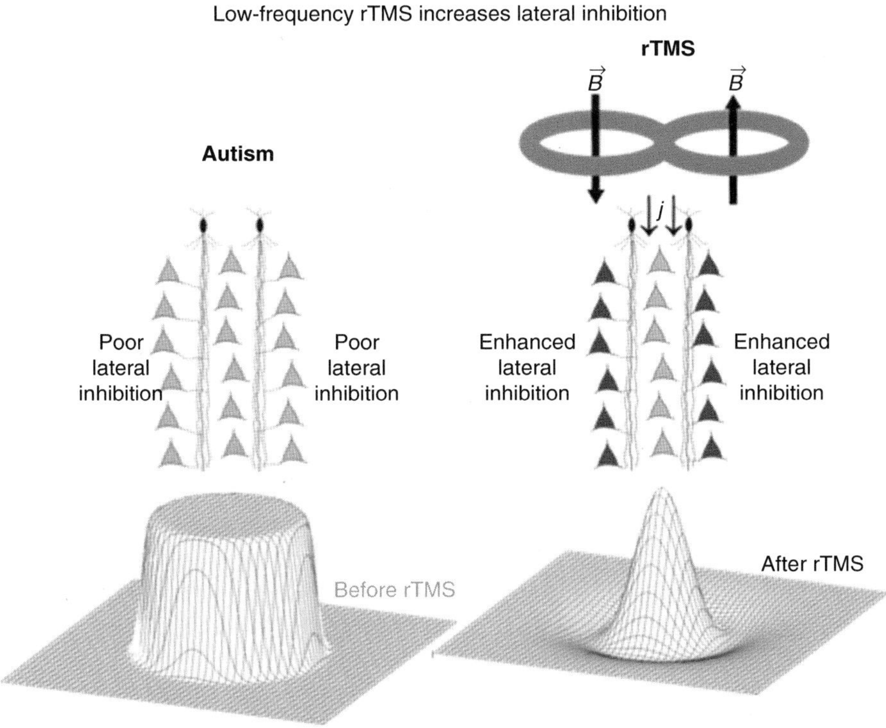

Fig. 12.9 Low-Frequency rTMS increases lateral inhibition. *Left panel* shows typical minicolumns consisting of vertical chairns of pyramidal cells surrounded by inactive double bouquest cells. *Right panel* shows how repetitive low frequency TMS activates the double bouquet cells that provide the lateral inhibition. Autistic brains lack proper lateral inhibition (Courtesy of Dr. Manuel F. Casanova)

as to whether microstimulation has the specificity and reliability required to control behavior on a fine scale, or whether it only weakly biases the tendency for certain behavioral alternatives in a probabilistic manner.

Cognitive Neural Prosthetics

A cognitive neural prosthesis (CNP) can be defined as an assistive device that utilizes high-order brain signals to restore the normal brain function to a person with neurological deficits [169, 170]. Prosthetics may be useful to a large population of patients, including those suffering from Alzheimer's disease, schizophrenia, autism, and drug addiction. Development of neural decoders for such prosthetics requires an understanding of brain microcircuits [158] and their relationship to cognition [73, 74]. CNPs can be interfaced to brain substitution systems (prosthetic limbs, percept/memory chips) and communication devices [171]. CNPs use cortical and subcortical signals that reflect such cognitive functions as decision-making, executive control, attention, and working memory [73, 74, 172]. The CNPs utilize: (i) signals recorded from the higher-order brain areas (like the prefrontal cortex) and feedback signals received from external devices; (ii) invasive (electrical) or noninvasive (magnetic) stimulation to inject signals in the brain [72, 153]; (iii) controllers with MIMO relations [28] to process information and drive microstimulation; (iv) extracted information from the brain that is decoded by neural decoding algorithms [173, 174]; (v) assistive devices, such as computers, brain chips, communication systems, speech generators, prosthetic limbs, etc. [167].

Memory Prosthetics

A recurring question in neuroscience inquires whether a neural prosthetics can restore memory. Berger and colleagues [52, 60] demonstrated, for the first time in rodents and then in nonhuman primates, that a neural prosthesis is capable to identify/manipulate in real-time the encoding process that can restore and even enhance cognitive mnemonic processes. The idea is to block the ability to form long-term memories by using pharmacological agents that disrupt neural circuitry between the two subfields of the hippocampus, CA1 and CA3, which interact to create the long-term memory engram. By employing an artificial hippocampal system based on the multiple-input, multiple-output (MIMO) model [52, 172, 173], one could duplicate the pattern of interaction between CA3-CA1, by monitoring neural activity in cells recorded by the electrode array, and then playing back the same pattern on the same array. Long-term memory capability was restored in the pharmacologically blocked rats/monkeys following activation of an electronic device, programmed to duplicate memory-encoding ability for a specific memory item (i.e. which lever to pull) in rat tests or which target to select (in monkeys). Thus, if a prosthetic memory device is implanted in animals with a normal, functioning hippocampus, the device could actually strengthen memory.

Berger and collaborators duplicated the rodent results in monkeys, with the aim of eventually creating prostheses that might help human sufferers of Alzheimer's disease, stroke, or injury. To this end, the MIMO model [60, 168, 173] was applied in the primate prefrontal cortex. Ensemble firing patterns of up to 16 prefrontal neurons were recorded using a system for wireless recording [117] of neural ensemble activity in monkeys. Firing patterns were analyzed by a MIMO model to provide coefficients for prediction of layer 5 output from layer 2/3 input. A custom built 8-channel wireless stimulator (Triangle BioSystems Inc. Durham, NC) delivered patterns of electrical pulses to layer 5 electrodes. Stimulation patterns were derived from predicted Layer 5 activity by online MIMO analysis of layer 2/3 neural activity during the match target presentation in the task. Results show that behavioral performance on stimulated trials was significantly improved compared to non-stimulated trials and behavioral latency to match target response was significantly reduced on stimulation trials [117, 168]. In addition, this study demonstrates feasibility of implementing a compact wireless neural prosthesis in nonhuman primates.

Executive Control Prosthetics

The neural prostheses approach holds out the promise of assisting individuals who are unable to move but who are capable of making movement plans. Musallam et al. (2004) have shown how monkeys learn to control the location of a computer cursor by merely thinking about movements [174]. An executive prosthesis may ba able to even correct in real time a decision making process [175]. The key aspect is that a decision making signal is "rising" to a threshold (increase/buildup) when the preferred option is selected or falling down (decrease) for a non-preferred option. Signals are recorded, decoded and interpreted so that the optimal option is selected. When the decision signal is not optimal, and error signal instructs the stimulator to apply a micro-current in the appropriate brain region (for example, in the prefrontal cortical layer 2/3, layer 5 or caudate if either sensory evidence is weak, the selection signal is weak, or else if the decision bias is weak) and the decision signal may be corrected in real time

Advanced Technologies

Nanotechnology

To understand the vast complexity of brain circuitry and its emergent functions, neuroscientists have zoomed into the details of neural microcircuits and suggested that brain communicates in a nanotech language [176]. Nanotechnology is based on the manipulations of matter on the atomic, molecular and supra-molecular level. During the last decade or so, a number of successful applications of nanotechnological methods to basic neuroscience and to medical practice emerged [177–179]. Development of novel nanotechnologies include biomaterials for neural regeneration [180, 181], characterization of biophysical features of neural cells [182], advances in molecular genetics of neurons [183], new insights into the function of neural microcircuits [184, 185] and their degeneration using animal models [186]. Furthermore, research on graphene and silicon based nanomaterials and/or devices, high density nanofabricated neural probes, integrated neural sensors, carbon nanotubes use in neural interfacing applications and other approaches that have already proven feasible for brain machine interfaces [187, 188].

Nanotechnology, as a rapidly evolving field, provides simple, practical and reproducible tools to investigate the nervous system in health and disease. Among these tools are nanoparticle-based sensors that detect biochemical and physiological properties of neurons and glia, and generate signals proportionate to physical, chemical and/or electrical changes in single cells, tissues, and whole organisms. The most commonly used sensors are those composed of quantum dots (QDs), carbon materials (C-dots, graphene and nanodiamonds) and gold nanoparticles [189, 195]. These sensors have been designed to quantify molecular entries such as intracellular and extracellular pH, oxygen, glucose, redox, electrical activity, changes in calcium concentrations, protein dimerization, and enzymatic activities. Scientists have made significant progress in developing artificial nanoparticle-based sensors, but several challenges remain. To illustrate this, we review work using nanoparticle-based sensors to detect changes in nerve cells and microglia when exposed to harmful signals or subjected to stress. Specifically, we focus on the many hurdles involved in developing artificial nanoparticle-based sensors, highlighting both their advantages and limitations.

MEA Technology

Multi-Electrode Array (MEA) technologies are playing a key role in brain machine interfaces and neuroprosthetics [190–192]. Carbon nanotubes [193, 194], in particular, have an arsenal of properties (electrical, mechanical, and chemical) that make them very promising materials for applications in MEAs neuroscience. There are two forms of carbon nanotubes (CNTs) efficiently used in MEAs: single-wall carbon nanotubes (SWCNTs) or nested multiwall carbon nanotubes (MWCNTs). A new electrode is based on "structurally controlled nanowires," for neurophysiological measurements in vivo [195]. This electrode has a sensing part made of a thin metal layer deposited on epitaxial grown GaP nanowires. Suyatin et al. (2013) realized the first functional CNW-based electrode [185]. Also, Suzuki et al. (2013) developed MEA chips of planar CNTs that can measure both the electrophysiological responses (such as action potentials and field postsynaptic potentials) and the release of the dopamine neurotransmitter [189]. These MEA chips are useful for various applications such as drug screening and toxicity, in vitro stem cell differentiation, synaptic plasticity, or pathogenic processes associated with stroke, epilepsy, Alzheimer's and other neurodegenerative diseases. Moreover, multi-walled carbon nanotubes MEAs have the advantage of decreased physical size of microelectrode with increased impedance and decreased charge-transfer capability [196, 197]. Figure 12.10 provides an illustration of various MEA technologies involving graphene/carbon nanotubes that record spikes or local field potentials [198–220].

Multiplexed High Density MEAs

Neural probes based on silicon, Du et al. (2011) employed nanofabricated, high-density electrical leads that can read out multichannel data. MEA uses an application-specific integrated circuit to intensify signals, multiplexing functions and band-pass filtering [198]. Multiplex high density devices with a fully integrated low noise, 64-channel system can perform high spatial resolution extracellular measurements and weighs just 330 mg [198]. Viventi et al. (2011) integrated "ultrathin and flexible silicon nanomembrane transistors" into a MEA [199], enabling "dense arrays" of thousands of amplified and multiplexed sensors to be connected with fewer wires.

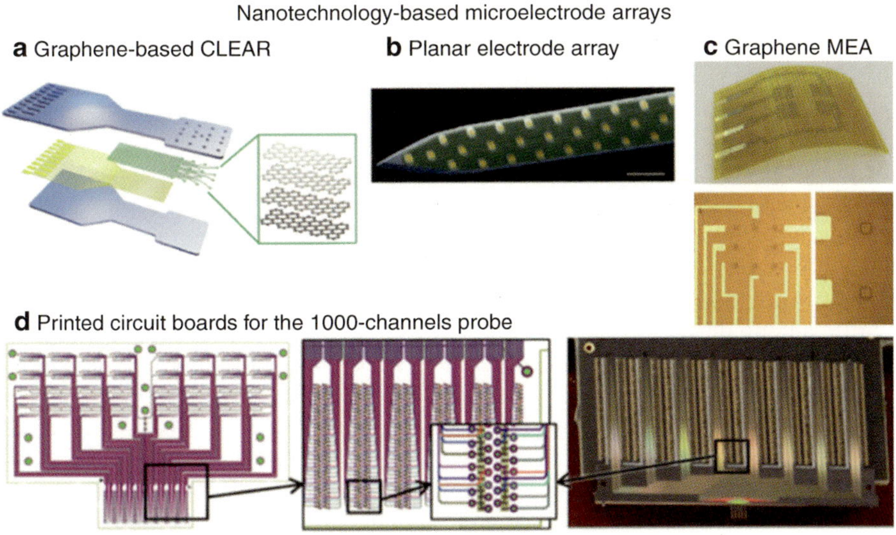

Fig. 12.10 Multielectrode arrays. (**a**) Graphene-based carbon-layered electrode array device construction showing the layered structures (With permission © MacMillan Publishers [219]) (**b**) Nanofabricated planar electrode array for high-density neuronal voltage recording. False-color SEM image of a portion of a 64-channel array patterned on a silicon substrate. Scale bar = 50 μm (Modified with permission ©PLOS One [198]) (**c**) Description of graphene electrodes. (*a*) Schematic illustration of a flexible graphene neural electrode array. Patterned graphene electrodes are in contact with Au contact pads to interface with the data acquisition system. (*b*) Microscope image of an 8-electrode hippocampal slice array. The electrode size is 50 × 50 mm². (With permisson PLOS One [220]) (**d**) Printed circuit boards design schematics for the 1000-channel probe. The routing for the 1000-channel probe was broken into a comb-shaped multifinger design, of eight fingers with 128 pads each (photograph of the probe after wire bonding but before encapsulation) (With permission © IEEE [218])

Substrate-Integrated MEAs

Substrate-integrated MEAs seem to provide the finest approach to study brain circuitry, connectivity, neurophysiology, or pathology both in vivo and in vitro. MEAs add versatility to the real-time, long-term recording of chemical fluctuations in the extra-cellular micro-environment along with neurophysiological activity while being minimally invasive [200–202]. These MEAs can monitor the organization of neural network, its neuronal excitability, and synaptic plasticity, together with drug responses.

Nanotechnology Based Brain Machine Interfaces

Latest developments in nanomaterials generated new avenues for highly advanced systems to interface the human brain [182]. Nanotechnology is employing macromolecular approaches to implants that mimic the "biologic topology" and take into account the surface interaction of biologic cells. Combinations of neural cells with micro-implants can become the platform of stable bio-hybrid interfaces. Artificial synapses in neuromorphic circuits based on nanoscale memory devices provide novel circuit architectures that tolerate variability and/or defects [197]. Such memory elements based on carbon nanotubes (CNTs) may be used as "artificial synapses" combined with "conventional neurons" further "trained" to perform several functions (by applying a supervised learning algorithm). This approach has huge potential for application to parallel learning of several devices with more complex functions, because the same device can be trained to code successively any type combination of Boolean logic functions (3-inputs) despite variability among devices.

Carbon nanowires (used as interface material in contact with neurons) can deliver electrical stimulation to these cells and detect neuronal electrical activity [203]. In recent years, CNT substrates have been used to examine in vivo formation of neurons and neuronal networks during guided growth by artificial nano-scaled cues. Additionally, prostheses for monitoring brain activity were developed using interfaces based on nanotube architecture [204]. Thus, Fabbro et al. (2012) demonstrated the alteration of various hippocampal neurons responses by the CNT substrates in cultures [205]. This observation highlighted the exceptional ability of the CNT substrate to induce nerve tissue growth. CNT scaffolds promote the development of immature neurons isolated from the neonatal rat spinal cord and maintained in vitro by performing electrophysiological studies associated with gene expression analysis.

The potential for employing inter-laminar recording and micro-stimulation of cortical microcircuits with CNT-MEAs to build neural prostheses for repair and augmentation of cognitive function is now being considered. Thus, nanotechnology is instrumental to nanofabricate planar electrode arrays to be used in high-density neuronal voltage recording [195, 198]. Micro and nano-fabrication technologies raise the prospect for increasing the numbers of electrodes for smaller, less invasive implantable devices. A promising nano-array for brain microcircuits is the new planar electrode array [199, 206], which is configured on a crystalline, ceramic, or polymer support structure. Recording neural firing with 3-dimensional microelectrode arrays [207] represents a major advance in brain activity mapping techniques, by providing a tool to demonstrate how intra and inter-laminar/regional neural circuits cooperate together to process relevant information. Building prosthetic minicolumns as basic modules to repair the damaged cortical tissue will become a valuable approach for cognitive neuroprosthetics [185]. This may be accomplished by designing artificial minicolumns that can be inserted by minor surgery into the human brain, or the use of nanowire contacts to place a device with minicolumn function within the damaged circuitry [208, 209]. Moreover, neural enhancement approaches may be applied to inter-laminar microcircuits across the entire cortex [168].

Wireless Stimulation of Cognitive Prosthetics

Latest advances in sensor technology, targeting the development of non-invasive and implantable wireless BMI-systems (combined with brain stimulation), are suggesting that BMI-related strategies will play an increasing role in neurorehabilitation of stroke [210], sensorimotor functions [211, 212]. A super multi-channel recording system was developed by Suzuki et al., [213] in which 4096 channels of Electrocorticogram (ECoG) signal can be amplified and transmitted to outside the body by using an Ultra Wide Band (UWB) wireless system. Neural chips with wireless stimulation for memory [36] and/or decision making [73, 74, 114, 115, 117] propose that an error signal instructs the wireless microstimulator to apply a microcurrent in the right brain region and the decision signal should be corrected in real time.

Neural Chips

Converging technologies exploit the synergies between neuroscience, psychology, computer sciences, engineering and nanotechnology to build the largest IBM chip in a brain inspired computer (www.research.ibm.com/articles/brain-chip.shtml). The chip consumes merely 70 milliwatts, and is capable of 46 billion synaptic operations per second, per watt (i.e. a synaptic supercomputer in hand). Similar to the brain—the neuromorphic chip has a parallel, distributed, modular, scalable, fault-tolerant, flexible architecture that integrates computation, communication, and memory and has no clock. The neurosynaptic chips can be tiled to create vast, scalable neuromorphic systems [215]. The brain-inspired chip can be used in combination with other cognitive computing technologies to create systems that learns, reason and help humans make better decisions. Moreover, the neuromorphic structure of these chips can solve a broad class of problems from sensory neuroscience to cognition, and has the potential to revolutionize the computer industry by integrating its brain-inspired capability into devices with computational constraints in speed and power. These neuromorphic systems using spikes as inputs and outputs have the ability to process in real time, high-dimensional, noisy sensory data, with several orders of magnitude less power than the conventional computers. It is envisioned a new generation of field-adaptable neurosynaptic computers capable of online learning [215].

Future Directions

Future research is targeting the mapping of the brain and mind with nanotechnology. In 2013 the BRAIN initiative was launched by the USA - the world's biggest project to map the brain and understand the human mind by combining neuroscience with nanotechnology. New devices based on nanotechnology (minimally invasive and noninvasive) and spintronix (nanomagnetism or micromagnetism) or quantum dots, as well as nano-TMS and 3D nano-magnetic imaging based on tunneling magnetoresistance are emerging. This will yield the knowledge necessary to understand the mind and cure its devastating disorders.

Conclusion

The advancement of neural technology is providing new therapeutic approaches to improve mental performance for patients with cognitive disorders. By developing stimulation systems with minimally invasive and noninvasive ability it allows manipulatation of cognitive and behavioral performance. Electro-stimulation therapies become instrumental in modifying (improving) memory and cognition including working memory, decision-making and executive control by enhancing cognitive performance. The use of various neuroprosthetic devices and technologies developed recently has multiple clinical applications to human brain disorders. The ultimate goal should be to develop devices that patients can learn to control without external intervention.

References

1. Parent A. Aldini's Essay on Galvanism. Can J Neurol Sci. 2004;31(4):576–84.
2. Aldini J. Essai théorique et expérimental sur le galvanisme, avec une série d'expériences faites devant des commissaires de l'Institut national de France, et en divers amphithéâtres anatomiques de Londres. Paris: Fournier Fils; 1804.
3. Fritsch G, Hitsig E. On the electrical excitability of the cerebrum. Archiv für Anatomie, Physiologie, und Wissenscahftliche Medicin. 1870;37:300–32.
4. Ferrier D. The functions of the brain. London: Smith, Elder & Co; 1886.
5. Penfield W, Perot P. The brain's record of auditory and visual experience. A Final Summary and Discussion. Brain. 1963;86:595–696.
6. Stamm JS, Rosen SC. Electrical stimulation and steady potential shifts in prefrontal cortex during delayed response performance by monkeys. Acta Biol Exp (Warsz). 1969;29(3):385–99.
7. Geddes LA. History of Magnetic Stimulation of the Nervous System. J Clin Neurophysiol. 1991;8(1):3–9.
8. Barker AT, Jalinous R, Freeston IL. Non-invasive magnetic stimulation of human motor cortex. The Lancet. 1985;325(8437):1106–7.
9. Albert DJ. The effect of spreading depression on the consolidation of learning. Neuropsychologia. 1966;4:49–64.
10. Merton PA, Morton HB. Stimulation of the cerebral cortex in the intact human subject. Nature. 1980;285(5762):227.
11. Christie MJ, Williams JT, North RA. Electrical coupling synchronizes subthreshold activity in locus coeruleus neurons in vitro from neonatal rats. J Neurosci. 1989;9:3584–9.
12. Alvarez VA, Chow CC, Van Bockstaele EJ, Williams JT. Frequency-dependent synchrony in locus ceruleus: role of electrotonic coupling. Proc Natl Acad Sci U S A. 2002;99:4032–6.

13. Opris I, Barborica A, Ferrera VP. Effects of electrical microstimulation in monkey frontal eye field on saccades to remembered targets. Vision Res. 2005a;45(27):3414–29.
14. Opris I, Barborica A, Ferrera VP. Microstimulation of dorsolateral prefrontal cortex biases saccade target selection. J Cogn Neurosci. 2005b;17(6):893–904.
15. Wegener SP, Johnston K, Everling S. Microstimulation of monkey dorsolateral prefrontal cortex impairs antisaccade performance. Exp Brain Res. 2008;190(4):463–73.
16. Popa I, Donos C, Barborica A, Opris I, Mălîia MD, Ene M, Ciurea J, Mîndruţă I. Intrusive thoughts elicited by direct electrical stimulation during stereo-electroencephalography. Front. Neurol. 2016. http://dx.doi.org/10.3389/fneur.2016.00114.
17. Opris I, Popa IL, Casanova MF. Prefrontal cortical microcircuits of executive control. Chapter 10. In: Manuel F, editor. Recent advances on the modular organization of the cerebral cortex. Dordrecht: Casanova and Ioan Opris, Springer; 2015. p. 157–79.
18. Carter ME, Yizhar O, Chikahisa S, Nguyen H, Adamantidis A, et al. Tuning arousal with optogenetic modulation of locus coeruleus neurons. Nat Neurosci. 2010;13:1526–33.
19. Ohayon S, Grimaldi P, Schweers N, Tsao DY. Saccade modulation by optical and electrical stimulation in the macaque frontal eye field. J Neurosci. 2013;33:16684–97.
20. Dai J, Brooks DI, Sheinberg DL. Optogenetic and electrical microstimulation systematically bias visuospatial choice in primates. Curr Biol. 2014;24:63–9.
21. Tehovnik EJ. Electrical stimulation of neural tissue to evoke behavioral responses. J Neurosci Methods. 1996;65:1–17.
22. Gerits A, Farivar R, Rosen BR, Wald LL, Boyden ES, Vanduffel W. Optogenetically induced behavioral and functional network changes in primates. Curr Biol. 2012;22:1722–6.
23. Cavanaugh J, Monosov IE, McAlonan K, Berman R, Smith MK, et al. Optogenetic inactivation modifies monkey visuomotor behavior. Neuron. 2012;76:901–7.
24. Jazayeri M, Lindbloom-Brown Z, Horwitz GD. Saccadic eye movements evoked by optogenetic activation of primate V1. Nat Neurosci. 2012;15:1368–70.
25. Diester I, Kaufman MT, Mogri M, Pashaie R, Goo W, Yizhar O, Ramakrishnan C, Deisseroth K, Shenoy KV. An optogenetic toolbox designed for primates. Nat Neurosci. 2011;14(3):387–97. doi:10.1038/nn.2749.
26. Dai J, Ozden I, Brooks DI, Wagner F, May T, Agha NS, Brush B, Borton D, Nurmikko AV, Sheinberg DL. Modified toolbox for optogenetics in the nonhuman primate. Neurophotonics. 2015;2(3):031202. doi:10.1117/1.NPh.2.3.031202.
27. Gold JI, Shadlen MN. Representation of a perceptual decision in developing oculomotor commands. Nature. 2000;404(6776):390–4.
28. Vlachos A, Müller-Dahlhaus F, Rosskopp J, Lenz M, Ziemann U, Deller T. Repetitive magnetic stimulation induces functional and structural plasticity of excitatory postsynapses in mouse organotypic hippocampal slice cultures. J Neurosci. 2012;32(48):17514–23.
29. Demirtas-Tatlidede A, Vahabzadeh-Hagh AM, Pascual-Leone A. Can noninvasive brain stimulation enhance cognition in neuropsychiatric disorders? Neuropharmacology. 2013;64:566–78.
30. Slotema CW, Blom JD, Hoek HW, Sommer IE. Should we expand the toolbox of psychiatric treatment methods to include Repetitive Transcranial Magnetic Stimulation (rTMS)? A meta-analysis of the efficacy of rTMS in psychiatric disorders. J Clin Psychiatry. 2010 Jul;71(7):873–84.
31. Hallett M. Transcranial magnetic stimulation: a primer. Neuron. 2007;55:187–99.
32. Neuling T, Wagner S, Wolters CH, Zaehle T, Herrmann CS. Finite-element model predicts current density distribution for clinical applications of tDCS and tACS. Front Psych. 2012;3:83.
33. Davis NJ, Van Koningsbruggen MG. "Non-invasive" brain stimulation is not non-invasive. Front. Syst. Neurosci. 2013;7:76.
34. Bauer RH, Fuster JM. Delayed-matching and delayed-response deficit from cooling dorsolateral prefrontal cortex in monkeys. Q J Exp Psychol B. 1976;90:293–302.

35. Funahashi S, Bruce CJ, Goldman-Rakic PS. Mnemonic coding of visual space in the monkey's dorsolateral prefrontal cortex. J Neurophysiol. 1989;61:331–49.
36. Fuster JM, Alexander GE. Neuron activity related to short-term memory. Science. 1971;173:652–4.
37. Funahashi S, Bruce CJ, Goldman-Rakic PS. Dorsolateral prefrontal lesions and oculomotor delayedresponse performance: evidence for mnemonic "scotomas". J Neurosci. 1993;13:1479–97.
38. Miller EK, Li L, Desimone R. Activity of neurons in anterior inferior temporal cortex during a short-term memory task. J Neurosci. 1993;13:1460–78.
39. Chafee MV, Goldman-Rakic PS. Matching patterns of activity in primate prefrontal area 8a and parietal area 7ip neurons during a spatial working memory task. J Neurophysiol. 1998;79:2919–40.
40. Curtis CE, D'Esposito M. Persistent activity in the prefrontal cortex during working memory. Trends Cogn Sci. 2003;7:415–23.
41. Curtis CE, Rao VY, D'Esposito M. Maintenance of spatial and motor codes during oculomotor delayed response tasks. J Neurosci. 2004;24:3944–52.
42. D'Esposito M. From cognitive to neural models of working memory. Phil Trans R Soc B. 2007;362:761–72.
43. Gazzaley A, Rissman J, Desposito M. Functional connectivity during working memory maintenance. Cogn Affect Behav Neurosci. 2004;4:580–99.
44. George MS, Nahas Z, Kozel FA, Goldman J, Molloy M, Oliver N. Improvement of depression following transcranial magnetic stimulation. Curr Psychiatry Rep. 1999;1(2):114–24.
45. Mondino M et al. Can transcranial direct current stimulation (tDCS) alleviate symptoms and improve cognition in psychiatric disorders? World J Biol Psychiatry. 2014;15(4):261–75.
46. Casanova MF, Sokhadze E, Opris I, Wang Y, Li X. Autism spectrum disorders: linking neuropathological findings to treatment with transcranial magnetic stimulation. Acta Paediatr. 2015;104(4):346–55. doi:10.1111/apa.12943.
47. Sokhadze EM, El-Baz AS, Sears LL, Opris I, Casanova MF. rTMS neuromodulation improves electrocortical functional measures of information processing and behavioral responses in autism. Front Syst Neurosci. 2014;8:134. doi:10.3389/fnsys.2014.00134.
48. Fitzsimmons NA, Drake W, Hanson TL, Lebedev MA, Nicolelis MA. Primate reaching cued by multichannel spatiotemporal cortical microstimulation. J Neurosci. 2007;7(21):5593–602.
49. Churchland MM, Shenoy KV. Delay of movement caused by disruption of cortical preparatory activity. J Neurophysiol. 2007;97(1):348–59.
50. Logothetis NK, Augath M, Murayama Y, Rauch A, Sultan F, Goense J, Oeltermann A, Merkle H. The effects of electrical microstimulation on cortical signal propagation. Nat Neurosci. 2010;13(10):1283–91.
51. Salzman CD, Newsome WT. Neural mechanisms for forming a perceptual decision. Science. 1994;264:231–7.
52. Berger TW, Hampson RE, Song D, Goonawardena A, Marmarelis VZ, Deadwyler SA. A cortical neural prosthesis for restoring and enhancing memory. J Neural Eng. 2011;8(4):046017.
53. Selimbeyoglu A, Parvizi J. Electrical stimulation of the human brain: perceptual and behavioral phenomena reported in the old and new literature. Front Hum Neurosci. 2010;4:1–11.
54. Ruffini G, Wendling F, Merlet I, Molaee-Ardekani B, Mekonnen A, Salvador R, Soria-Frisch A, Grau C, Dunne S, Miranda PC. Transcranial current brain stimulation (tCS): models and technologies. IEEE Trans Neural Syst Rehabil Eng. 2013;21(3):333–45.
55. Westerberg CE, Florczak SM, Weintraub S, Mesulam MM, Marshall L, Zee PC, Paller KA. Memory improvement via slow-oscillatory stimulation during sleep in older adults. Neurobiol Aging.2015 pii: S0197–4580(15)00295-X. doi: 10.1016/j.neurobiolaging.2015.05.014.
56. Nitsche MA, Cohen LG, Wassermann EM, Priori A, Lang N, Antal A, Paulus W, Hummel F, Boggio PS, Fregni F, Pascual-Leone A. Transcranial direct current stimulation: State of the art 2008. Brain Stimul. 2008;1(3):206–23.

57. Carandini M, Churchland AK. Probing perceptual decisions in rodents. Nat Neurosci. 2013;16(7):824–31.
58. Hanks TD, Ditterich J, Shadlen MN. Microstimulation of macaque area LIP affects decision-making in a motion discrimination task. Nat Neurosci. 2006;9(5):682–9.
59. Cohen MR, Newsome WT. What electrical microstimulation has revealed about the neural basis of cognition. Curr Opin Neurobiol. 2004;14:169–77.
60. Hampson RE, Song D, Opris I, Santos LM, Shin DC, Gerhardt GA, Marmarelis VZ, Berger TW, Deadwyler SA. Facilitation of memory encoding in primate hippocampus by a neuroprosthesis that promotes task-specific neural firing. J Neural Eng. 2013;10(6):066013.
61. Opris I, Santos LM, Song D, Berger TW, Gerhardt GA, Hampson RE, Deadwyler SA. Prefrontal cortical microcircuits bind perception to executive control. Sci Rep. 2013;3:2285. doi:10.1038/srep02285.
62. Berthier ML, Pulvermüller F. Neuroscience insights improve neurorehabilitation of poststroke aphasia. Nat Rev Neurol. 2011;7(2):86–97. doi:10.1038/nrneurol.2010.201.
63. Galletta EE, Rao PR, Barrett AM. Transcranial magnetic stimulation (TMS): potential progress for language improvement in aphasia. Top Stroke Rehabil. 2011;18(2):87–91.
64. Hecht D, Walsh V, Lavidor M. Transcranial direct current stimulation facilitates decision making in a probabilistic guessing task. J Neurosci. 2010;30(12):4241–5.
65. Kuehne M, Heimrath K, Heinze HJ, Zaehle T. Transcranial direct current stimulation of the left dorsolateral prefrontal cortex shifts preference of moral judgments. PLoS One. 2015;10(5):e0127061. doi:10.1371/journal.pone.0127061.
66. Penolazzi B, Bergamaschi S, Pastore M, Villani D, Sartori G, Mondini S. Transcranial direct current stimulation and cognitive training in the rehabilitation of Alzheimer disease: A case study. Neuropsychol Rehabil. 2014;7:1–19.
67. Penfield W, Boldrey E. Somatic motor and sensory represen¬tation in the cerebral cortex of man as studied by electrical stimulation. Brain. 1937;60:389–443.
68. Penfield W, Jasper HH. Epilepsy and the functional anatomy of the human brain. London: J. & A. Churchill; 1954.
69. Penfield W. Some mechanisms of consciousness discovered during electrical stimulation of the brain. Proc Natl Acad Sci U S A. 1958;44:51–66.
70. Penfield W. The electrode, the brain and the mind. Z Neurol. 1972;201:297–309.
71. Minamoto T, Azuma M, Yaoi K, Ashizuka A, Mima T, Osaka M, Fukuyama H, Osaka N. The anodal tDCS over the left posterior parietal cortex enhances attention toward a focus word in a sentence. Front Hum Neurosci. 2014;8:992.
72. Jeon SY, Han SJ. Improvement of the working memory and naming by transcranial direct current stimulation. Ann Rehabil Med. 2012;36(5):585–95.
73. Boggio PS, Khoury LP, Martins DC, Martins OE, de Macedo EC, Fregni F. Temporal cortex direct current stimulation enhances performance on a visual recognition memory task in Alzheimer disease. J Neurol Neurosurg Psychiatry. 2009;80(4):444–7.
74. Giglia G, Brighina F, Rizzo S, Puma A, Indovino S, Maccora S, Baschi R, Cosentino G, Fierro B. Anodal transcranial direct current stimulation of the right dorsolateral prefrontal cortex enhances memory-guided responses in a visuospatial working memory task. Funct Neurol. 2014;29(3):189–93.
75. Metuki N, Sela T, Lavidor M. Enhancing cognitive control components of insight problems solving by anodal tDCS of the left dorsolateral prefrontal cortex. Brain Stimul. 2012;5(2):110–5.
76. Otal B, Olma MC, Flöel A, Wellwood I. Inhibitory non-invasive brain stimulation to homologous language regions as an adjunct to speech and language therapy in post-stroke aphasia: a meta-analysis. Front Hum Neurosci. 2015;9:236.
77. Elsner B, Kugler J, Pohl M, Mehrholz J. Transcranial direct current stimulation (tDCS) for improving aphasia in patients with aphasia after stroke. Cochrane Database Syst Rev. 2015;5:CD009760.

78. Santarnecchi E, Polizzotto NR, Godone M, Giovannelli F, Feurra M, Matzen L, Rossi A, Rossi S. Frequency-dependent enhancement of fluid intelligence induced by transcranial oscillatory potentials. Curr Biol. 2013;23(15):1449–53.
79. Grabner RH, Rütsche B, Ruff CC, Hauser TU. Transcranial direct current stimulation of the posterior parietal cortex modulates arithmetic learning. Eur J Neurosci. 2015; doi:10.1111/ejn.12947.
80. Nitsche MA, Nitsche MS, Klein CC, Tergau F, Rothwell JC, Paulus W. Level of action of cathodal DC polarisation induced inhibition of the human motor cortex. Clin Neurophysiol. 2003;114(4):600–4.
81. Cerruti C, Schlaug G. Anodal transcranial direct current stimulation of the prefrontal cortex enhances complex verbal associative thought. J Cogn Neurosci. 2009;21(10):1980–7.
82. Bennabi D. Transcranial direct current stimulation for memory enhancement: from clinical research to animal models. Front Syst Neurosci. 2014;8:159.
83. Clemens B, Jung S, Zvyagintsev M, Domahs F, Willmes K. Modulating arithmetic fact retrieval: a single-blind, sham-controlled tDCS study with repeated fMRI measurements. Neuropsychologia. 2013;51(7):1279–86.
84. Underwood E. 2016. http://www.sciencemag.org/news/2016/04/cadaver-study-casts-doubts-how-zapping-brain-may-boost-mood-relieve-pain.
85. Rossini P, Rossi S. Transcranial magnetic stimulation: diagnostic, therapeutic, and research potential. Neurology. 2007;68(7):484–8.
86. Zangen A, Roth Y, Voller B, Hallett M. Transcranial magnetic stimulation of deep brain regions: Evidence for efficacy of the H-Coil. Clin Neurophysiol. 2005;116(4):775–9.
87. Bersani FS, Minichino A, Enticott PG, et al. Deep transcranial magnetic stimulation as a treatment for psychiatric disorders: a comprehensive review. Eur Psychiatry (Review). 2013;28(1):30–9.
88. Rapinesi C, Bersani FS, Kotzalidis GD, Imperatori C, Del Casale A, Di Pietro S, Ferri VR, Serata D, Raccah RN, Zangen A, Angeletti G, Girardi P. Maintenance deep transcranial magnetic stimulation sessions are associated with reduced depressive relapses in patients with unipolar or bipolar depression. Front Neurol. 2015;6:16.
89. Sokhadze E, Baruth JM, Sears L, Sokhadze GE, El-Baz AS, Casanova MF. Prefrontal neuromodulation using rTMS improves error monitoring and correction functions in autism. Appl Psychophysiol Biofeedback. 2012;37(2):91–102.
90. Di Lazzaro V, Ziemann U. The contribution of transcranial magnetic stimulation in the functional evaluation of microcircuits in human motor cortex. Front Neural Circuits. 2013;7:18. doi:10.3389/fncir.2013.00018.
91. Weise D, Mann J, Ridding M, Eskandar K, Huss M, Rumpf JJ, Di Lazzaro V, Mazzone P, Ranieri F, Classen J. Microcircuit mechanisms involved in paired associative stimulation-induced depression of corticospinal excitability. J Physiol. 2013;591(19):4903–20.
92. Opris I, Ferrera VP. Modifying cognition and behavior with electrical microstimulation: implications for cognitive prostheses. Neurosci Biobehav Rev. 2014;47:321–35.
93. Opris I, Barborica A, Ferrera VP. A gap effect during microstimulation in the prefrontal cortex of monkey. Exp Brain Res. 2001;138:1–7.
94. Balan P, Ferrera VP. Effects of gaze shifts on maintenance of spatial memory in macaque frontal eye field. J Neurosci. 2003;23:5446–54.
95. Hanes DP, Schall JD. Neural control of voluntary movement initiation. Science. 1996;274:427–30.
96. Schall JD. On building a bridge between brain and behavior. Annu Rev Psychol. 2004; doi:10.1146/annurev.psych.55.090902.141907.
97. Schlag Rey M, Schlag J, Dassonville P. How the frontal eye field can impose a saccade goal on superior colliculus neurons. J Neurophysiol. 1992;67:1003–5.
98. White 3rd RL, Snyder LH. Subthreshold microstimulation in frontal eye fields updates spatial memories. Exp Brain Res. 2007;181(3):477–92.

99. Lenartowicz A, Escobedo-Quiroz R, Cohen JD. Updating of context in working memory: an event-related potential study. Cogn Affect Behav Neurosci. 2010;10(2):298–315.
100. Barborica A, Ferrera VP. Estimating invisible target speed from neuronal activity in monkey frontal eye field. Nat Neurosci. 2003;6:66–74.
101. Goldberg ME, Bruce CJ. Primate frontal eye fields . III. Maintenance of a spatially accurate saccade signal. J Neurophysiol. 1990;64(2):489–508.
102. Lisberger SG, Ferrera VP. Vector averaging for smooth pursuit eye movements initiated by two moving targets in monkeys. J Neurosci. 1997;17(19):7490–502.
103. Umeno MM, Goldberg ME. Spatial processing in the monkey frontal eye field I. Predictive visual responses. J Neurophysiol. 1997;78:1373–83.
104. Quaia C, Optican LM, Goldberg ME. The maintenance of spatial accuracy by the perisaccadic remapping of visual receptive fields. Neural Netw. 1998;11:1229–40.
105. Mountcastle VB. Modality and topographic properties of single neurons of cat's somatic sensory cortex. J Neurophysiol. 1957;20:408–34.
106. Mountcastle VB. The columnar organization of the n eocortex. Brain. 1997;120:701–22.
107. Shepherd G, Grillner S. Handbook of brain microcircuits. New York: Oxford University Press; 2010.
108. Opris I, Bruce CJ. Neural circuitry of judgment and decision mechanisms. Brain Res Brain Res Rev. 2005;48(3):509–26.
109. Szentagothai J. The 'module-concept' in cerebral cortex architecture. Brain Res. 1975;95: 475–96.
110. Constantinople CM, Bruno RM. Deep cortical layers are activated directly by thalamus. Science. 2013;340(6140):1591–4.
111. Buxhoeveden DP, Casanova MF. The minicolumn hypothesis in neuroscience. Brain. 2002;125:935–51.
112. Casanova MF, El-Baz A, Switala A. Laws of conservation as related to brain growth, aging, and evolution: symmetry of the minicolumn. Front Neuroanat. 2011;5:66.
113. Moxon KA, Leiser SC, Gerhardt GA, Barbee KA, Chapin JK. Ceramic-based multisite electrode arrays for chronic single-neuron recording. IEEE Trans Biomed Eng. 2004;51:647–56.
114. Opris I, Hampson RE, Stanford TR, Gerhardt GA, Deadwyler SA. Neural activity in frontal cortical cell layers: evidence for columnar sensorimotor processing. J Cogn Neurosci. 2011;23:1507–21.
115. Opris I, Hampson RE, Gerhardt GA, Berger TW, Deadwyler SA. Columnar processing in primate pFC: Evidence for executive control microcircuits. J Cogn Neuro. 2012a;24(12):2334–47.
116. Opris I, Fuqua JL, Huettl P, Gerhardt GA, Berger TW, Hampson RE, Deadwyler SA. Closing the loop in primate prefrontal cortex: Inter-laminar processing. Front Neural Circuits. 2012b;6:88. doi:10.3389/fncir.2012.00088.
117. Hampson RE, Gerhardt GA, Marmarelis VZ, Song D, Opris I, Santos LM, Berger TW, Deadwyler SA. Facilitation and restoration of cognitive function in primate prefrontal cortex by a neuroprosthesis that utilizes minicolumn-specific neural firing. J Neural Eng. 2012;9(5):056012.
118. Opris I, Santos LM, Gerhardt GA, Song D, Berger TW, Hampson RE, Deadwyler SA. Distributed encoding of spatial and object categories in primate hippocampal microcircuits. Front Neurosci. 2015;9:317. doi:10.3389/fnins.2015.00317.
119. Opris I, Casanova MF. Prefrontal cortical minicolumn: from executive control to disrupted cognitive processing. Brain. 2914;137(7):1863–75. doi:10.1093/brain/awt359.
120. Opris I, Fuqua JL, Gerhardt GA, Hampson RE, Deadwyler SA. Prefrontal cortical recordings with biomorphic MEAs reveal complex columnar-laminar microcircuits for BCI/BMI implementation. J Neurosci Methods. 2015;244:104–13.
121. Opris I, Gerhardt GA, Hampson RE, Deadwyler SA. Disruption of columnar and laminar cognitive processing in primate prefrontal cortex following cocaine exposure. Front Syst Neurosci. 2015;9:79. doi:10.3389/fnsys.2015.00079.

122. Riddle DR, Lichtenwalner RJ. In: Riddle DR, editor. Neurogenesis in the adult and aging brain brain aging: models, methods, and mechanisms (frontiers in neuroscience). Boca Raton: CRC Press; 2007.
123. Blanke O, Landis T, Seeck M. Electrical cortical stimulation of the human prefrontal cortex evokes complex visual hallucinations. Epilepsy Behav. 2000;1:356–61.
124. Lobel E, Kahane P, Leonards U, Grosbras M, Lehericy S, Le Bihan D, Berthoz A. Localization of human frontal eye fields: anatomical and functional findings of functional magnetic resonance imaging and intracerebral electrical stimulation. J Neurosurg. 2001;95:804–15.
125. Jacobs JV, Lou JS, Kraakevik JA, Horak FB. The supplementary motor area contributes to the timing of the anticipatory postural adjustment during step initiation in participants with and without Parkinson's disease. Neuroscience. 2009;164(2):877–85.
126. Bolzoni F, Bruttini C, Esposti R, Castellani C, Cavallari P. Transcranial direct current stimulation of SMA modulates anticipatory postural adjustments without affecting the primary movement. Behav Brain Res. 2015;291:407–13.
127. Chassagnon S, Minotti L, Kremer S, Hoffmann D, Kahane P. Somatosensory, motor, and reaching/grasping responses to direct electrical stimulation of the human cingulate motor areas. J Neurosurg. 2008;109(4):593–604.
128. Talairach J, Bancaud J, Geier S, Bordas-Ferrer M, Bonis A, Szikla G, Rusu M. The cingulate gyrus and human behaviour. Electroencephalogr Clin Neurophysiol. 1973;34:45–52.
129. Desmurget M, Reilly KT, Richard N, Szathmari A, Mottolese C, Sirigu A. Movement intention after parietal cortex stimulation in humans. Science. 2009;324(5928):811–3.
130. Rochas V, Gelmini L, Krolak-Salmon P, Poulet E, Saoud M, Brunelin J, Bediou B. Disrupting pre-SMA activity impairs facial happiness recognition: an event-related TMS study. Cereb Cortex. 2013;23(7):1517–25. doi:10.1093/cercor/bhs133.
131. Osaka N, Osaka M, Kondo H, Morishita M, Fukuyama H, Shibasaki H. An emotion-based facial expression word activates laughter module in the human brain: a functional magnetic resonance imaging study. Neurosci Lett. 2003;340(2):127–30.
132. Sperli F, Spinelli L, Pollo C, Seeck M. Contralateral smile and laughter, but no mirth, induced by electrical stimulation of the cingulate cortex. Epilepsia. 2006;47(2):440–3.
133. Choi JC, Kim J, Kang E, Lee JM, Cha J, Kim YJ, Lee HG, Choi JH, Yi DJ. Brain mechanisms of pain relief by transcutaneous electrical nerve stimulation: A functional magnetic resonance imaging study. Eur J Pain. 2015; doi:10.1002/ejp.696.
134. Tsubokawa T, Katayama Y, Ueno Y, Moriyasu N. Evidence for involvement of the frontal cortex in pain-related cerebral events in cats: increase in local cerebral blood flow by noxious stimuli. Brain Res. 1981;217(1):179–85.
135. Cohen Kadosh R, Soskic S, Iuculano T, Kanai R, Walsh V. Modulating neuronal activity produces specific and long-lasting changes in numerical competence. Curr Biol. 2010;20(22):2016–20. doi:10.1016/j.cub.2010.10.007.
136. Coffman BA, Clark VP, Parasuraman R. Battery powered thought: enhancement of attention, learning, and memory in healthy adults using transcranial direct current stimulation. Neuroimage. 2014;85(Pt 3):895–908.
137. Bennabi D, Pedron S, Haffen E, Monnin J, Peterschmitt Y, Van Waes V. Transcranial direct current stimulation for memory enhancement: from clinical research to animal models. Front Syst Neurosci. 2014;8:159.
138. Chi RP, Snyder AW. Brain stimulation enables the solution of an inherently difficult problem. Neurosci Lett. 2012;515(2):121–4. doi:10.1016/j.neulet.2012.03.012.
139. Wokke ME, Talsma LJ, Vissers ME. Biasing neural network dynamics using non-invasive brain stimulation. Front Syst Neurosci. 2015;8:246. doi:10.3389/fnsys.2014.00246.
140. Fregni F, Boggio PS, Nitsche M, Pascual-Leone A. Transcranial direct current stimulation. Br J Psychiatry. 2005;186:446–7.
141. Keeser D, Meindl T, Bor J, Palm U, Pogarell O, Mulert C, Brunelin J, Möller HJ, Reiser M, Padberg F. Prefrontal transcranial direct current stimulation changes connectivity of resting-state networks during fMRI. J Neurosci. 2011a;31(43):15284–93.

142. Keeser D, Padberg F, Reisinger E, Pogarell O, Kirsch V, Palm U, Karch S, Möller HJ, Nitsche MA, Mulert C. Prefrontal direct current stimulation modulates resting EEG and event-related potentials in healthy subjects: a standardized low resolution tomography (sLORETA) study. Neuroimage. 2011b;55(2):644–57.
143. Padberg F, George MS. Repetitive transcranial magnetic stimulation of the prefrontal cortex in depression. Exp Neurol. 2009;219(1):2–13.
144. Salinas FS, Narayama S, Zhang W, Fox PT, Szabó SA. Repetitive transcranial magnetic stimulation elicits rate-dependent brain network responses in non-human primates. Brain Stimul. 2013; doi:10.1016/j.brs.2013.03.002.
145. Broadbent HJ, Van Den Eynde F, Guillaume S, Hanif EL, Stahl D, David AS, Campbell IC, Schmidt U. Blinding success of rTMS applied to the dorsolateral prefrontal cortex in randomised sham-controlled trials: a systematic review. World J Biol Psychiatry. 2011;12(4):240.
146. Chi RP, Snyder AW. Facilitate insight by non-invasive brain stimulation. PLoS One. 2011;6(2):e16655.
147. George MS, Taylor JJ, Short B. Treating the depressions with superficial brain stimulation methods. Handb Clin Neurol. 2013;116:399–413.
148. Hovington CL, McGirr A, Lepage M, Berlim MT. Repetitive transcranial magnetic stimulation (rTMS) for treating major depression and schizophrenia: a systematic review of recent meta-analyses. Ann Med. 2013;45(4):308–21.
149. Sokhadze E, El-Baz A, Baruth J, Mathai G, Sears L, Casanova M. Effects of low frequency repetitive transcranial magnetic stimulation (rTMS) on gamma frequency oscillations and event-related potentials during processing of illusory figures in autism. J Autism Dev Disord. 2009;39:619–34.
150. Casanova M, Baruth J, El-Baz A, Tasman A, Sears L, Sokhadze E. Repetitive transcranial magnetic stimulation (rTMS) modulates event-related potential (ERP) indices of attention in autism. Transl Neurosci. 2012;3(2):170–80.
151. Baruth J, Casanova M, El-Baz A, Horrell T, Mathai G, Sears L, Sokhadze E. Low-frequency repetitive Transcranial Magnetic Stimulation modulates evoked-gamma frequency oscillations in autism spectrum disorders. J Neurother. 2010;14(3):179–94.
152. George MS, Nahas Z, Lisanby SH, Schlaepfer T, Kozel FA, Greenberg BD. Transcranial magnetic stimulation. Neurosurg Clin N Am. 2003;14(2):283–301.
153. George MS. Transcranial magnetic stimulation for the treatment of depression. Expert Rev Neurother. 2010;10(11):1761–72. doi:10.1586/ern.10.95.
154. Aleman A. Use of repetitive transcranial magnetic stimulation for treatment in psychiatry. Clin Psychopharmacol Neurosci (Review). 2013;11(2):53–9.
155. Lefaucheur JP et al. Evidence-based guidelines on the therapeutic use of repetitive transcranial magnetic stimulation (rTMS). Clin Neurophysiol. 2014;125(11):2150–206.
156. George MS, Post RM. Daily left prefrontal repetitive transcranial magnetic stimulation for acute treatment of medication-resistant depression. Am J Psychiatry. 2011;168(4):356–64.
157. Berlim MT, Van den Eynde F, Jeff Daskalakis Z. Clinically meaningful efficacy and acceptability of low-frequency repetitive transcranial magnetic stimulation (rTMS) for treating primary major depression: a meta-analysis of randomized, double-blind and sham-controlled trials. Neuropsychopharmacology. 2013;38(4):543–51.
158. Hamidi M, Slagter HA, Tononi G, Bradley Postle BR. Repetitive transcranial magnetic stimulation affects behavior by biasing endogenous cortical oscillations. Front Integr Neurosci. 2009;3:14.
159. Rubenstein JLR, Merzenich MM. Model of autism: increased ratio of excitation/inhibition in key neural systems. Genes Brain Behav. 2003;2:255–67.
160. Vlamings PH, Jonkman LM, Hoeksma MR, van Engeland H, Kemner C. Reduced error monitoring in children with autism spectrum disorder: an ERP study. Eur J Neurosci. 2008;28:399–406. doi:10.1111/j.1460-9568.2008. 06336.
161. Bogte H, Flamma B, van der Meere J, van Engeland H. Post-error adaptation in adults with high functioning autism. Neuropsychologia. 2007;45(8):1707–14.

162. Henderson H, Schwartz C, Mundy P, Burnette C, Sutton S, Zahka N, Pradella A. Response monitoring, the error-related negativity, and differences in social behavior in autism. Brain Cogn. 2006;61(1):96–109.
163. Daly JJ, Huggins JE. Brain-computer interface: current and emerging rehabilitation applications. Arch Phys Med Rehabil. 2015;96(3 Suppl):S1–7.
164. Grau C, Ginhoux R, Riera A, Nguyen TL, Chauvat H, Berg M, Amengual JL, Pascual-Leone A, Ruffini G. Conscious brain-to-brain communication in humans using non-invasive technologies. PLoS One. 2014;9(8):e105225.
165. Chen CH, Ho MS, Shyu KK, Hsu KC, Wang KW, Lee PL. A noninvasive brain computer interface using visually-induced near-infrared spectroscopy responses. Neurosci Lett. 2014;580:22–6.
166. Grosse-Wentrup M, Mattia D, Oweiss K. Using brain-computer interfaces to induce neural plasticity and restore function. J Neural Eng. 2011;8(2):025004.
167. Lebedev MA, Nicolelis MA. Brain-machine interfaces: past, present and future. Trends Neurosci. 2006;29(9):536–46.
168. Opris I. Inter-laminar microcircuits across the neocortex: repair and augmentation. Front. Syst. Neurosci. 2013;7:80. doi:10.3389/fnsys.2013.00080.
169. Andersen RA, Hwang EJ, Mulliken GH. Cognitive neural prosthetics. Annu Rev Psychol. 2010;61:169–90. C1-3
170. Nicolelis MA. Actions from thoughts. Nature. 2001;409(6818):403–7.
171. Bach-y-Rita P, Kercel WS. Sensory substitution and the human-machine interface.Trends. Cognit Sci. 2003;7(12):541–6.
172. Kim SP, Sanchez JC, Rao YN, Erdogmus D, Carmena JM, Lebedev MA, Nicolelis MA, Principe JC. A comparison of optimal MIMO linear and nonlinear models for brain-machine interfaces. J Neural Eng. 2006;3(2):145–61.
173. Song D, Chan RH, Marmarelis VZ, Hampson RE, Deadwyler SA, Berger TW. Nonlinear modeling of neural population dynamics for hippocampal prostheses. Neural Netw. 2009;22(9):1340–51.
174. Musallam S, Corneil BD, Greger B, Scherberger H, Andersen RA. Cognitive control signals for neural prosthetics. Science. 2004;305(5681):258–62.
175. Poli R, Valeriani D, Cinel C. Collaborative brain-computer interface for aiding decision-making. PLoS One. 2014;9(7):e102693.
176. Garbayo E, Estella-Hermoso de Mendoza A, Blanco-Prieto MJ. Diagnostic and therapeutic uses of nanomaterials in the brain. Curr Med Chem. 2014;21(36):4100–31.
177. Gibney E. Injectable brain implant spies on individual neurons. Nature. 2015;522(7555):137–8.
178. Chhabra R, Tosi G, Grabrucker AM. Emerging use of nanotechnology in the treatment of neurological disorders. Curr Pharm Des. 2015;21:3111–30.
179. Angle MR, Cui B, Melosh NA. Nanotechnology and neurophysiology. Curr Opin Neurobiol. 2015;32:132–40.
180. Zhu W, O'Brien C, O'Brien JR. Zhang LG.3D nano/microfabrication techniques and nanobiomaterials for neural tissue regeneration. Nanomedicine (Lond). 2014;9(6):859–75.
181. Monaco AM, Giugliano M. Carbon-based smart nanomaterials in biomedicine and neuroengineering. Beilstein J Nanotechnol. 2014;5:1849–63.
182. Stieglitz T. Restoration of neurological functions by neuroprosthetic technologies: future prospects and trends towards micro-, nano-, and biohybrid systems. Acta Neurochir Suppl. 2007;97(Pt 1):435–42.
183. Silva GA. Nanotechnology applications and approaches for neuroregeneration and drug delivery to the central nervous system. Ann N Y Acad Sci. 2010;1199:221–30.
184. Spira ME, Hai A. Multi-electrode array technologies for neuroscience and cardiology. Nat Nanotechnol. 2013;8(2):83–94.
185. Vidu R, Rahman M, Mahmoudi M, Enachescu M, Poteca TD, Opris I. Nanostructures: a platform for brain repair and augmentation. Front Syst Neurosci. 2014;8:91.

186. Brunello CA, Jokinen V, Sakha P, Terazono H, Nomura F, Kaneko T, Lauri SE, Franssila S, Rivera C, Yasuda K, Huttunen HJ. Microtechnologies to fuel neurobiological research with nanometer precision. J Nanobiotechnology. 2013;11:11.
187. Jiang C, Li L, Hao H. Carbon nanotube yarns for deep brain stimulation electrode. IEEE Trans Neural Syst Rehabil Eng. 2011 Dec;19(6):612–6.
188. Keefer EW, Botterman BR, Romero MI, Rossi AF, Gross GW. Carbon nanotube coating improves neuronal recordings. Nat Nanotechnol. 2008;3(7):434–9.
189. Suyatin DB, Wallman L, Thelin J, Prinz CN, Jorntell H, Samuelson L, et al. Nanowire-based electrode for acute in vivo neural recordings in the brain. PLoS One. 2013;8:e56673. doi:10.1371/journal.pone. 0056673.
190. Hai A, Shappir J. Spira ME Long-term, multisite, parallel, in-cell recording and stimulation by an array of extracellular microelectrodes. J Neurophysiol. 2010 Jul;104(1):559–68.
191. Nam Y, Wheeler BC. In vitro microelectrode array technology and neural recordings. Crit Rev Biomed Eng. 2011;39(1):45–61.
192. Patrick E, Sankar V, Rowe W, Sanchez JC, Nishida T. An implantable integrated low-power amplifier-microelectrode array for brain-machine interfaces. Conf Proc IEEE Eng Med Biol Soc. 2010;2010:1816–9.
193. Hwang JY, Shin US, Jang WC, Hyun JK, Wall IB, Kim HW. Biofunctionalized carbon nanotubes in neural regeneration: a mini-review. Nanoscale. 2013;5(2):487–97.
194. David-Pur M, Bareket-Keren L, Beit-Yaakov G, Raz-Prag D, Hanein Y. All-carbon-nanotube flexible multi-electrode array for neuronal recording and stimulation. Biomed Microdevices. 2014;16(1):43–53.
195. Xie C, Hanson L, Xie W, Lin Z, Cui B, Cui Y. Noninvasive neuron pinning with nanopillar arrays. Nano Lett. 2010;10:4020–4.
196. Suzuki I, Fukuda M, Shirakawa K, Jiko H, Gotoh M. Carbon nanotube multi-electrode array chips for noninvasive real-time measurement of dopamine, action potentials, and postsynaptic potentials. Biosens Bioelectron. 2013;49:270–5.
197. Gacem K, Retrouvey J-M, Chabi D, Filoramo A, Zhao W, Klein J-O, et al. Neuromorphic function learning with carbon nanotube based synapses. Nanotechnology. 2013;24:384013.
198. Du J, Blanche TJ, Harrison RR, Lester HA, Masmanidis S. Multiplexed, high density electrophysiology with nanofabricated neural probes. PLoS One. 2011;6:e26204.
199. Viventi J, Kim D-H, Vigeland L, Frechette ES, Blanco JA, Kim Y-S, et al. Flexible, foldable, actively multiplexed, high-density electrode array for mapping brain activity in vivo. Nat Neurosci. 2011;14:U1599–605.
200. Wise KD. Integrated sensors, MEMS, and microsystems: reflections on a fantastic voyage. Sens Actuators A Phys. 2007;136:39–50.
201. Chang-Hsiao C, Shih-Chang C, Yu-Tao L, Yen-Chung C, Shih-Rung Y, Da-Jeng Y. Three-dimensional flexible microprobe for recording the neural signal. J Micro. 2010;9:031007.
202. Amaral J, Pinto V, Costa T, Gaspar J, Ferreira R, Paz E, et al. Integration of TMR sensors in silicon microneedles for magnetic measurements of neurons. IEEE Trans Magn. 2013;49:3512–5.
203. Malarkey EB, Parpura V. Carbon nanotubes in neuroscience. In: Czernicki Z, Baethmann A, Ito U, Katayama Y, Kuroiwa T, Mendelow D, editors. Brain Edema XIV. Vienna: Springer; 2010. p. 337–41.
204. Stankova L, Fraczek-Szczypta A, Blazewicz M, Filova E, Blazewicz S, Lisa V, et al. Human osteoblast-like MG 63 cells on polysulfone modified with carbon nanotubes or carbon nanohorns. Carbon. 2014;67:578–91.
205. Fabbro A, Bosi S, Ballerini L, Prato M. Carbon nanotubes: artificial nanomaterials to engineer single neurons and neuronal networks. ACS Chem Nerosci. 2012;3:611–8.
206. Alivisatos AP, Andrews AM, Boyden ES, Chun M, Church GM, Deisseroth K, et al. Nanotools for neuroscience and brain activity mapping. ACS Nano. 2013;7:1850–66.
207. Zorzos AN, Scholvin J, Boyden ES, Fonstad CG. Threedimensional multiwaveguide probe array for light delivery to distributed brain circuits. Opt Lett. 2012;37:4841–3.

208. Bokara KK, Kim JY, Lee YI, Yun K, Webster TJ, Lee JE. Biocompatability of carbon nanotubes with stem cells to treat CNS injuries. Anat Cell Biol. 2013;46:85–92.
209. Marmarelis VZ, Shin DC, Song D, Hampson RE, Deadwyler SA, Berger TW. On parsing the neural code in the prefrontal cortex of primates using principal dynamic modes. J Comput Neurosci. 2014;36:321–37.
210. Soekadar SR, Birbaumer N, Slutzky MW, Cohen LG. Brain-machine interfaces in neurorehabilitation of stroke. Neurobiol Dis. 2014. pii: S0969–9961(14)00371–4. doi: 10.1016/j.nbd.2014.11.025.
211. Schwarz DA, Lebedev MA, Hanson TL, Dimitrov DF, Lehew G, Meloy J, Rajangam S, Subramanian V, Ifft PJ, Li Z, Ramakrishnan A, Tate A, Zhuang KZ, Nicolelis MA. Chronic, wireless recordings of large-scale brain activity in freely moving rhesus monkeys. Nat Methods. 2014;11(6):670–6. doi:10.1038/nmeth.2936.
212. Zippo AG, Romanelli P, Torres Martinez NR, Caramenti GC, Benabid AL, Biella GE. A novel wireless recording and stimulating multichannel epicortical grid for supplementing or enhancing the sensory-motor functions in monkey (*Macaca fascicularis*). Front Syst Neurosci. 2015;9:73. doi:10.3389/fnsys.2015.00073.
213. Suzuki T, Ando H, Yoshida T, Sawahata H, Kawasaki K, Hasegawa I, Matsushita K, Hirata M, Yoshimine T, Takizawa K. Super multi-channel recording systems with UWB wireless transmitter for BMI. Conf Proc IEEE Eng Med Biol Soc. 2014;2014:5208–11.
214. Merolla PA, Arthur JV, Alvarez-Icaza R, Cassidy AS, Sawada J, Akopyan F, Jackson BL, Imam N, Guo C, Nakamura Y, Brezzo B, Vo I, Esser SK, Appuswamy R, Taba B, Amir A, Flickner MD, Risk WP, Manohar R, Modha DS. Artificial brains. A million spiking-neuron integrated circuit with a scalable communication network and interface. Science. 2014;345(6197):668–73.
215. Simonite T. New form of memory could advance. Brain-Inspired Computers. 2014. http://www.technologyreview.com/news/533526/new-form-of-memory-could-advance-brain-inspired-computers/.
216. Wei W, Song Y, Fan X, et al. Simultaneous recording of brain extracellular glucose, spike and local field potential in real time using an implantable microelectrode array with nanomaterials. Nanotechnology. 2016;27(2016):114001. doi:10.1088/0957-4484/27/11/114001.
217. Kuzum D, Rakesh G, Jeyasingh D, Lee B, Philip Wong H-S. Nanoelectronic programmable synapses based on phase change materials for brain-inspired computing. Nano Lett. 2016;12(5):2179–86. doi:10.1021/nl201040y.
218. Scholvin J, Kinney JP, Bernstein JG, Moore-Kochlacs C, Kopell N, Fonstad CG, Boyden ES. Close-packed silicon microelectrodes for scalable spatially oversampled neural recording. IEEE Trans Biomed Eng. 2016;63(1):120–30.
219. Park D-W, Schendel AA, Mikael S, Brodnick SK, Richner TJ, Ness JP, et al. Graphene-based carbon-layered electrode array technology for neural imaging and optogenetic applications. Nat Commun. 2014;5:5258. doi:10.1038/ncomms6258.
220. Kuzum D, Takano T, Shim E, Reed JC, Juul H, Richardson AG, et al. Transparent and flexible low noise graphene electrodes for simultaneous electrophysiology and neuroimaging. Nat Commun. 2014;5:5259. doi:10.1038/ncomms6259.

Chapter 13
Neuromodulation of Consciousness Disorders

Ana Ciurea, Jean Ciurea, and Ioan Opris

Abstract Some patients may develop an altered state of consciousness (coma, vegetative state, minimal consciousness state) following traumatic and other brain injuries. While the cause of their altered consciousness may be well documented in most cases, the precise underlying mechanisms mediating the altered consciousness and its treatment are yet to be discovered. Several hypotheses have been put forward on how the level of consciousness can be improved; all are based on the principle that an injured brain needs to reconnect its disrupted areas. To address this need, several neuromodulation therapies (using invasive and noninvasive stimulation) may serve this purpose. Invasive therapies use chronic electrodes for stimulation, while non-invasive therapies employ transcranial magnetic stimulation (TMS), transcranial direct current stimulation (tDCS) and somato-sensitive stimulation (SSS). The purpose of this chapter is to critically analyze the progress of these therapeutic methods and to review what is still needed to improve the impaired conscious states.

Keywords Consciousness • Awareness • Disturbance • Vegetative state • Neuromodulation • Therapy • TMS • tDCS

A. Ciurea
Neurology Department, Carol Davila University of Medicine and Pharmacy, Bucharest, Romania

Physics Department, University of Bucharest, Bucharest, Romania

J. Ciurea
Neurosurgery Department, Bagdasar-Arseni Hospital, Bucharest, Romania

I. Opris (✉)
Miami Project to Cure Paralysis, Department of Neurological Surgery, University of Miami, Miami, FL, USA
e-mail: ioanopris.phd@gmail.com

A. Majid (ed.), *Electroceuticals*, DOI 10.1007/978-3-319-28612-9_13

Introduction

A conscious state is when a subject is *awake* and *aware* of his or her own existence, sensations, thoughts, feelings and surroundings. The origin of the word "consciousness" is Latin and represents an association between the words "con" meaning "with" and "scio", meaning "to know". The terms "conscious" and "consciousness" were used for the first time in the seventeenth century and continued ever since [1]. On the other end, the antonym for this term is "unconscious". An altered state of consciousness [2] can occur after traumatic and other brain injuries and is a state of "perturbed" consciousness that spans the two opposing concepts. The altered state of consciousness is more difficult to classify since the defining elements involve both *objective* criteria [3], referring to patient's particularity, and *subjective* criteria [4], depending on the observer's training and experience. The altered consciousness state of the brain is a major and complex problem that needs to be tackled by both medical practitioners and researchers, to find new treatments that will serve to improve the lives of these individuals.

Although the causes of altered consciousness are usually well documented [4], the detailed mechanisms that underlie the malfunction are not well known. Several hypotheses for improving the level of consciousness in trauma patients have been proposed. All are based on the principle that an injured brain needs to reconnect its disrupted circuits. It is well documented that an initial lesion has evolving potential, to cause secondary damage, which may result in a deleterious cascade [5]. The recognition of specific disturbance patterns and its therapy may be followed by a good outcome in some cases [6]. To address this need, several neuromodulation therapies (using invasive and noninvasive stimulation) have been developed and studied to serve this purpose [7, 8]. Invasive therapies use chronic electrodes for stimulation, while non-invasive therapies employ transcranial magnetic stimulation (TMS, [9]), transcranial direct current stimulation (tDCS, [10]) and somato-sensitive stimulation (SSS, [11, 12]).

In this chapter we critically analyze and evaluate the progress of the therapeutic methods and review what is still needed to improve consciousness in conditions like coma, vegetative state, minimally conscious states by using electrical stimulation.

General Overview and Rationale

General overview and rationale for using electrical stimulation approach to reverse or improve impaired consciousness.

Brain Electrical Activity

The brain has spontaneous bioelectrical activity which is differentially modulated. The effects of electric fields on humans and animals have been studied since antiquity and have been used as therapies for hundreds of years for uses such as pain alleviation. In the nineteenth century, Volta and Galvani paved the way for modern approaches by conducting experiments with animals. A key aspect of brain electrical activity is the electrical charge of the cell membrane which is responsive to external electromagnetic manipulation.

Understanding the interaction of the external electromagnetic field with living matter, and particularly with the neurons in the brain, is crucial for understanding brain functions, including conscious states.

Brain electrical activity was first observed by Hans Berger in Jena, Germany in 1929. He demonstrated that currents produced by neurons in the brain can be recorded with electrodes on the scalp. The relevance of this electrical activity to consciousness, and coma have been debated and studied ever since [13].

Anatomical Localization of Consciousness

At the beginning of the twentieth century, Constantin von Economo observed the epidemics of *encephalita letargica*. He hypothesized that the place of consciousness is in the upper brainstem and posterior hypothalamus, based on his observations in post-mortem exploration of the patients brains [14]. In 1929 Frederic Bremer identified sections of feline brain in the upper mesencephalon plane that induced deep sleep [15]. Inspired by Bremer, Moruzzi and Magoun (1949) went on to describe the "ascending reticular activating system" (see Fig. 13.1) in the mesencephalon. When stimulated, this structure produced improvement on EEG in drowsy animals [16]. In recent years, brain research advanced and revealed a more complex anatomo-functional structure that includes the reticular formation [17, 18] and the neocortical microcircuits [19–25] that support the conscious state. A "consciousness network" in the brain has also been proposed and includes precuneus, anterior cingulate, temporo-parietal junction and central thalamus [26].

There have also been attempts to hypothetically explain consciousness. One is the global neuronal workspace model of consciousness where a "sudden self-amplifying process leads to a global brain-scale pattern of activity" and is based on neuronal structure [27, 28]. Another attempt is grounded on information integration and modular connectivity. Entropy and information is evaluated and "transformed" into a personal "subjective complexity" [29]. Global theories by Penrose and Hameroff are invoking the quantum physics theory. According to this view a putative quantum structure is located inside the neuron's tubules [30, 31]. Based on a holographic encoding of the nodes of interference patterns capable of containing the information about the environment, Pribram described the 'quanta of information'. He has hypothesized a relationship among entropy, chaotic attractors and the organization of consciousness concept [32]. Searle has categorized neuroscience approaches in consciousness as building block models or unified field models. Information about environment is fractioned and dispersed to specialized neuronal units of the multimodal sensory input. Local coincidence detectors assess fractionated activity by comparing exogenous sensory specific and substantially endogenous non-sensory specific influences on the neurons [33]. Congruence in these comparators transforms these fragmented sensations to fragmented

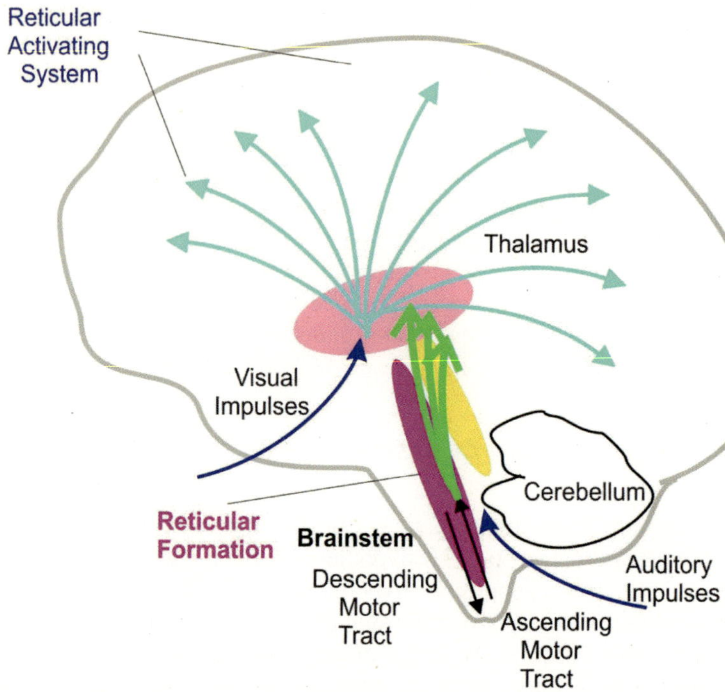

Fig. 13.1 Reticular activating system showing the visual impulses, the reticular formation, the brain stem, the ascending sensory tracts, the descending motor tracts, the spinal cord, the auditory impulses and the cerebellum. Midline brain structures that make up the consciousness system, also known as the neuronal correlates of consciousness. The temporal lobe plays a particularly essential role in understanding impaired consciousness in epileptic seizures

perceptions, and greatly enhances synchronized output from each ensemble. Neural activity from multiple brain areas is integrated to produce a unified perceptual experience, known as the "binding problem" [34].

Coma

Coma word comes from the Greek word κῶμα *koma*, meaning "deep sleep"). Coma is a state of unconsciousness in which a person: cannot be awakened; fails to respond normally to painful stimuli, light, or sound; lacks a normal wake-sleep cycle; and does not initiate voluntary actions [34, 35]. The possible subsequent outcome of coma is as follows: 1. death, 2. recovery or 3. vegetative state/minimally conscious state. Causes of coma are multiple and include post-concussive states, hypoxia, ischaemia, subarachnoid blood, seizures, hyponatremia or hypernatremia, hyperglycemia, hypoglycemia, hypercalcemia, post-seizure state, intoxication, drugs, hypercarbia, organ failure, encephalitis, etc. [35, 36].

Persistent Vegetative State (VS)

Patients are unware of self and of the environment, they sleep wake cycles, but without any voluntary activity or interaction. They may, however, retain reflexes, eat and have bowel and bladder continence. The clinical course and outcome of a persistent vegetative state depends on its cause. Three categories of disorder can cause such a state: acute traumatic and non-traumatic brain injuries, degenerative and metabolic brain disorders, and severe congenital malformations of the nervous system [37, 38].

In 2010, the European Task Force on Disorders of Consciousness decided that VS should be called "Unresponsive Wakefulness Syndrome" (UWS) based mainly on negative connotation of the expression "vegetative state" [39]. The outcome of VS /UWS is a matter of scientific debate [40]. Some authors have found that age greater than 39 years and bilateral absence of cortical components of middle latency auditory evoked potentials were significantly associated with deterioration [41]. Due to inconclusive results of experimental treatment approaches for VS/UWS, there is a tendency of nihilism towards these patients.

The Minimally Conscious State (MCS)

The Minimally Conscious State (MCS) terminology was introduced to describe patients showing more than reflex motor behavior (when they were previously in VS /UWS) but are still unable to communicate. Clinical examination of these individuals consists of examining: (1) command following, (2) intelligible verbalization, (3) discernible yes–no signals (regardless of accuracy), (4) specific responses to selective environmental stimuli, e.g. visual pursuit in front of a mirror [42]. Based on the complexity of the patients' behavior, MCS was further divided in:

- MCS+ command following or intention, intelligible verbalization or gestural or verbal yes/no responses;
- MCS- shows minimal behavioral interaction with non-reflex movements such as: orientation of noxious stimuli, pursuit eye movements in direct response to moving or salient stimuli; movements or affective behaviors in appropriate response to relevant environmental stimuli [43].

Locked in Syndrome

The subject is awake and aware but unable to move. This syndrome is not a consciousness disturbance and must be recognized by the examiner as a differential diagnosis when assessing altered conscious states.

Outcome Scales

The Glasgow Coma Scale and Glasgow Outcome Score

To evaluate altered consciousness and coma, the Glasgow Coma Scale (GCS) and Glasgow Outcome Score (GOS) have proved useful, mainly for head injured patients. Due to their simplicity and standardization, they are suitable for communication amongst paramedics, nurses and physician/surgeons. Using motor responses to commands or pain, eye opening, and verbal response, Teasdale and Jennett developed the GCS and it is now one of the most widely used and accepted tools for consciousness disorders (Table 13.1) [44, 45]. There are some limitations, e.g., especially when applied to children [46].

A reliable tool for assessing severely injured patients is the GOS. It contains five levels from death, persistent vegetative state, severe, moderate and low disability.

The GOS is widely used for assessing outcome in head injured patients [47]. Its simplicity has made it controversial but be used for long time prognosis [48].

Behavioral Tests and Functional Imagery in Consciousness Assessment

Several other behavioral assessment scales are also used for evaluating disorders of consciousness (DOC). The Coma Recovery Scale-Revised (CRS-R), Sensory Stimulation Assessment Measure (SSAM), Wessex Head Injury Matrix (WHIM), Western Neuro Sensory Stimulation Profile (WNSSP), Sensory Modality Assessment Technique (SMART), Disorders of Consciousness Scale (DOCS), and Coma/Near-Coma Scale (CNC) are examples. It is generally acceptable that CRS-R is the only scale to address most advanced criteria, when assessing DOC. CRS has emerged from the need to fulfill requirements of both clinical and research practices. Even so, it has limitations due to absence of behavioral criteria necessary to diagnose the minimally conscious state. When properly applied, CRS

Table 13.1 Glasgow Coma Scale

Level	1	2	3	4	5	6
Eye	Does not open eyes	Opens eyes in response to painful stimuli	Opens eyes in response to voice	Opens eyes spontaneously	N/A	N/A
Verbal	Makes no sounds	Incomprehensible sounds	Utters inappropriate words	Confused, disoriented	Oriented, converses normally	N/A
Motor	Makes no movements	Extension to painful stimuli (decerebrate response)	Abnormal flexion to painful stimuli (decorticate response)	Flexion / Withdrawal to painful stimuli	Localizes painful stimuli	Obeys commands

allows one to discriminate between minimally conscious states from those in the vegetative states [49].

Functional imaging tools include functional magnetic resonance imaging, (MRI), positron emission tomography (PET), single-photon emission computed tomography (SPECT). They are often used to determine the level of consciousness based on specific brain activities revealed by these methods. In VS, "rudiments" of consciousness not being detected by the patient's bedside evaluation may exist and functional magnetic resonance imaging obtained by activation of dedicated cortical areas may demonstrate it. [50–52].

Painful stimuli produce PET patterns of activation in minimally conscious states [53]. In one VS patient, task specific activation was observed, unequivocally, demonstrating consciousness in the absence of obvious clinical behavioral signs of consciousness. Interestingly, the patient subsequently recovered although the full extent of recovery is not described [54]. Functional neuroimaging is not enough for the diagnosis of vegetative state but it is increasingly clear that it can be used as an additive tool in this regard. Quantitative measurements of brain activity—in particular, activations beyond primary sensory cortices, are positively correlated with 'good recovery' from the vegetative state [55].

EEG is a continuous method of monitoring patients and is less expensive then fMRI and PET and brings functional information about the brain Spectral analysis of alpha/theta frequencies proved useful in differentiating patients with disorders of consciousness [56]. Coupling TMS and EEG assesses the reaction of the brain to magnetic pulse exploring the connectivity between different areas [57]. A perturbation complexity index (PCI; 58), assigns a numerical value of the brain's complex activity patterns capacity. In VS versus MCS, the low index reflects lower levels of connectivity [58].

A good example of controlled reversibility of consciousness is coma induced by general anesthesia. Emery Brown and team observed loss of consciousness during propofol general anesthesia. They hypothesized the following as causes for producing this effect: i) the loss of communication within the frontal cortical thalamo–cortical circuits [60], while, ii) the propofol-induced slow oscillations may correspond to a state of functional isolation between cortical areas [61]. The authors observed seizure–like highly structured oscillations, which are associated with unconsciousness [62], and could be a mechanism for anesthetic-induced unconsciousness. These highly structured oscillations could be responsible for the disruption of integrated information processing within the brain [63], as well as anterior–posterior cortical feedback [64, 65], both of which are considered crucial for conscious processing [66]. Meanwhile, it is important to stress that coma induced by anesthesia is totally reversible and based on other mechanisms than in, e.g. post-trauma injured brain [67–70].

Figure 13.2 depicts the transition from consciousness to unconsciousness and the return to conscious state. The initiation of discovery on how to regain and improve consciousness by electrical neuromodulation is the merit of Moruzzi and Magoun (1949), who achieved waking of the drowsy cat by stimulating the ascending reticular activating system [16].

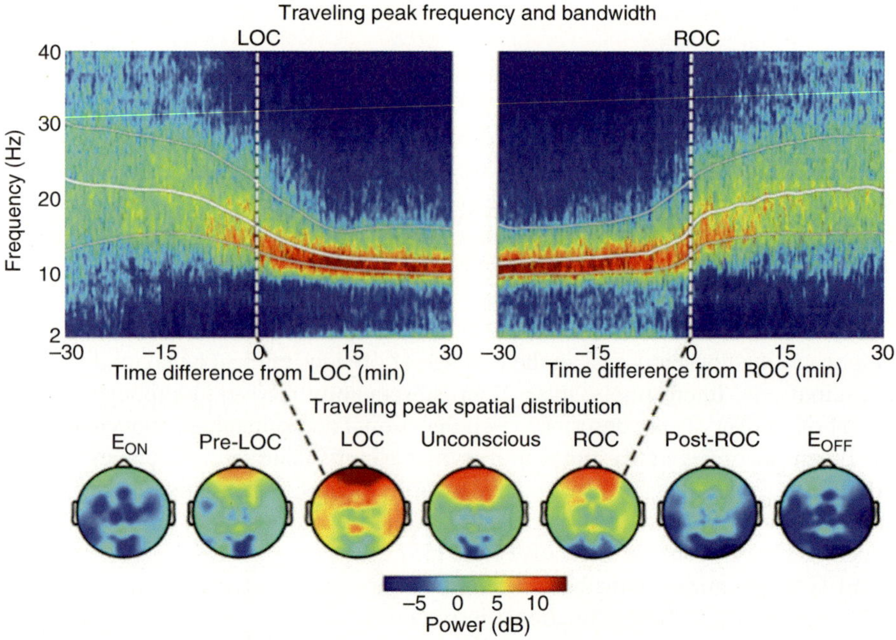

Fig. 13.2 Time course of the traveling peak, the continuous transformation in median frequency and bandwidth spanning the gamma, beta, and alpha bands during the transitions into and out of unconsciousness. (**a**) Group-level spectrograms computed between 2 and 40 Hz for a single frontal channel (approximately Fz, nearest-neighbor Laplacian reference), aligned with respect to LOC (*Left*) and ROC (*Right*) and normalized by the baseline spectrum. The 25th, median, and 75th percentiles within this frequency range are overlaid in white. The median represents the center frequency of the traveling peak, while the interquartile range (i.e., the difference between the 75th and 25th percentiles) represents the bandwidth of the traveling peak. (**b**) Spatial distribution of power at the median frequency at different behavioral end points. Pre-LOC is the midpoint between EON and LOC. Unconscious refers to the midpoint between LOC and ROC. Post-LOC is the midpoint between ROC and EOFF (With permission from Purdon et al. [69])

Therapeutic Strategies Based on Pathophysiology

A legitimate question one may ask is "What should a therapy accomplish?" Since we do not understand the underpinnings of consciousness yet, there are some observation elements that may allow to ground the therapy actions on an empiric basis. Bellow we describe several steps that a therapy may need to accomplish.

(a) Secondary lesions controls. Destruction of brain tissue is followed by brain swelling, high intracranial pressure and insufficient blood supply to the affected area. This disturbance induces a number of processes including decreased oxygen, altered ion balance, glutamate alterations, and apoptosis [59]. The main therapeutic strategy seems to reduce or stop this cascade in order to preserve the undamaged tissue and limit secondary lesions. Since the primary brain lesion may induce secondary lesions, limiting this secondary damage is a crucial therapeutic strategy

(b) To keep pathways functional. Based on the principle that unused brain pathways and connections are lost in time, an early start of rehabilitation is a sound option. Let us use two examples, a famous virtuoso violin soloist and an athlete training for the Olympic games. Due to some unhappy circumstances, they have to stop their rehearsals and training. Both will decline in their performances. Rehabilitation and neuro-modulation are targeting this functional aspect of behavior. However, these procedures may interfere and be confused with natural healing. Understanding the mechanisms of consciousness and its neuromarkers could help to differentiate the two. If a stimulated patient in a vegetative state is waking-up as a prolonged post-effect of stimulation, he/she is in a reversible vegetative state; if no waking effect is observed the subject falls into an irreversible vegetative state. This means that stimulation could be seen as a triage tool between reversible and irreversible states.

(c) The 'default network' activity. The 'default network' is represented by brain structures identified on functional magnetic resonance imaging connectivity analyses that show more activity at rest than during attention-demanding executive tasks. They are in the posterior-cingulate/precuneus, the anterior cingulate/mesiofrontal cortex and the temporo-parietal junctions. This network may be identified in the resting state of healthy volunteers in the absence of any task. While functional connectivity patterns predict the level of consciousness and recovery outcome in acquired brain injuries [71], the integrity of the resting-state connectivity pattern is negatively correlated with the degree of clinical consciousness impairment, as demonstrated in the study by Vanhaudenhuyse et al. [72]. Restauration by stimulation of this resting state activity placed in above mentioned areas could become an improving marker of certain therapy measures. Thus, electrical stimulation of a small brain area in the Claustrum reversibly disrupts consciousness. [73]

(d) Neuroplasticity. Neuroplasticity is the ability of nervous system to adapt to new environmental changes and on repetitive input, particularly, at synaptic and neuronal level. This is accomplished in a dynamic manner [74]. The term was coined by Jerzy Konorski, a Polish neurophysiologist during 1940's [75]. The "use-induced" plasticity is a remarkable concept, developed by Hebb (1949), reflecting brain response to different events whereby the repeated and persistent stimulation of presynaptic cell modifies the response of the postsynaptic cell [76]. "Let us assume that the persistence or repetition of a reverberatory activity (or "trace") tends to induce lasting cellular changes that add to its stability. When an axon of cell A is near enough to excite a cell B and repeatedly or persistently takes part in firing it, some growth process or metabolic change takes place in one or both cells such that A's efficiency, as one of the cells firing B, is increased" [76]. Damage of the brain structure is followed by a structural and functional reorganization, enabling survival, when possible.

Neural Plasticity can appear when:

- *Dormant neural pathways are activated by the removal of the inhibition* [77]
- *There is modified neuronal membrane excitability* [78]
- *A strengthening or weakening of active synapses may be induced by the process of long-term potentiation* (LTP) *or long-term depression* (LTD, [79])
- *Morphological changes may be induced by long term potentiation consisting of multiple synapses between a single axon terminal and a dendrite* [80].

Overview of the Clinical Therapeutic Data

Invasive therapies use chronic implanted electrodes for stimulation, while non-invasive therapies employ transcranial magnetic stimulation (TMS), transcranial current stimulation (tDCS) and median nerve stimulation. We will critically analyze the progress of the therapeutic methods that are currently used or being evaluated for the treatment of consciousness disturbance.

A review of literature on vegetative state reveals a relatively small number of cases with a myriad of therapy methods, many of them in the early stage of exploration. (Due to non-uniformity of cases and small numbers per center, prospective random studies for standardized therapy is difficult, if not impossible, to conduct).

These cases include:

1. Chemical, electromagnetic and either non-invasive methods, such as somatosensitive stimulation, speech and music stimulation and transcranial magnetic stimulation, etc.,
2. Invasive methods, such as chronic electrodes for stimulation of different targets in the brain and spine. Most of them are based on the principle supporting the view that an injured brain needs a reconnection of its disrupted areas or circuits.

Stimulation

Transcutaneous Nerve Stimulation

Median Nerve Stimulation

The fact that the spino-reticular tract synapses with neurons of the ascending reticular activating system makes the median nerve a possible ‘pathway to the brain (from the dorsal root ganglia there are projections to the posterior horn of the medulla and from there to thalamus and other brain areas). The right side is chosen since the majority of subjects are right handed. The median nerve was stimulated to prevent spastic contraction of the hand in comatosed patients. Subsequently, an improvement (accelerated awakening) was observed in acute and chronic states of coma [81]. Rubber electrodes were placed on palmar surface of the wrist. The stimulation impulses were asymmetrically biphasic, with amplitude of 15–20 milliamps with a pulse width of 300 μs at 40 Hz for 20 s. The level of stimulation was 1.5 of motor threshold, which is less than what produces pain. Total time of stimulation was 8–12 h/day, for a mean of 3 weeks. There were no changes in heart rate, respiration, systemic arterial pressure and intracranial pressure. When stimulation started early after coma, the positive effects were recorded earlier. Longer periods of coma or vegetative state may necessitate months or even years of stimulation (unpublished data from the lead author).

A patient in post-anoxic VS for 6 months was stimulated from the right median nerve. After 3 months of treatment, he showed improved visual pursuit and fixation, better posture, swallowing and phonation. The proponents of median nerve stimulation stress that therapy has to be initiated early because brain atrophy is in progress and it may be too late to achieve a recovery of brain function at a later stage. It is suggested that some months or even years are needed in the chronic stimulation setup. Possible mechanisms of median nerve stimulation are: increased cerebral blood flow, increased levels of dopamine and norepinephrine, and activation of Broca's area [82, 83]. The usefulness of median nerve stimulation in patients with severe traumatic brain injury is determined on the basis of changes in cerebrospinal fluid dopamine, and cerebral blood flow increases up after this procedure [11].

Spinal Cord Stimulation or Dorsal Column Stimulation

Spinal cord stimulation (SCS) is currently used for the treatment of pain. It has also proved effective in 214 patients who had been in VS due to trauma, anoxia or stroke. In a prospective uncontrolled and nonrandomized observational study for 20 consecutive years (1986–2005). Electrodes were placed epidurally in space between C2 and C4. Stimulation parameters were 2.0–3.0 V; frequency: 70 Hz; pulse width: 120 μs for 15 min on/15 min off during daytime only, without reaching the motor threshold. When included in the study, the duration of the VS was at least 1 year in traumatic cases and at least 3 months in non-traumatic cases. Clinical results were evaluated using an efficacy scale designed by the investigators to fulfill the needs of the study based on detecting signs of awareness of self and surrounding. Excellent and positive clinical results were reported in 109 of the 201 patients (54%); but results were better in patients below the age of 35, those of PVS of traumatic origin and those patients with regional cerebral blood flow over 20 mL/100 g/min. Possible mechanisms for improvement are: increases in the regional cerebral blood flow via brainstem pathways, increases in the levels of neurotransmitters and neuromodulators, and enhances of sympathetic activity, promoting neuroplasticity in the central nervous system, stimulation of the undamaged, nonspecific pathways, activates residual functional cortical areas [84]. In a previous study performed by the same team, clinical improvement included ability to follow commands, interaction with family and self-feeding that occurred in 42% of cases [85]. The majority (3/4) of patients had severe head injury. Improvement was much better in this category than in the vascular and hypoxic injury. Patients who were less than 40 years. of age (particularly those in their early 30s) did much better than those over 50s. More improvement was observed results when stimulation started earlier. Deep brain lesions and cortical atrophy disqualified patients for stimulation [86].

Deep Brain Stimulation (DBS)

Deep brain stimulation consists of the implantation of small cylindrical electrodes serially placed in the deep structure of the brain. Precise placement is accomplished by neuro-navigation or by stereotactic methods. A subcutaneous implantable pulse generator is composed of a long life battery or a rechargeable one and the hardware and software producing electrical stimuli adapted to patient needs by telemetry from outside the skin and by placing the remote control on it. The titration of energy is done by specialized medical personal following specific protocols. This tuning is obtained by frequency, current, pulse width and polarity selection.

DBS has been used for treatment of different neurological disease like Parkinson disease and dystonia, but also in psychiatric disorders and obesity. The surgical technique is not fundamentally different from what is already a routine in neurosurgical practice. It consists of a preplan for identification of a vessel free path to the target identified by MRI morphology and anatomical atlases. Sudden stop of stimulation may induce severe deprivation syndrome and special precaution must be taken to prevent it. Since DBS is more frequently used in Parkinson disease, valuable clinical and experimental information may be extrapolated to DOC where the number of cases is smaller. Based on neurophysiology studies there were attempts to treat patients presenting with coma, VS, and MCS by stimulating the mesencephalon-diencephalic junction starting with the second half of last century. An optimistic arousal response of stimulated patients was observed. An improvement was recorded in stimulated patients but not consistently supported with the behavioral scales and statistics [87].

Hassler [88] is a distinguished neuroanatomist who decided to stimulate the pallidum and the lateropolar nucleus of the contralateral thalamus. The results of neuromodulation on behavioral and EEG arousal are evoking earlier experiments of Moruzzi and Magoon [88]. Ten years later another case was reported, this time, an upper brain stem infarction followed by a deep coma where the left thalamic reticular nucleus was stimulated [89]. During mid 80's and early 90's there were reports coming from France and oriented on prolonged traumatic unconsciousness thalamic stimulation [90, 91]. The Japanese's vast experience with deep brain stimulation in vegetative state is also reported [92, 93].

One of the largest series ($n = 21$) of DBS in VS stimulated patients, targeted the mesencephalic reticular formation (two patients) and centromedian-parafascicularis nucleus complex ($n = 19$ cases). Eight of the patients recovered from VS. All eight presented a desynchronization on continuous EEG frequency analysis. The authors' conclusion is that patient selection might be done on the basis of electrophysiological criteria [94]. It is worth to mention that a negative result in a patient implanted in the left thalamus 6 month after trauma, who did not show signs of improvements after other 6 month of stimulation [95].

DBS may act differently based on the phase of treatment: initial, acute and chronic [96–98]. Also DBS may increase synaptic activity inducing the improvement of pharmacological effects in patients with preserved large-scale integrative cerebral networks [99]. The anatomical pathway underlying this approach is between the midbrain reticular formation and thalamic intralaminar nuclei which are theoretically the main connections to the upper cortical levels [100]. Fibers connecting striatum to thalamus and cortex are medium spiny striatal neurons and are responsible for action potentials [101]. Neuroplasticity appears within seconds and minutes after stimulation started and may persist to longer times after it is interrupted [102, 103]. The stimulation effects persist after stimulation has stopped. A proposed mechanism of action during central thalamic stimulation is frontal lobe activation [104]. Presumably, premotor area acts on attention [105–107]. Cortical and thalamic activity is controlled by the "arousal system" affected in coma and other deficits of consciousness [108].

Anterior cingulate cortex is involved in tasks requiring high vigilance [109]. Arousal regulation may be controlled by dialog between thalamus and anterior cingulate cortex. DBS can act as compensation to affected neuronal circuits in the brain [8]. A desynchronization in neuronal populations could be a desirable effect during DBS [110]. The best documented case of DBS for DOC is a patient who suffered from traumatic brain injury who developed minimally cognitive state, MCS. After 6 years he was implanted for thalamic stimulation. Bilateral anterior intra-laminar nuclei in central thalamus were targeted. A double-blind alternating crossover study of 6 months showed that neuromodulation induced behavioral responsiveness. Based on Coma Recovery Scale-Revised scores (motor, communication and arousal subscales), the authors found that the frequency of cognitively mediated behaviors increased during the 'on' state of DBS compared with the 'off' state of DBS. An improvement was recorded in purposeful upper extremity limb movement and oral feeding [111]. Regrettably, it is a single case; team and others did not replicate this success. These obviate the high grade of complexity and difficulty in this domain. A great responsibility is taken by those who actively involve taking the risk of failure. Due to the high costs of the procedure, effect on professional prestige due to negative results, most neurosurgeons prefer to send patients to rehab centers. On the other side, the accumulation of knowledge is promising and points to future avenues for investigation. The methods described above are invasive and associated with surgical risks and complications [112], and are also expensive. However, many patients in MCS will live unacceptable terrible lifes post injury for whom this could be the only option to improve.

Extradural Cortical Stimulation

Penfield and his team introduced cortical stimulation in the 1950s. It has become a frequently used investigational approach for treating patients with epilepsy and Parkinson's disease among others. The method consists of implanting electrodes over or into cortex, and then injecting electrical currents through these electrodes

[113, 114]. Based on a similar approach, Canavero reported a promising clinical response in VS patients after epidural cortical stimulation [115]. It must be considered that cortical neurons activating thresholds by surface placed electrodes depend on many elements, e.g. polarity, electrode shape and configuration, current, waveform, cortical columns and layers. It has been demonstrated that bipolar electrode configurations are more effective at confining the modulatory effects of stimulation to regions directly below the electrode. Subthreshold changes in neurons can induce modulatory effects. Placement of electrodes in bipolar configurations influences differently produced effects. Location of neurons on gyrus or in the depth of the sulcus will make a difference in reactivity threshold, being higher for deep neurons [116].

The effects of stimulation may appear far from electrode placement due to effects on fibers traveling through brain and spine. Direct activation of sparse, distributed populations of cortical neurons by electrical microstimulation is responsible for this effect [117–122]. It is important to identify the optimal areas for implantation to obtain best results and avoid adverse effects. Epidural placement is less invasive than cortical or intra-parenchymal electrodes. However, it has the disadvantage that the current must pass through meningeal layer and cerebrospinal fluid where it loses energy and focus. The new generation of electrodes may surpass the invasiveness disadvantage, being less destructive and better tolerated. A promising compromise will be implanting electrodes at epi and subdural levels to fulfill the therapy's requirements. These approaches are associated with an improvement in specificity and selectivity of stimulation. Shaping of electromagnetic fields within surface and in depth of the brain is complicated by existence of gyri, sulci, and white matter. Neuronal populations are affected by different electrical gradients. Newly developed surface electrodes are flexible and foldable making possible a better adaptability to individual morphological characteristics [123–126]. Newly designed electrodes as well as current steering technology are promising in a translational perspective, from hearing prosthetics to cortical stimulation [127]. A caveat with stimulation of the cortex is that it has a higher risk of inducing seizures. Cortical stimulation in clinical trials for Parkinson's disease, for example, reported seizures in about 50% of the patients [128].

Translational Methods in Perspective

Direct current (DC) and alternating current (AC) diagnostics and therapy consist in application of electric currents to the surface of the head, under different labels such as electrotherapy, electroanesthesia, and electrosleep. The purpose is to inject electrical energy into the brain through surface electrodes. Using an experimental approach employing a head shaped electrolytic tank and theoretical techniques using three concentric spheres presenting different resistances corresponding to brain, skull, and scalp, the authors [129] demonstrated that:

1. "The total current passing through the cranial cavity when the electrodes lie on the scalp (near the centers of the occipital and frontal bones) is about 45 percent of that applied.

2. With the electrode placement above maximum current, density in the cortex just under the electrode relates in the ratio of 3:1 to minimum current density at the point in the brain farthest from the electrode.
3. The range of current densities (in the brain) in the plane perpendicular to the line between the electrodes and midway between them is 1.3 to 1.
4. With a current-electrode spacing of 5 cm, a substantial portion of the current entering the brain is localized in the cortex under the electrodes. At closer spacing, the shunting effect of the scalp predominates.
5. From the theoretic model, good estimates of the effects of electrode placement, of the detailed distribution of current in the head, skull thickness, scalp thickness, and head size can be made."

The model was validated on monkey brain invasively and humans noninvasively [129].

The great advantage of current is that the effects may be reversible, faster than drugs, and more easily titrated. Also, currents injected in periphery may reach higher levels or as electricity if nerves are behaving like double way routes. Median nerve stimulation already presented and established as a transcutaneous electrical nerve stimulation therapy (TENS), is based on large brain projection. Extrapolating, there are other nerves, especially cranial nerves, able to fulfill large brain projection with similar possibilities, e.g. trigeminal nerve. Characterized by their low impedance, acupuncture points could become efficient portal for introducing currents and avoiding skin high resistance.

Transcranial Direct Current Stimulation (tDCS)

When using transcranial direct current stimulation, the current flows from the negative electrode known as cathode to the positive electrode known as anode [130]. It is a noninvasive method also referred to as polarization of the brain. It consists of sessions of 10 min or more with injection of tiny currents of 0.5–2 mA [10]. A sponge electrode with a surface of 25 cm^2 soaked in saline or conductive gel is placed on the scalp after meticulous cleaning. The injected current value is 0.08 mA/sq. cm. Smaller electrode surface is 1.4 cm^2 and the current's value is about 1.43 mA/cm^2. They present a higher focalization of the injected currents [131, 132]. Pyramidal cells respond with facilitation when they are stimulated by the anode, and the cathode induces inhibition by hyperpolarization [10]. There is an abundance of data showing that functional connectivity [19–25, 133, 134] increases post stimulation with direct current not only locally but in the whole brain including: (1) reorganizing the intrinsic functional architecture of the human primary motor cortex [135]; (2) modulation of large-scale brain networks [136]; (3) changes in brain connectivity by prefrontal transcranial direct current stimulation of subject's resting state [137, 138].

Development of biomarkers able to demonstrate the effects of stimulation and targeted injection of currents are major challenges [139, 140]. Longer stimulation sessions are inducing more persisting effects, but this can be associated with seizure risks [141]. The injected current must not exceed the threshold level and the total amount must be maintained in safety parameters. As a consequence, this will determine a change in spontaneous neuronal activity and excitability [142].

Positioning of the electrodes on the scalp frequently uses 10–20 EEG for placement. Personalized arrangement of electrodes seems crucial for focalization of stimulation and the algorithm should include previous functional neuroimaging information. Regular EEG electrodes are not appropriate for the stimulation. EEG recordings are used for evaluation of the stimulation effects but they cannot be performed during stimulation due to interferences. However, EEG recording and high density tDCS have been performed simultaneously in a pilot study [143]. On the other hand, current stimulation can be carried out simultaneously with fMRI examination, making possible a direct observation of the effects produced by neuromodulation [144]. This is due to high technological progress,

Transcranial Alternative Current Stimulation (tACS)

When compared with direct current stimulation, alternative current stimulation is less studied and applied. Indeed, the source of DC could be a battery, with associated wires, a measurement instrument and a power regulator, whereas an alternative current generator is more complicated and the procedure is associated with pain during stimulation. It has been shown that electrical stimulation through intact scalp, skull, dural cover and CSF was difficult due to high electrical resistance and high amount of energy to be injected, and also induced pain reactions in subjects [145]. When compared with brain implanted electrodes, the spatial resolution is less precise, the injected energy is higher and the time necessary to obtain results is longer. However, tACS has advantages such as producing no iontophoretic effects, since polarity is not the key point as in tDCS, and because a different mechanism of action on neural membranes induces easier reversibility. The tACS effect begins when the Na- channels of neuronal membranes start to open. This induces a cascade influx of Na- ions into the cell which induces membrane depolarization. From subthreshold stimulation to depolarization must be an exponential effect. Prolonged alternative current stimulation may have a cumulative effect on certain neuronal structures inducing more intense aftereffects. High frequency tACS produced a weak depolarization of the cell membrane in cultured rat neurons [146]. The upper end of human physiological oscillation is 640 Hz for thalamus and 1 kHz for small periependimar cells. Frequency ranges of 80–200 Hz (ripples) have been associated with plasticity processes [147].

tACS may possess the capacity to induce cortical networks, enabling local and remote areas' synchronization or desynchronization. Correlations between the stimulation duration threshold and neuroplastic effects which can be measured when using shorter stimulation durations are under study [148]. It has been showed that neurons exposed to weak electrical fields are capable of synchronizing [149]. Generally, the stimulation is a subthreshold excitation. A direction of depolarization is not occurring. A possible mechanism of action of tACS is on sodium channels [150]. Another possible mechanism of action of tACS is consolidation of learning and memory by excitability enhancement. Indeed there are studies showing that an excitability enhancement is a condition for learning by inducing strengthening of synapses/long-term potentiation by modifying NMDA-receptor efficacy [151, 152].

Concluding, current stimulation is noninvasive, selective, painless and demonstrated reversible excitability modulation. Also it is cheap, portable, repeatable and easy to standardize. The transcranial injection of weak AC looks like a promising tool for clinical studies on neuroplasticity. The main focus must be on how to obtain durable clinical effects after weak current application. This should be possible with large scale research including neuroscientists, experimental and clinical specialists, and industry. Alternative current stimulation is used for median nerve stimulation, and invasively in deep brain and spinal cord stimulation.

Transcranial Magnetic Stimulation (TMS)

Transcranial magnetic stimulation (TMS) was introduced in 1985 as a method to evaluate global cortical excitability and motor pathway integrity. The principle is of electromagnetic induction [9, 153]. A brisk rise of magnetic field is followed by a slow fall. The effect is similar to injecting current by wire, but non-invasive. This method consists in sudden discharge of an electromagnetic pulse by a coil placed above the targeted nervous tissue where eddy currents are inducing membrane depolarization.

Coils are circular or figure-eight shaped, the latter with higher focalization and lesser energy consumption required for production of eddy currents. This device can be handheld, or for more precision, can be manipulated by a robotic arm controlled by a neuronavigational system. This enables repetitive and standardized targeting in the brain, spine or peripheral nerves. After the measurement of the motor threshold, representing the minimum level of energy able to produce a muscle contraction on electromyographic recording (EMG), this stimulation can be applied to brain, spine, peripheral nerves for diagnostic and/or therapy.

Currently available stimulators are generating a magnetic field of 1.5 T. The magnetic field passes perpendicularly through skin, bone, and cerebrospinal fluid to induce eddy current in the cortex. The effects are dependent on the shape of cells, orientation of the fibers, local homogeneity and wave form. The effects can be excitatory or inhibitory. If a group of pyramidal cells is depolarized, then a muscle contraction corresponding topographically is observed and may be recorded by electromyography. This could be useful mainly in neurosurgery for mapping of the brain surface. Stimulation may be performed in a single pulse, repeated and preprogramed in one or more sessions. Frequency dependent effects are different as follows: more than 3 Hz is facilitatory, less than 1 Hz is inhibitory. Repetitive TMS on main motor aria can induce robust excitatory effects over 30 min post-stimulation [154].

There is a risk of seizure post TMS [155], but it can be controlled by safety recommendations [156]. TMS is used in clinical applications for medication resistant depression and stroke motor recovery. There are some observations that may ground application to conscious disturbances.

The left dorsolateral prefrontal cortex is inhibited in depression as functional neuroimaging has revealed [157]. Repeated transcranial stimulation (Fig. 13.3) on ipsilateral or opposite hemisphere may induce a dysfunction correction [158]. Stroke is a killer for affected neurons, but dormant neurons may be able to recover. The functional consequence of stroke is diaschisis, a severe disruption in whole brain connectivity. TMS may bring improvement in these cases [159–163]. Repetitive TMS on the primary motor area can induce robust excitatory effects over 30 min post-stimulation [154]. Unfortunately, TMS devices are heavy, voluminous, expensive and not suitable for personal use, suggesting the need for refined alternatives using micro-magnetic approaches.

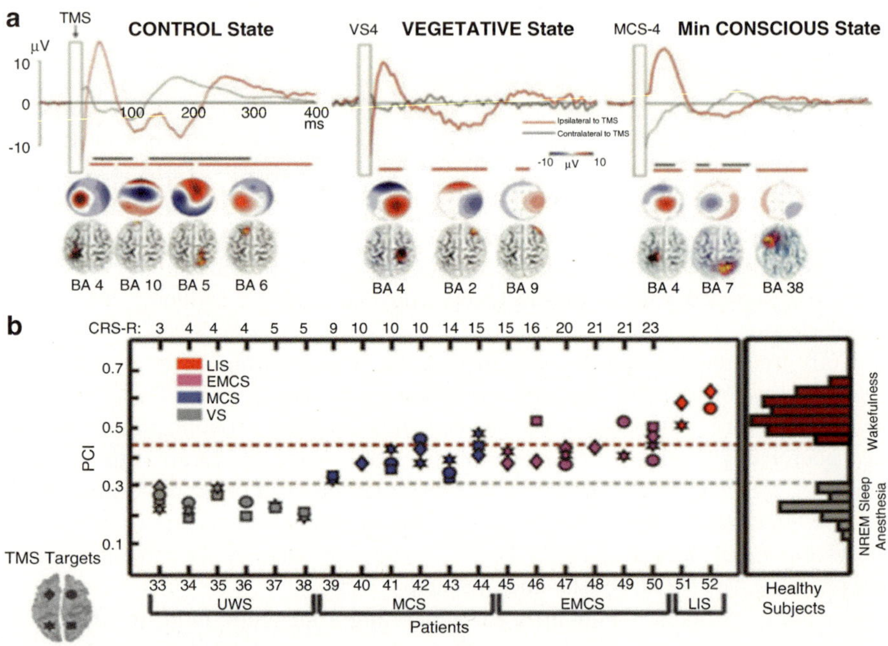

Fig. 13.3 (**a**) TMS-evoked potentials, TEPs recorded in VS, MCS patients and healthy controls. TEPs recorded from C3 and C4 following stimulation of the left or right M1 in VS and MCS patients. The control panel indicates the grand average TEPs obtained in five healthy controls stimulated above the left primary motor cortex (M1; C3). For all patients and the control group, the presented TEPs were recorded from the closest electrode to the hot-spot (ipsilateral to TMS – *red line*) and from the corresponding electrode on the contralateral hemisphere (*black line*). The hot-spot is indicated with a black dot. The responses obtained during the sham condition were point-by-point subtracted from those obtained during the real TMS. The significant time-windows (i.e., EEG signal exceeding three standard deviations of the pre-stimulus activity for at least 20 ms) are separately indicated for the ipsilateral electrode with a horizontal red line and for the electrodes contralateral to the TMS hot-spot with a black line (With permission from Ragazzoni et al. [177], https://creativecommons.org/licenses/by/4.0/). (**b**) The perturbational Complexity Index. PCI values in severely brain-injured patients. PCI progressively increases from unresponsive wakefulness (*UWS*) to minimally conscious (*MCS*) and to recovery of functional communication (*EMCS*). PCI attains levels of healthy awake subjects in LIS patients. *CRS-R* Coma Recovery Scale-Revised (With permission from Gosseries et al. [178])

Discussion

Neuromodulation is defined as the long term activation, inhibition and modification or regulation of nervous system activity. The most frequent used forms of neuromodulation are electrical, electromagnetic, optogenetic and chemical. Improvements of patients presenting with DOC, with or without recovery of social or clinical intervention, may take place within the first 3 months after non-traumatic cerebral accidents and after 12 months after traumatic ones. Survival beyond 10 years remains unusual – albeit depending on the level of medical and nursing care [164]. However, subjects with late spontaneous recoveries [165, 166] or after invasive interventional treatments (e.g., Schiff et al., 2007) make it impossible to establish temporally fixed periods for recovery. Since knowledge on mechanisms underlying recovery of consciousness is limited, the explanatory attempts remain speculative for now. For example, functions of "dormant neurons" and cerebral plasticity potential in DOC patients are overlooked. Hypothetical mechanisms such as neurogenesis, axonal sprouting and neurite growth, are difficult to translate from experimental studies and limited in clinical practice.

It is important to understand why some patients improve and others do not; this needs to be studied in further clinical studies. Optimal design for future investigations must fulfill the following requirements: prospective cohort studies or double-blind placebo-controlled studies; carefully established safety guidelines for stimulation protocols, revised and updated; electrode characteristics have to maintain injected charge densities within safe limits; and seizure prevention.

New Directions

Development of new electrodes for recording and modulation is an important future direction [167]. Improved spatial targeting may be obtained by different shaped electrodes with radial extensions [168]. Another pathway for neuromodulation is the bloodstream. It consists of placing catheters in very tiny blood vessels of the brain to serve as high precision delivery channels for energy and substances. An intra-capillary electrode can record and modulate the area when surgically placed in the parenchyma [169]. Nanotechnology is producing submicronic components which can be assembled into recording and modulation implantable systems in a minimally invasive manner. Energy sources for these systems are designed to use local energy: nanogenerators based on the metabolism of glucose extracted from blood, heat based devices, and pressure wave piezoelectric devices [170, 171]. Another promising domain is microdialysis, where neurochemical monitoring systems may be associated with human (DBS, deep brain stimulation) surgery. Based on electrochemical techniques and validated by preclinical models, this new method has demonstrated the successful monitoring of changes in various neurotransmitter systems in vivo with high temporal and spatial resolution. The electrochemical recording is of paramount importance for elucidating different aspects of human neurophysiology and to discover new therapies. Wireless Instantaneous Neurotransmitter Concentration Sensing (WINCS) is a new system that combines rapid scan voltammetry and fixed potential amperometry with wireless telemetry for electrochemical recording and analysis. It has demonstrated high temporal and spatial resolution in detecting changes in tissue. The analyzed substances include dopamine, adenosine, glutamate, serotonin, and histamine. Neurochemical monitoring in humans represents a new approach to understanding the neurophysiology of the central nervous system [172]. This approach has the advantage of allowing an on-line correlation between behavioral changes, secondary to neuromodulation and neurochemical fast reactions. Indeed, major advantages are small spatial resolution and infrasecond temporal response. Nanoelectrodes will be able to monitor neurotransmitters in real time.

Another promising direction is carbon based advanced materials such as diamond-like carbon, carbon nanofibers, and carbon nanotubes. The diameter of nanotube is less than 100 nm and the length can vary from hundreds of nanometers to many micrometers. They present special characteristics extending the application area. The open ends have a very fast electron transfer rate while the side wall has isolation properties, which makes them particularly promising for neuromodulation application. Meanwhile electrochemical signals can be picked up at the open end and transported to the other end for capture and analysis. Encapsulation of carbon nanofibers in SiO2 or Parylene produces semiconductor properties which can be mass produced at low price. Fibers and tubes directly grown on top of tetrahedral amorphous carbon produced superior electrodes performance. The stable water window of these sensors enables detection of a wide range of neurotransmitters, as well as capability of supporting higher potentials without suffering degradation [173]. These fabrication processes with low cost of carbon derived products make them affordable in many applications.

Since light is an electromagnetic field, it can be used with high specificity dependent on wave length using another important method which is optogenetics; this consists in transfecting genes in neurons making possible the identification of the polarization status of the cell or activating it using a certain color with a laser beam. Presently, the method is limited to experimental environments [174]. A nonhuman primate brain is the model system closest to the human brain. Experimental validation of optogenetic technologies in monkeys is a critical preclinical step on the translational path of new generation cell-type-specific neural modulation therapies. This will facilitate understanding of brain circuits and controlling brain regions at the millisecond timescale [175]. Figure 13.4 illustrates the optogenetics implementation in nonhuman primates. Optogenetics is becoming a state-of-the-art method for making causal connections between brain activity and behavior. Light-based mind control could one day be made to work in humans for therapeutic purposes.

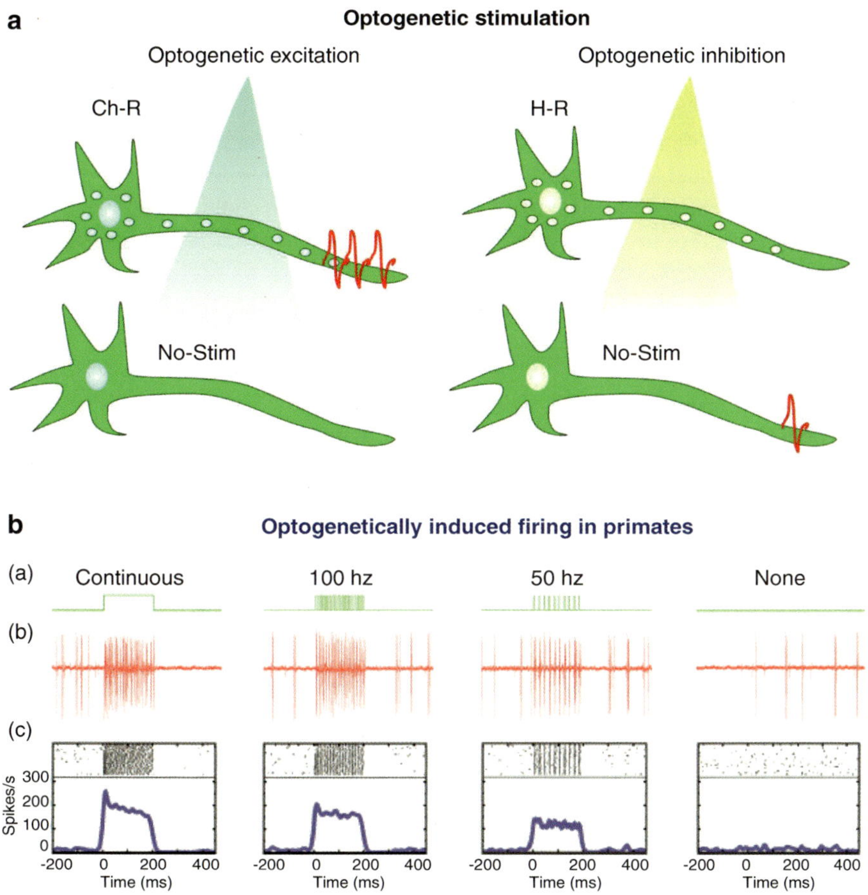

Fig. 13.4 (**a**) Illustration of optogenetic stimulation. (**b**) Example of optogenetic modulation. Each column represents a different stimulation frequency. From top to bottom, we show: *(a)* a schematic of the pulse train delivered to the laser at each stimulation frequency, *(b)* the raw spike train from one randomly picked trial for each frequency, and *(c)* the raster and the spike density functions (With permission from Dai et al. [176])

Conclusion

DOC clinical therapy approaches are explorative at best at the moment. Attempts to improve the level of consciousness of patients in the different stages of DOC have shown some promise. Assessing experimental and clinical studies' effectiveness is still in development. Better understanding of brain function and large randomized trials are necessary. Improved knowledge and processes on how novel techniques are identified and characterized and how they can be optimized to induce long- lasting effects are needed. Early neuromodulation could overlap on spontaneous recovery (natural history) and be confused as a therapeutic effect. Furthermore, neuromodulation can become a triage tool between different states, such as persistent and reversible vegetative state. The problem of treating patients in a vegetative state remains unresolved and is still a huge clinical problem.

Spinal cord stimulation (SCS), deep brain stimulation and median TENS (transcutaneous electrical neurostimulation), seem promising in some studies, suggesting that further research is needed. Median nerve stimulation could provide an efficient peripheral portal for neuromodulation of central nervous system. Noninvasive interventions are preferred over those that are invasive. They exhibit many advantages such as the ease to implement, with less risks, fewer liability concerns and lower cost than invasive devices.

Future research should also focus on identifying specific neuromarkers though it is a formidable challenge. The reversibility versus irreversibility of consciousness needs to be determined. Natural healing must be augmented and major losses could be replaced by intelligent prosthetic devices. Intelligent neuromodulation is possible by using closed loop stimulation. This will involve strict patient inclusion criteria based on protocols, biomarkers able to define the present status compared with past, and flexible changes in modulation parameters by a control algorithm for more efficient and affective outcomes. This will need better information input and better sensors, hardware, software, and rechargeable power sources based on the regenerated energy from the glycolytic processes. Complexity and results in treatment of DOC need a coordinated effort for the acquisition of knowledge on consciousness and its deficiency.

Acknowledgment Ana Ciurea was supported by the strategic grant POSDRU/159/1.5/S/133652, "Integrated system to improve the quality of doctoral and postdoctoral research in Romania and promotion of the role of science in society "co-financed by the European Social Fund within the Sectorial Operational Program Human Resources Development 2007–2013. Authors thank Dr. Cheryl Ann Sexton for reading and editing the manuscript.

References

1. Lewis CS. Studies in words. Cambridge: Cambridge University Press; 1960.
2. Boly M, Massimini M, Tononi G. Theoretical approaches to the diagnosis of altered states of consciousness. Prog Brain Res. 2009;177:383–98.
3. Bodien YG, Carlowicz CA, Chatelle C, Giacino JT. Sensitivity and specificity of the coma recovery scale-revised total score in detection of conscious awareness. Arch Phys Med Rehabil. 2015;97(3):490–492.e1.
4. Toth A. Chapter 24. Magnetic resonance imaging application in the area of mild and acute traumatic brain injury: implications for diagnostic markers?In: Kobeissy FH PhD, editor. Brain neurotrauma: molecular, neuropsychological, and rehabilitation aspects. Boca Raton (FL): CRC Press; 2015.
5. Auxéméry Y. Mild traumatic brain injury and postconcussive syndrome: a re-emergent questioning. Encephale. 2012;38(4):329–35.
6. Ng YS, Chua KS. States of severely altered consciousness: clinical characteristics, medical complications and functional outcome after rehabilitation. NeuroRehabilitation. 2005;20(2): 97–105.

7. Lefaucheur JP, André-Obadia N, Antal A, Ayache SS, Baeken C, Benninger DH, et al. Evidence-based guidelines on the therapeutic use of repetitive transcranial magnetic stimulation (rTMS). Clin Neurophysiol. 2014;125(11):2150–206.
8. Johnson MD, Vitek JL, McIntyre CC. Pallidal stimulation that improves parkinsonian motor symptoms also modulates neuronal firing patterns in primary motor cortex in the MPTP-treated monkey. Exp Neurol. 2009;219(1):359–62.
9. Barker AT, Jalinous R, Freeston IL. Non-invasive magnetic stimulation of human motor cortex. Lancet. 1985;1(8437):1106–7.
10. Nitsche MA, Cohen LG, Wassermann EM, Priori A, Lang N, Antal A, et al. Transcranial direct current stimulation. State of the art. Brain Stimul. 2008;1(3):206–23.
11. Liu JT, Wang CH, Chou IC, Sun SS, Koa CH, Cooper E. Regaining consciousness for prolonged comatose patients with right median nerve stimulation. Acta Neurochir Suppl. 2003;87:11–4.
12. Izumi H, Karita K. Somatosensory stimulation causes autonomic vasodilatation in cat lip. J Physiol. 1992;450:191–202.
13. Berger H. Über das Elektrenkephalogramm des Menschen. Arch Psychiatr Nervenkr. 1929;87(1):527–70.
14. Demetriades AK. From encephalitis lethargica to cerebral cytoarchitectonics: the polymath talent of Constantin von Economo (1876-1931), pioneer neuroanatomist, neurophysiologist and military aviator. Medizinhist J. 2012;57(4):232–6.
15. Kerkhofs M, Lavie P. Frédéric Bremer (1892-1982): a pioneer in sleep research. Sleep Med Rev. 2000;4(5):505–14.
16. Moruzzi G, Magoun HW. Brain stem reticular formation and activation of the EEG. Electroencephalogr Clin Neurophysiol. 1949;1:455–73.
17. Steriade M. Arousal: revisiting the reticular activating system. Science. 1996;272(5259):225–6.
18. Magoun HW. An ascending reticular activating system in the brainstem. Ama Arch NeurPsych. 1952;67(2):145–54.
19. Mountcastle VB. The columnar organization of the neocortex. A comprehensive review of the literature indicating the modular architecture of the cortex. Brain. 1997;120(4):701–22.
20. Opris I, Hampson RE, Stanford TR, Gerhardt GA, Deadwyler SA. Neural activity in frontal cortical cell layers: evidence for columnar sensorimotor processing. J Cogn Neurosci. 2011;23:1507–21.
21. Opris I, Hampson RE, Gerhardt GA, Berger TW, Deadwyler SA. Columnar processing in primate pFC: evidence for executive control microcircuits. J Cogn Neurosci. 2012;24(12):2334–47.
22. Opris I, Fuqua JL, Huettl P, Gerhardt GA, Berger TW, Hampson RE, Deadwyler SA. Closing the loop in primate prefrontal cortex: inter-laminar processing. Front Neural Circuits. 2012;6:88. doi:10.3389/fncir.2012.00088.
23. Opris I, Santos LM, Song D, Berger TW, Gerhardt GA, Hampson RE, Deadwyler SA. Prefrontal cortical microcircuits bind perception to executive control. Sci Rep. 2013;3:2285. doi:10.1038/srep02285.
24. Opris I, Casanova MF. Prefrontal cortical minicolumn: from executive control to disrupted cognitive processing. Brain. 2014;137(7):1863–75. doi:10.1093/brain/awt359.
25. Opris I, Bruce CJ. Neural circuitry of judgment and decision mechanisms. Brain. Res Rev. 2005;48:509–28.
26. Laureys S, Faymonville ME, Ferring M. Differences in brain metabolism between patients in coma, vegetative state, minimally conscious state and locked-in syndrome. Neuroimage. 2001;13(6):806.
27. Dehaene S, Changeux JP, Naccache L, Sackur J, Sergent C. Conscious preconscious and subliminal processing: attestable taxonomy. Trends Cogn Sci. 2006;10:204–11.
28. Dehaene S, Naccache L. Towards a cognitive neuroscience of consciousness: basic evidence and a work space framework. Cognition. 2001;79:1–37.
29. Tononi G. An information integration theory of consciousness. BMC Neurosci. 2004;5:42.
30. Penrose R. Shadow of the mind. Oxford: Oxford University Press; 1994.

31. Hameroff SR, Penrose R. Quantum computation in brain micro-tubules? The Penrose-Hameroff "Orch OR" model of consciousness. Philos Trans R Soc Lond A. 1998;356:1869–96.
32. Pribram KH. Brain and perception: holonomy and structure in figural processing. Hillsdale: Lawrence Erlbaum Associates; 1991.
33. Searle JR. Consciousness. Annu Rev Neurosci. 2000;23:557–78.
34. Weyhenmyeye JA, Gallman EA. Rapid review neuroscience 1st ed. Mosby Elsevier. 2007. p. 177–79.
35. Kandel ER, Jessell TM, Schwartz JH. Principles of neural science. New York: McGraw-Hill; 2000. p. 901.
36. Posner JB, Saper CB, Schiff ND, Plum F. Plum and posner's diagnosis of stupor and coma. Oxford/New York: Oxford University Press; 2007. p. 41.
37. The Multi-Society Task Force on PVS. Medical aspects of Persistent Vegetative State (First of two parts). N Engl J Med. 1994;330(21):1499–508.
38. The Multi-Society Task Force on PVS. Medical aspects of Persistent Vegetative State (Second of two parts). N Engl J Med. 1994;330(22):1572–9.
39. Laureys S, Celesia GG, Cohadon F, Lavrijsen J, León-Carrión J, Sannita WG, et al. Unresponsive wakefulness syndrome: a new name for the vegetative state or apallic syndrome. European Task Force on Disorders of Consciousness. BMC Med. 8:68.
40. Dolce G, Quintieri M, Serra S, Lagani V, Pignolo L. Clinical signs and early prognosis in vegetative state: a decisional tree, datamining study. Brain Inj. 2008;22:617–23.
41. Luaute J, Maucort-Boulch D, Tell L, Quelard F, Sarraf T, et al. Long-term outcomes of chronic minimally conscious and vegetative states. Neurology. 2010;75:246–52.
42. Giacino JT, Ashwal S, Childs N, Cranford R, Jennett B, Katz DI, et al. The minimally conscious state: definition and diagnostic criteria. Neurology. 2002;58:349–53.
43. Bruno MA, Vanhaudenhuyse A, Thibaut A, Moonen G, Laureys S. From unresponsive wakefulness to minimally conscious PLUS and functional locked-in syndromes: recent advances in our understanding of disorders of consciousness. J Neurol. 2011;258(7):1373–84.
44. Teasdale GM, Jennett B. Assessment of coma and impaired consciousness. A practical scale. Lancet. 1974;2:81–4.
45. Jennett B, Teasdale G, Braakman R, et al. Predicting outcome in individual patients after severe head injury. Lancet. 1976;1:1031–4.
46. Lieh-Lai MW, Theodorou AA, Sarnaik AP, Meert KL, Moylan PM, Canady AI. Limitations of the Glasgow Coma Scale in predicting outcome in children with traumatic brain injury. J Pediatr. 1992;120(2):195–9.
47. Jennett B, Bond M. Assessment of outcome after severe brain damage. Lancet. 1975;1(7905):480–4. doi:10.1016/s0140-6736(75)92830-5.
48. Woischneck D, Firsching R. Efficiency of the Glasgow Outcome Scale (GOS): score for the long-term follow-up after severe brain injuries. Acta Neurochir Suppl. 1998;71:138–41.
49. Seel RT, Sherer M, Whyte J, Katz DI, Giacino JT, Rosenbaum AM, et al. Assessment scales for disorders of consciousness: evidence-based recommendations for clinical practice and research. Arch Phys Med Rehabil. 2010;91:1795–813.
50. Schiff ND, Rodriguez-Moreno D, Kamal A, et al. fMRI reveals large-scale network activation in minimally conscious patients. Neurology. 2005;64:514–23.
51. Monti MM, Coleman MR, Owen AM. Neuroimaging and the vegetative state: resolving the behavioral assessment dilemma? Disorders of Consciousness. Ann N Y Acad Sci. 2009;1157:81–9.
52. Coleman MR, Davis MH, Rodd JM, Robson T, Ali A, Owen AM, Pickard JD. Towards the routine use of brain imaging to aid the clinical diagnosis of disorders of consciousness. Brain. 2009;132:2541–52.
53. Boly M, Faymonville ME, Schnakers C, Peigneux P, Lambermont B, Phillips C, et al. Perception of pain in the with PET activation: an observational study. Lancet Neurol. 2008;7:1013–20.
54. Demertzi A, Laureys S, Boly M. Coma persistent vegetative states and diminished consciousness. In: Banks WP, editor. Encyclopedia of consciousness, vol. 1. Amsterdam: Elsevier; 2009. p. 147–56.

55. Monti M, Laureys S, Owen A. The vegetative state. Br Med J. 2010;341:292–6.
56. Lechinger J, Chwala Schlegel N, Fellinger R, Donis J, Michitsch G, Pichler G. Mirroring of a simple motor behavior in disorders of consciousness. Clin Neurophysiol. 2013;124:27–34.
57. Rosanova M, Gosseries O, Casarotto S, Boly M, Casali AG, Bruno MA, et al. Recovery of cortical effective connectivity and recovery of consciousness in vegetative patients. Brain. 2012;135:1308–20.
58. Casali AG, Gosseries O, Rosanova M, Boly M, Sarasso S, Casali KR, et al. A theoretically based index of consciousness in dependent of sensory processing and behavior. Sci Transl Med. 2013;5:198ra105.
59. Giza CC, Hovda DA. The neurometabolic cascade of concussion. J Athl Train. 2001;36(3):228–35.
60. Ching S, Cimenser A, Purdon PL, Brown EN, Kopell NJ. Thalamocortical model for a propofol-induced alpha-rhythm associated with loss of consciousness. Proc Natl Acad Sci U S A. 2010;107(52):22665–70.
61. Imas OA, Ropella KM, Ward BD, Wood JD, Hudetz AG. Volatile anesthetics disrupt frontal-posterior recurrent information transfer at gamma frequencies in rat. Neurosci Lett. 2005;387(3):145–50.
62. Blumenfeld H. Epilepsy and the consciousness system: transient vegetative state? Neurol Clin. 2011;29(4):801–23.
63. Alkire MT, Hudetz AG, Tononi G. Consciousness and anesthesia. Science. 2008;322(5903):876–80.
64. Ku SW, Lee U, Noh GJ, Jun IG, Mashour GA. Preferential inhibition of frontal-toparietal feedback connectivity is a neurophysiologic correlate of general anesthesia in surgical patients. PLoS One. 2011;6(10):e25155.
65. Boly M, Moran R, Murphy M, Boveroux P, Bruno M-A, Noirhomme Q, Ledoux D, et al. Connectivity changes underlying spectral EEG changes during propofol-induced loss of consciousness. J Neurosci. 2012;32(20):7082–90.
66. Dehaene S, Changeux JP. Experimental and theoretical approaches to conscious processing. Neuron. 2011;70(2):200–27.
67. Brown EN, Lydic R, Schiff ND. General anesthesia sleep and coma. N Engl J Med. 2010;363:2638–50.
68. Mukamel EA et al. A transition in brain state during propofol-induced unconsciousness. J Neurosci. 2014;34:839–45.
69. Purdon PL et al. Electroencephalogram signatures of loss and recovery of consciousness from propofol. Proc Natl Acad Sci U S A. 2013;110:E1142–51.
70. Wong KF et al. Statistical modeling of behavioral dynamics during propofol-induced loss of consciousness. J Neurosci Methods. 2014;227:65–74.
71. Wu X, Zou Q, Hu J, Tang W, Mao Y, Gao L, et al. Intrinsic functional connectivity patterns predict consciousness level and recovery outcome in acquired brain injury. J Neurosci. 2015;35(37):12932–46.
72. Vanhaudenhuyse A, Noirhomme Q, Tshibanda LJ, Bruno MA, Boveroux P, Schnakers C, et al. Default network connectivity reflects the level of consciousness in non-communicative brain-damaged patients. Brain. 2010;133:161–71.
73. Koubeissi MZ, Bartolomei F, Beltagy A, Picard F. Electrical stimulation of a small brain area reversibly disrupts consciousness. Epilepsy Behav. 2014;37:32–5.
74. Butefisch CM. Neurobiological bases of rehabilitation. Neurol Sci. 2006;27(Suppl. 1):18–23.
75. Zielinski K. Jerzy Konorski on brain associations. Acta Neurobiol Exp (Wars). 2006;66:75–90.
76. Hebb DO. The organization of behavior. New York: Wiley & Sons; 1949.
77. Jacobs KM, Donoghue JP. Reshaping the cortical motor map by unmasking latent intracortical connections. Science. 1991;251:944–7.
78. Halter JA, Carp JS, Wolpaw JR. Operantly conditioned motoneuron plasticity: possible role of sodium channels. J Neurophysiol. 1995;73:867–71.

79. Hess G, Aizenman CD, Donoghue JP. Conditions for the induction of long term potentiation in layer II/III horizontal connections of the rat motor cortex. J Neurophysiol. 1995;75:1765–78.
80. Buchs N, Nikonenko P, Bron CR, Muller D. LTP promotes formation of multiple spine synapses between a single axon terminal and a dendrite. Nature. 1999;402:421–5.
81. van Dijk KR, Scherder EJ, Scheltens P, Sergeant JA. Effects of transcutaneous electrical nerve stimulation (TENS) on non-pain related cognitive and behavioural functioning. Rev Neurosci. 2002;13(3):257–70.
82. Cooper EB, Scherder EJ, Cooper JB. Electrical treatment of reduced consciousness: experience with coma and Alzheimer's disease. Neuropsychol Rehabil. 2005;15:389–405.
83. Moriya T, Hayashi N, Sakurai A, Utagawa A, Kobayashi Y, Yajima K, et al. Prevention of vegetation after severe head trauma and stroke by combination therapy of cerebral hypothermia and activation of immune-dopaminergic nervous system. Soc Treat Coma. 2000;6:133–47.
84. Kanno T, Morita I, Yamaguchi S, Yokoyama T, Kamei Y, Anil SM, Karagiozov KL. Dorsal column stimulation in persistent vegetative state. Neuromodulation. 2009;12:33–8.
85. Kanno T, Kamei Y, Yokoyama T. Effects of dorsal spinal cord stimulation (DCS) on reversibility of neuronal function—experience of treatment for vegetative states. Pacing Clin Electrophysiol. 1989;12:733–8.
86. Kanno T, Kamei Y, Yokoyama T. Treating the vegetative state with dorsal column stimulation. Soc Treat Coma. 1992;1:67–75.
87. McLardy T, Ervin F, Mark V, Scoville W, Sweet W. Attempted inset-electrodes-arousal from traumatic coma: neuropathological findings. Trans Am Neurol Assoc. 1968;93:25–30.
88. Hassler R, Ore GD, Dieckmann G, Bricolo A, Dolce G. Behavioural and EEG arousal induced by stimulation of in a patient with posttraumatic apallic syndrome. Electroencephalogr Clin Neurophysiol. 1969;27:306–10.
89. Sturm V, Kuhner A, Schmitt HP, Assmus H, Stock G. Chronic electrical stimulation of the thalamic unspecific activating system in a patient with coma due to midbrain and upper brain stem infarction. Acta Neurochir. 1979;47:235–44.
90. Cohadon F. Deep brain stimulation in cases of prolonged traumatic unconsciousness. In: Lazorthes Y, ARM U, editors. Neurostimulation: an overview. New York: Futura Publishers; 1985. p. 247–50.
91. Deliac P, Richer E, Berthomieu J, Paty J, Cohadon F, Bensch C. Electrophysiological development under thalamic stimulation of post-traumatic persistent vegetative states. Apropos of 25 cases. Neurochirurgie. 1993;39:293–303.
92. Tsubokawa T, Yamamoto T, Katayama Y, Hirayama T, Maejima S, Moriya T. Deep brain stimulation in a persistent vegetative state: follow-up results and criteria for selection of candidates. Brain Inj. 1990;44:315–27.
93. Hosobuchi Y, Yingling C. The treatment of prolonged coma with neurostimulation. In: Devinsky O, Beric A, Dogali M, editors. Electrical and magnetic stimulation of the brain and spinal cord. New York: Raven Press. Ltd; 1993. p. 247–52.
94. Yamamoto T, Katayama Y, Kobayashi K, Oshima H, Fukaya C, Tsubokawa T. Deep brain stimulation for the treatment of vegetative state. Eur J Neurosci. 2010;32(7):1145–51.
95. Matsuda W, Matsumura A, Komatsu Y, Yanaka K, Nose T. Awakenings from persistent vegetative state: report of three cases with parkinsonism and brain stem lesions on MRI. J Neurol Neurosurg Psychiatry. 2003;74:1571–3.
96. McIntyre CC, Grill WM, Sherman DL, Thakor NV. Cellular effects of deep brain stimulation: model-based analysis of activation and inhibition. J Neurophysiol. 2004;91(4):1457–69.
97. Ranck Jr JB. Which elements are excited in electrical stimulation of mammalian central nervous system: a review. Brain Res. 1975;98(3):417–40.
98. Kringelbach MLN, Jenkinson N, Owen SLF, Aziz TZ. Translational principles of deep brain stimulation. Nat Rev Neurosci. 2007;8(8):623–35.
99. Schiff ND. Central thalamic deep-brain stimulation in the severely injured brain: rationale and proposed mechanisms of action. Ann N Y Acad Sci. 2009;1157:101–16.

100. Steriade M, Glenn LL. Neocortical and caudate projections of intralaminar thalamic neurons and their synaptic excitation from midbrain reticular core. J Neurophysiol. 1982;48: 352–71.
101. Grillner S, Hellgren J, Menard A, Saitoh K, Wikstrom MA. Mechanisms for selection of basic motor programs—roles for the striatum and pallidum. Trends Neurosci. 2005;28:364–70.
102. Vitek JLT, Hashimoto T, Peoples J, DeLong MR, Bakay RA. Acute stimulation in the external segment of the globus pallidus improves parkinsonian motor signs. Mov Disord. 2004;19((8)):907–15.
103. Yianni JPG, Bain PG, Gregory RP, Nandi D, Joint C, Scott RB, et al. Post-operative progress of dystonia patients following globus pallidus internus deep brain stimulation. Eur J Neurol. 2003;10(3):239–47.
104. Norman DA, Shallice T. Attention to action: willed and automatic control of behaviour. In: Davidson RJ, Schwartz GE, Shapiro D, editors. Consciousness and self-regulation. New York: Plenum Press; 1986. p. 1–14.
105. Rizzolatti G, Riggio L, Dascola I, Umilta C. Reorienting attention across the horizontal and vertical meridians: evidence in favor of a premotor theory of attention. Neuropsychologia. 1987;25:31–40.
106. Schlag-Rey M, Schlag J. Visuomotor functions of central thalamus in monkey. I. Unit activity related to spontaneous eye movements. J Neurophysiol. 1984;51:1149–74.
107. Schlag J, Schlag-Rey M. Visuomotor functions of central thalamus in monkey. II. Unit activity related to visual events, targeting, and fixation. J Neurophysiol. 1984;51:1175–95.
108. Parvizi J, Damasio AR. Neuroanatomical correlates of brainstem coma. Brain. 2003;126:1524–36.
109. Paus T. Time-related changes in neural systems underlying attention and arousal during the performance of an auditory vigilance task. J Cogn Neurosci. 1997;9:392–408.
110. Wilson CJB, Beverlin 2nd B, Netoff T. Chaotic desynchronization as the therapeutic mechanism of deep brain stimulation. Front Syst Neurosci. 2011;5:50.
111. Schiff ND, Giacino JT, Kalmar K, Victor JD, Baker K, Gerber M, et al. Behavioural improvements with thalamic stimulation after severe traumatic brain injury. Nature. 2007;448:600–3.
112. Giacino J, Fins JJ, Machado A, Schiff ND. Central thalamic deep brain stimulation to promote recovery from chronic posttraumatic minimally conscious state: challenges and opportunities. Neuromodulation. 2012;15:339–49. doi:10.1111/j.1525-140.00458.x.
113. Penfield W, Jasper H. Epilepsy and the functional anatomy of the human brain. Boston: Little Brown; 1954.
114. Ciurea A, Mindruta I, Al C, Ciurea J, Barborica A, Donos C, Casanova MF, Opris I. Chapter 15. Modular signatures and neural avalanches in epileptic brain networks. In: Casanova MF, Opris I, editors. Recent Advances on the Modular Organization of the Cerebral Cortex. Netherlands: Springer; 2015. p. 271–95.
115. Canaverno S, Massa-Micon B, Cauda F, Montanaro E. Bifocal extradural cortical stimulation-induced recovery of consciousness in the permanent post-traumatic vegetative state. J Neurol. 2009;256:834–6.
116. Wongsarnpigoon A, Grill WM. Computer-based model of epidural motor cortex stimulation: effects of electrode position and geometry on activation of cortical neurons. Clin Neurophysiol. 2012;123(1):160–72.
117. Histed MHV, Bonin V, Reid RC. Direct activation of sparse, distributed populations of cortical neurons by electrical microstimulation. Neuron. 63((4)):508–22.
118. Opris I, Barborica A, Ferrera VP. Effects of electrical microstimulation in monkey frontal eye field on saccades to remembered targets. Vision Res. 2005;45(27):3414–29.
119. Opris I, Barborica A, Ferrera VP. Microstimulation of dorsolateral prefrontal cortex biases saccade target selection. J Cogn Neurosci. 2005;17(6):893–904.
120. Opris I, Ferrera VP. Modifying cognition and behavior with microstimulation: implications for cognitive prostheses. Neurosci Biobehav Rev. 2014;47:321–35.

121. Opris I, Barborica A, Ferrera VP. On the gap effect during microstimulation in the prefrontal cortex of monkey. Exp Brain Res. 2001;138:1–7.
122. Hampson RE, Gerhardt GA, Marmarelis VZ, Song D, Opris I, Santos LM, Berger TW, Deadwyler SA. Facilitation and restoration of cognitive function in primate prefrontal cortex by a neuroprosthesis that utilizes minicolumn-specific neural firing. J Neural Eng. 2012;9(5):056012.
123. Viventi J, Kim DHL, Vigeland L, Frechette ESJA, Blanco JA, Kim YS, et al. Flexible, foldable, actively multiplexed, high-density electrode array for mapping brain activity in vivo.
124. Vidu R, Rahman M, Mahmoudi M, Enachescu M, Poteca TD, Opris I. Nanostructures: a platform for brain augmentation. Front Syst Neurosci. 2014;8:91.
125. Opris I, Fuqua JL, Gerhardt GA, Hampson RE, Deadwyler SA. Prefrontal cortical recordings with biomorphic MEAs reveal complex columnar-laminar microcircuits for BCI/BMI implementation. J Neurosci Methods. 2015;244:104–13.
126. Opris I. Inter-laminar microcircuits across the neocortex: repair and augmentation. Research topic: "augmentation of brain function: facts, fiction and controversy". Lebedev MA, Opris I, Casanova MF, editors. Front Syst Neurosci. 2013;7:80.
127. Bonham BH, Litvak LM. Current focusing and steering: modeling, physiology and psychophysics. Hear Res. 2008;242(1–2):141–53.
128. Seijo FJ, Alvarez-Vega MA, Gutierrez JC, Fdez-Glez F, Lozano B. Complications in subthalamic nucleus stimulation surgery for treatment of Parkinson's disease. Review of 272 procedures. Acta Neurochir. 2007;149(9):867–75.
129. Rush S, Driscoll DA. Current distribution in the brain from surface electrodes. Anesth Analg. 1968;47(6):717–23.
130. Zaghi S, Acar M, Hultgren B, Boggio PS, Fregni F. Noninvasive brain stimulation with low-intensity electrical currents: putative mechanisms of action for direct and alternating current stimulation.
131. Datta A, Bansal V, Diaz J, Patel J, Reato D, Bikson M. Gyri precise head model of transcranial direct current stimulation: improved spatial focality using a ring electrode versus conventional rectangular pad. Brain Stimul. 2009;2(4):201–7.
132. Parazzini M, Fiocchi S, Rossi E, Paglialonga A, Ravazzani P. Transcranial direct current stimulation: estimation of the electric field and of the current density in an anatomical human head model. IEEE Trans Biomed Eng. 2011;58(6):1773–80.
133. Opris I, Gerhardt GA, Hampson RE, Deadwyler SA. Disruption of columnar and laminar cognitive processing in primate prefrontal cortex following cocaine exposure. Front Syst Neurosci. 2015;9:79. doi:10.3389/fnsys.2015.00079.
134. Opris I, Santos LM, Gerhardt GA, Song D, Berger TW, Hampson RE, Deadwyler SA. Distributed Encoding of Spatial and Object Categories in Primate Hippocampal Microcircuits. Front Neurosci. 2015;9:317.
135. Polania R, Paulus W, Nitsche MA. Reorganizing the intrinsic functional architecture of the human primary motor cortex during rest with non-invasive cortical stimulation. PLoS One. 2012;7(1):e30971.
136. Pena-Gomez C, Sala-Lonch R, Junque C, Clemente IC, Vidal D, Bargallo N, et al. Modulation of large-scale brain networks by transcranial direct current stimulation evidenced by resting-state functional MRI. Brain Stimul. 5((3)):252–63.
137. Keeser D, Meindl T, Bor J, Palm U, Pogarell O, Mulert C, et al. Prefrontal transcranial direct current stimulation changes connectivity of resting-state networks during fMRI. J Neurosci. 2011;31(43):15284–93.
138. Dmochowski JP, Datta A, Bikson M, Su Y, Parra LC. Optimized multi-electrode stimulation increases focality and intensity at target. J Neural Eng. 2011;8(4):046011.
139. Sadleir RJ, Vannorsdall TD, Schretlen DJ, Gordon B. Target optimization in transcranial direct current stimulation. Front Psychiatry. 2012;3:90.
140. Clark VP, Coffman BA, Mayer AR, Weisend MP, Lane TD, Calhoun VD. TDCS guided using fMRI significantly accelerates learning to identify concealed objects. Neuroimage. 2012;59(1):117–28.

141. Brunoni AR, Nitsche MA, Bolognini N, Bikson M, Wagner T, Merabet L, et al. Clinical research with transcranial direct current stimulation (tDCS): challenges and future directions. Brain Stimul. 2012;5(3):175–95.
142. Nitsche MA, Paulus W. Excitability changes induced in the human motor cortex by weak transcranial direct current stimulation. J Physiol. 2000;527(Pt 3):633–9.
143. Faria P, Fregni F, Sebastiao F, Dias AI, Leal A. Feasibility of focal transcranial DC polarization with simultaneous EEG recording: preliminary assessment in healthy subjects and human epilepsy. Epilepsy Behav. 2012;25(3):417–25.
144. Antal A, Bikson M, Datta A, Lafon B, Dechent P, Parra L, et al. Imaging artifacts induced by electrical stimulation during conventional fMRI of the brain. Neuroimage. 2012;85(pt 3):1040–7.
145. Merton PA, Morton HB. Stimulation of the cerebral cortex in the intact human subject. Nature. 1980;285:227.
146. Schoen I, Fromherz P. Extracellular stimulation of mammalian neurons through repetitive activation of Na – channels by weak capacitive currents on a silicon chip. J Neurophysiol. 2008;100:346–57.
147. Grenier F, Timofeev I, Steriade M. Focal synchronization of ripples (80–200 Hz) in neocortex and their neuronal correlates. J Neurophysiol. 2001;86:1884–98.
148. Terney D, Chaieb L, Moliadze V, et al. Increasing human brain excitability by transcranial high-frequency random noise stimulation. J Neurosci. 2008;28(52):14147–55.
149. Francis JT, Gluckman BJ, Schiff SJ. Sensitivity of neurons to weak electric fields. J Neurosci. 2003;23:7255–61.
150. Bromm B. Die Natrium-Gleichrichtung der unterschwellig erregten Membran in der quantitative Formulierung der Ionentheorie. Pflugers Arch. 1968;302:233–44.
151. Bennett MR. The concept of long term potentiation of transmission at synapses. Prog Neurobiol. 2000;60:109–37.
152. Rioult-Pedotti MS, Friedman D, Hess G, Donoghue JP. Learning induced LTP in neocortex. Science. 2000;290:533–6.
153. Wagner T, Valero-Cabre A, Pascual-Leone A. Noninvasive human brain stimulation. Annu Rev Biomed Eng. 2007;9:527–65.
154. Huang YZ, Edwards MJ, Rounis E, Bhatia KP, Rothwell JC. Theta burst stimulation of the human motor cortex. Neuron. 2005;45:201–6.
155. Wassermann EM. Risk and safety of repetitive transcranial magnetic stimulation: report and suggested guidelines from the International Workshop on the Safety of Repetitive Transcranial Magnetic Stimulation, June 5–7,1996. Electroencephalogr Clin Neurophysiol. 1998;108: 1–16.
156. Rossi S, Hallett M, Rossini PM, Pascual-Leone A. Safety ethical considerations and application guidelines for the use of transcranial magnetic stimulation in clinical practice and research. Clin Neurophysiol. 2009;120(12):2008–39.
157. Fitzgerald PB, Oxley TJ, Laird AR, Kulkarni J, Egan GF, Daskalakis ZJ. An analysis of functional neuroimaging studies of dorsolateral prefrontal cortical activity in depression. Psychiatry Res. 2006;148(1):33–45.
158. Pascual-Leone A, Rubio B, Pallardo F, Catala MD. Rapid-rate transcranial magnetic stimulation of left dorsolateral prefrontal cortex in drug resistant depression. Lancet. 1996;348(9022):233–7.
159. Mansur CG, Fregni F, Boggio PS, Riberto M, Gallucci-Neto J, Santos CM, et al. A sham stimulation-controlled trial of rTMS of the unaffected hemisphere in stroke patients. Neurology. 2005;64(10):1802–4.
160. Fregni F, Boggio PS, Valle AC, Rocha RR, Duarte J, Ferreira MJ, et al. A sham- controlled trial of a 5-day course of repetitive transcranial magnetic stimulation of the unaffected hemisphere in stroke patients. Stroke. 2006;37(8):2115–22.
161. Kim YH, You SH, Ko MH, Park JW, Lee KH, Jang SH, et al. Repetitive transcranial magnetic stimulation induced corticomotor excitability and associated motor skill acquisition in chronic stroke. Stroke. 2006;37(6):1471–6.

162. Chang WH, Kim YH, Bang OY, Kim ST, Park YH, Lee PK. Long-term effects of rTMS on motor recovery in patients after subacute stroke. J Rehabil Med. 2010;42(8):758–64.
163. Khedr EM, Abdel-Fadeil MR, Farghali A, Qaid M. Role of 1 and 3 Hz repetitive transcranial magnetic stimulation on motor function recovery after acute ischemic stroke. Eur J Neurol. 2009;16(12):1323–30.
164. Monti MM, Vanhaudenhuyse A, Coleman MR, Boly M, Pickard JD, Tshibanda L, et al. Willful modulation of brain activity in disorders of consciousness. N Engl J Med. 2010;362:579–89.
165. Voss HU, Uluc AM, Dyke JP, Watts R, Kobylarz EJ, BD MC, et al. Possible axonal regrowth in late recovery from the minimally conscious state. J Clin Invest. 2006;116:2005–11.
166. Estraneo A, Moretta P, Loreto V, Lanzillo B, Santoro L, Trojano L. Late recovery after traumatic, anoxic, or hemorrhagic long-lasting vegetative state. Neurology. 2010;75:239–45.
167. McCreery D, Lossinsky A, Pikov V, Liu X. Microelectrode array for chronic deep-brain microstimulation and recording. IEEE Trans Biomed Eng. 2006;53(4):726–37.
168. Keane M, Deyo S, Abosch A, Bajwa JA, Johnson MD. Improved spatial targeting with directionally segmented deep brain stimulation leads for treating essential tremor. J Neural Eng. 2012;9(4):046005.
169. Watanabe H, Takahashi H, Nakao M, Walton K, Llinas RR. Intravascular Neural Interface with Nanowire Electrode. Electron Commun Jpn. 2009;92:29–37.
170. Lee BY, Zhang J, Zueger C, Chung WJ, Yoo SY, Wang E, et al. Virus-based piezoelectric energy generation. Nat Nanotechnol. 2012;7:351–6.
171. Xu S, Qin Y, Xu C, Wei Y, Yang R, Wang ZL. Self-powered nanowire devices. Nat Nanotechnol. 2012;5:366–73.
172. Kasasbeh A, Lee K, Bieber A, Bennet K, Chang SY. Wireless neurochemical monitoring in humans. Stereotact Funct Neurosurg. Review. 2013;91(3):141–7. doi:10.1159/000345111.
173. Sainio S, Palomäki T, Tujunen N, Protopopova V, Koehne J, Kordas K, et al. Integrated carbon nanostructures for detection of neurotransmitters. Mol Neurobiol. 2015;52:859–66.
174. Deisseroth K. Optogenetics. Nat Methods. 2011;8(1):26–9.
175. Han X. Optogenetics in the nonhuman primate. Prog Brain Res. 2012;196:215–33.
176. Dai J, Ozden I, Brooks DI, et al. Modified toolbox for optogenetics in the nonhuman primate. Neurophotonics. 2015;2(3):031202.
177. Ragazzoni A, Veniero D, Pirulli C, Miniussi C. Vegetative versus minimally conscious states: a study using TMS-EEG sensory and event-related potentials. PLoS One. 2013;8(2):e57069. doi:10.1371/journal.pone.0057069.
178. Gosseries O, Thibaut A, Boly M, Rosanova M, Massimini M, Laureys S. Assessing consciousness in coma and related states using transcranial magnetic stimulation combined with electroencephalography. Ann Fr Anesth Reanim. 2014;33(2):65–71.

Printed by Printforce, the Netherlands